American University Studies

Series IX
History

Vol. 126

PETER LANG
New York • San Francisco • Bern
kfurt am Main • Berlin • Wien • Paris

Tisso

Fran

Antoinette Emch-Dériaz

Tissot

Physician of the Enlightenment

PETER LANG
New York • San Francisco • Bern
Frankfurt am Main • Berlin • Wien • Paris

Library of Congress Cataloging-in-Publication Data

Emch-Dériaz, Antoinette Suzanne.
    Tissot, physician of the Enlightenment / Antoinette Emch-Dériaz.
        p. cm. — (American university studies. Series IX, History ;
vol. 126)
        Includes bibliographical references and index.
        1. Tissot, S. A. D. (Samuel Auguste David), 1728-1797.
2. Physicians—Switzerland—Biography.   I. Title.   II. Series.
R566.T57E43   1992   610′.92—dc20   [B]   91-46129
ISBN 0-8204-1819-6   CIP
ISSN 0-0740-0462

Die Deutsche Bibliothek-CIP-Einheitsaufnahme

Emch-Dériaz, Antoinette:
Tissot : physician of the enlightenment / Antoinette Emch-Dériaz.—
New York; Berlin; Bern; Frankfurt/M.; Paris; Wien: Lang, 1992
    (American university studies : Ser. 9, History ; Vol. 126)
    ISBN 0-8204-1819-6
NE: American university studies / 09

The paper in this book meets the guidelines for permanence and
durability of the Committee on Production Guidelines for
Book Longevity of the Council on Library Resources.

Printed in the United States of America.

Table of Contents

Preface

Since 1839 when Eynard wrote *Essai sur la vie de Tissot* (a mostly biographical account), the eighteenth-century Swiss medical doctor has received such scant and superficial attention that even his first names have been misrepresented: Simon-André while his real ones are Samuel-Auguste. In the present study, I aimed at tracing Tissot's medical journey, intertwined as it was with the intellectual context of French speaking and Calvinist Switzerland. From this vista, a different picture of Tissot is drawn than the traditional portrait, etched from his most studied books (*Onanisme* and *Avis au peuple sur sa santé*), which presents him as a clever manipulator of favorite Enlightenment themes, a popularizer of others' ideas without much originality or even expertise on his own.[1]

Yet, beyond Eynard's *Essai* and the fragmented view based on the narrow perspective gained from two books, while Tissot had published twenty-five, lies a stronger personality and deeper medical philosophy revealed by the global reading of his published and unpublished works. This biography should not be read as a hagiographic work of rehabilitation; but as a presentation of the man and his milieu as complete as the preserved data allowed me, a historian aware of the special mentality and intricacies of eighteenth-century Switzerland. Any revisionist work has its dangers and pitfalls and I am grateful to several scholars for pointing out weaknesses and obscurities as well as the novel ideas which deserved more emphasis.

From the beginning of this project, I benefitted from the pertinent comments and questions of Dr. Elizabeth Fox- Genovese, my mentor and friend beyond our Rochester days; and of the help of Dr. Eugene D. Genovese who never let me get depressed by the obstacles raised on my path. Dr. Rémy G. Saisselin and Dr. Robert Joynt at the University of Rochester provided guidance in eighteenth-century studies and medical history. While I was a visiting scholar at the University of Pennsylvania, Dr. Charles E.

Rosenberg shared his vast knowledge of Buchan and other medical history topics and since then he has read the entire manuscript, offering many cogent comments. The supportive attitude of Dr. Ann La Berge (VPI) and Dr. Dora Weiner (UCLA) has meant as much to me as their questions which forced me to clarify my thoughts when I presented papers at meetings of the American Association for the History of Medicine. Dr. Matthew Ramsey (Vanderbilt) pointed out some apparent inconsistencies in the manuscript which had escaped me. Dr. Guenter B. Risse (UC/San Francisco) gave me steady support; he was a solid sounding board, bouncing back with ways to improve my work and its visibility.

On the other side of the Atlantic, Dr. Erwin H. Ackerknecht (Zurich) read a first draft and provided me with valuable directions for focussing my theme. Dr. Jean Starobinski (Geneva) helped me through the maze of obscure Swiss medical scholarship, and read several versions of the manuscript, offering me pertinent written comments and the valuable opportunity to present my findings in front of Swiss audiences. Dr. Jacques Roger (Paris/Sorbonne), by his enthusiasm for my project, helped me overcome the hurdles of transforming a dissertation into a book. Dr. Roy Porter (Wellcome Institute/ London) carefully read an earlier draft and spared no efforts to give me constructive information.

At Ole Miss, my colleagues Dr. Winthrop Jordan and Dr. Jeffrey Watt read the manuscript and provided me with suggestions to sharpen my argument. In Gainesville FL, while I was in the last stage of writing the present book, Ms Jeanne Weismantel gave me expert advice on the intricacies of a language I did not learn at my mother's knees.

While researching material, I received expert help from the curators of manuscript collections at the Bibliothèque publique et universitaire in Geneva, the Bibliothèque cantonale et universitaire in Lausanne, the Burgerbibliothek in Bern, the Zentral Bibliothek in Zurich, the Eleutherian Mills Historical Library, the American Philosophical Society Archives, and the Niedersaechsi- schelandesbibliothek in Hanover. A writing grant from the National Institutes of Health (National Library of Medicine LM 04313) is gratefully acknowledged.

Finally, I want to thank my family for their constant support while I was completing this work. First, my father Georges Dériaz who, never doubting that his daughter was as able as his three sons to study at the highest academic level, provided me with all the help possible to achieve my ambitions. Together with my mother Renée Dériaz-Bonnet, he always believed in me; though he never saw the end of my project, this book is dedicated to him. Second, my children Florence Emch-Bailey and René-Didier G. Emch who as teenagers and young adults showed patience and spontaneously took up household tasks while I was buried in my scholarly work. Third, my husband Gérard G. Emch who steadily since our 1950s college days has supported me emotionally and intellectually, even through the exigencies of a commuting marriage. Without him, I could not have persevered to the completion of the adventure.

To the memory of my father Georges Dériaz

Introduction

The intellectually fertile years of the second half of the eighteenth century, the Era of the Encyclopédie, generated open or covert questioning of a vast array of subjects. From domestic economy to the legitimacy of royal rule, from God's Creation to spontaneous generation, almost "no sacred cow" escaped the inquisitiveness of the eighteenth-century mind. This spirit provoked in the 1760s what French historians have come to call the "tournant des mentalités". This new mental attitude emanated from a stream of investigations whose source lay deep in the Renaissance's re-interpretation of the writings of the Ancients, fed in the seventeenth century on tributary thought from Baconian, Cartesian, or Newtonian scientific inquiries, which exploded the boundaries of the ancient world with the inventions of the telescope and microscope. This stream in the eighteenth century became a wide river of search for natural laws in all realms of life. It finally overflowed its banks in the French Revolution, seemingly sweeping away all traces of the old.

A changing world-view often implies a re-definition of basic premises. Medicine was no exception. In fact, medicine can be seen as the privileged locus of scrutiny and hope of a world in flux.[1] The "tournant des mentalités" bore heavily on medicine. Transformation of premises took place in medical theory, notably in Haller's research in physiology with his mono-causal conclusion of irritability; and in Sauvages' *Nosology* with his efforts at classification and rationalization, a quest for a natural order of diseases. Transformation of methods emerged in medical practice: percussion diagnosis with Auenbrugger, thermometry with de Haen, pathology with Morgagni. Transformation of both premises and methods fostered the new emphasis on clinical teaching that had begun with Boerhaave, and subsequently led to a re-definition of the role of hospitals.

The new mentality of secularization and modernity forced those in medicine to question assumptions on health. Health, once a state to be passively accepted, became a state to be cultivated and enjoyed. Early efforts to improve individual health led to the discovery that the well-being of the precious few was threatened by the conditions of the many. Private health could not be separated from public health.[2]

But why did this impatient desire for reform burst forth in the closing decades of the Ancien Régime? Built on patiently accumulated new understandings of natural, social, and economic processes, on heretofore unimaginable developments in agriculture, manufacturing, and trade, a new mentality of intervention and transformation challenged the old mentality of static order and resignation. This new mentality attained its clearest expression in the works of the Philosophes and the Encyclopedists who constituted a diverse group with wide interests. These thinkers addressed the economic, social, political, medical, and educational problems associated with the appearance of a new order, the banking, trading and manufacturing bourgeoisie which was gradually becoming distinct from the old nobility as much as from the old peasantry. The social groups that would, after the French Revolution, coalesce as a new class were already seeking to define themselves outside of the old orders of rich and poor, of dispensers and recipients of alms, of collectors of rent and taxable producers-providers of goods. The new bourgeoisie, sometimes impatiently, sometimes co-optingly, claimed a place for its special circumstances and endeavors in the Ancien Régime of Estates.[3]

The physicians, most of whom had traditionally belonged to the Third Estate, were drawn into taking an active part in the elaboration of the new order of society. They were few at first, yet influential beyond their numbers; for instance, the Chevalier de Jaucourt who wrote many of the *Encyclopédie* articles on medical subjects or Théophile de Bordeu who with the Montpellier School promoted vitalism, both fostered the modernization of medicine.

Therefore, in the spirit of the Annales School, carrying out the in-depth study of one particular recipient and proponent of the new mentality in the field of medicine, Samuel-Auguste-André-David Tissot (1728-1797), should bring more insight to the motivations as well as more light on the background of the eighteenth-century transformation of medicine. Tissot was chosen for the esteem and respect he had earned, as a practitioner, from his medical and lay contemporaries and for his influence as exponent and scribe of the new expectant medicine. Widely published and read in the eighteenth century, Tissot left voluminous personal papers in the form of original manuscripts, reading notes, and correspondence with the intellectual establishment and general public of Europe.

Tissot was a main actor in the renewal of medical thought during the closing decades of the Ancien Régime. In his published works, he contributed distinctively to the rethinking of medicine attendant upon social and economic changes and enlightened thoughts; he left in manuscript form extensive original contributions to the fields of medical teaching and care, and of public health; he also proposed a new role for physicians not only in their relations with their patients, but also in their interactions with political authorities. These concerns gradually led him toward a social conceptualization of health and medicine.

Tissot's career, which spanned almost the entire second half of the eighteenth century, consistently reflects his special background as a French-speaking Swiss from the Pays de Vaud (a subject land of the Republic of Bern) whose mother was from Geneva. He was thus privy to privileged avenues of thought and communication by virtue of the French-speaking and Protestant connections. Tissot's medical career can be divided, for reasons of conciseness, chronologically by the watershed of his teaching years at Pavia (1781-1783), and by subject-matter between his initial concern with the health of individuals, which he expanded in his thinking of "classes" of individuals, and his mature concern with what might be called the health of society, characterized by his emphasis on public hygiene.

Tissot's first paid appointment, as physician to the poor in Lausanne, gave him ample matter for reflection. From this experience, he drew correlations between sickness, poor health, and the ways or means of life for his poor as well as affluent patients. In his books, he especially discussed the threat external circumstances cast upon individual health; namely under- or over-nutrition; over-work and exhaustion which he saw of two kinds: physical for the people and mental for the intelligentsia; and boredom deriving from the lack of purposeful occupation for the well-to-do, an often neglected contributing circumstance to poor health.[4] He was among the first to denounce malnutrition and over-work as a factor, in the masses' poor health, tightly connected in a vicious circle to their poverty. He also left manuscripts on the health of women and children in which he linked their special constitutions to their specific diseases and needs for health and medical care.[5] Personal conditions influence health, and Tissot discussed how the knowledge and recognition of their importance by physician and patient alike are paramount to a sensible way of life conducive to good health.

His professorship at Pavia rendered Tissot particularly aware of the physician's role in an ever-expanding urbanized society. In his concern for the health of society, Tissot discussed the problem of educating a physician for the new task of promoting public hygiene and widening health care. Such a physician was to be aware of the threat to health that a city creates for its inhabitants, and he was to be ready to advise governments on the best measures to minimize the hazards of societal life. He voiced these concerns in a book on medical studies and in a manuscript on medical police, in both of which he defined a new role for the hospital.[6] Within this re-definition of the hospital's role there also appeared a new dimension in the interactions of physician and patient. Tissot advocated moving medicine away from a "science of discourse" about disease, with its seventeenth-century flights of Latin eloquence and specu-lation completely divorced from direct observation, to a "science of dialogue" in the vernacular between patient and physician corrobo-rated by direct observation and physical examination. Tissot thus abandoned the thought-experiment of Galileo and Pascal or the cogitations of the single mind exemplified by Descartes' *Discours de la méthode* and proposed to replace them in medicine with concrete observations and experiments and, above all, with a dialogue that can reach the root of the problem through an exchange, in the style of Diderot in his *Entretiens* or his *Rêve de d'Alembert*.[7]

Tissot's work exemplifies the tensions between peaceful reforms and revolution that characterized so much thought of the Enlight-enment, e.g. the Physiocrats.[8] In many instances, the implications of his thoughts and proposals were radical enough, although he himself never overtly espoused radical positions. These tensions appear in each of his books, beginning with his youthful darings in smallpox inoculation which he soberly buttressed with the aid of mathematicians such as Daniel Bernoulli who on this occasion introduced the emerging precision of statistics and probability calculus into the field of medicine.[9] Or when Tissot denounced onanism, i.e. masturbation, he did so in the name of medicine, health, and of new sensibilities, not of religion. Furthermore, he attacked luxury and the lenient, boring and permissive life that favored the debilitating habit, even denouncing as one of the causes the parents who relinquished their educational duties to servants or boarding schools.[10]

In *Avis au peuple sur sa santé*, he turned his attention to the "most useful part of society", but also complained of the people's credulity in the miraculous cure of quacks. For Tissot, hope and wealth were embodied in agriculture and in the people who tilled the soil. Implementing enlightened health care in the countryside would restore agriculture to a profitable level and would discourage the population from looking to domestic service or mercenary military enrollment to supplement their income, thus arresting the depopulation of the countryside that Tissot deplored. Here again, in denouncing mercenary domestic and military service, Tissot exemplified the tension between age-old patterns of service and the novelty of market-oriented production. He would again address this problem of production versus service in his next two books, *De la santé des gens de lettres* and *Essai sur les maladies des gens du monde*. He became the champion of good health to promote independence through a productive life. Throughout his career, Tissot resorted to medicine to bring dignity through self-sufficiency. He recognized that dignity through self-sufficiency, to which he added education to achieve full humanity, paved the road to democracy. But recoiling from the full implications of his medical theories, he always argued his points from a strictly medical vantage, not from a political position. For him, medical reasons should suffice to move politics in the right direction. He also understood the stressful demands that a polite society put upon the individual and he addressed the problem in *Traité des nerfs*; yet in the name of public health, Tissot promoted in *De la médecine civile* a "polished" environment to be accepted by a "honnête" society as a small price to pay toward a healthy happiness for all.

These same intentions are illustrated in his projected reforms of medical studies. Tissot wanted to retain Latin as the language *par excellence* of medicine only for classroom use and proposed to jettison scholastic Latin discourse in favor of Neo-Hippocratic observations of patients in the clinical wards of the hospital. For him, bedside observation was essentially complementary to and inseparable from the learning done in the classroom or the library. He described himself as an avid reader. And even without this explicit testimony, the extensive library he acquired, of which the catalog still exists, as well as his reading notes on his colleagues' books preserved in his personal papers, furnish ample proof of his knowledge of past and contemporary intellectual achievements. In his works Tissot created a special and unique blend from the influence of the Scottish Schools of medicine and of political economy, of Physiocratic thoughts and of Necker's benevolent charity workshops, of Rousseau's *Contrat Social* and Diderot's *Encyclopédie*.

The geographical and political location of Lausanne offered Tissot various contacts with foreign travellers and allowed him to be receptive to the main currents of the European intelligentsia, an open-mindedness reinforced by the duality of his early educational experience in the Pays de Vaud under the paternalistic subjection of the government of Bern, and his later schooling in Geneva, a city torn between aristocratic oligarchic rule and democratic dissent and demands. His choice of medicine as a career, rather than the family tradition of the ministry discloses the this-worldliness and unconventional orientation of his personality and faith, his bent toward the concrete rather than the esoteric. However, Tissot never allowed concreteness to become harshness. His up-bringing in the home of a country minister seems to have taught him to show empathy to the lowly.

Tissot's ability to absorb and synthesize the floating ideas of his age renders the assessment of his contributions to the field of medicine rather complex. He presents a mixed figure of traditional humoral medicine intertwined with the latest medical discoveries of his researcher colleagues. He defies characterization in his political or economic views; he seems to favor an agrarian community but subsumes the advance of industrialization in his call for public hygiene. By his full assimilation and embodiment of the new expectant medicine, with his mistrust of abusive heroic treatment and his commitment to more natural forms of regimen, Tissot was able to introduce this new medical venture into the emerging mentality so unobtrusively that the next century doctors who practiced the medicine he had preached only remembered the transcriber as the mere popularizer and old-fashioned adept of humoral medicine.[11]

In the nineteenth century, the understanding of these tensions was obscured because of the acceptance of some of their elements and complete rejection of others. Tissot's contributions were crowded out of the field of medical history. In one sense, he lived too long and impotently witnessed from behind the border of Old Regime Switzerland the sweeping changes that the French Revolution introduced in medicine and the inauguration (without his participation) of the medical venture he had called for.[12] In another sense, he did not live long enough to partake in the 1798 emancipation from the Bernese tutelage or to be able to achieve his role of mentor for health matters to the new political authorities of his native Pays de Vaud and, therefore, to implement his own social concept of medicine.

Nineteenth-century medicine was quick to disavow what seemed to be dead-end or dead-wood, or smelled of the Ancien Régime, and to acclaim only what was perceived as new or revolutionary. This same ex-centeredness which had served Tissot so well in the eighteenth century condemned him to rapid oblivion in the centralizing and nationalistic nineteenth century. He had to wait almost two centuries to have his works again acknowledged not only as representative of his age, but also as seminal for the next stage.[13]

In this respect too, Tissot offers an illuminating case-study for testing the enduring perception of the medicine of the Old Regime as static and repressive. Among many other authors, Michel Foucault has especially promoted this unilateral view and has thereby obscured not merely the kinds of change that occurred in the eighteenth century, in the use and purpose of the hospital, clinical teaching, and in the treatment of the insane and prisoners, but also the progressive and individualistic currents that characterized much eighteenth-century thought on public health. These currents frequently differed sharply from the repressive overtones in the cameralist views of Frank.[14] In fact, many French medical writings expressed an essentially democratic and individually motivated social conception of health, health care, public hygiene, and respect for human life in all its manifestations.[15] Tissot emerges all the more significant and interesting for his combination of elements of both currents. A close study of his writings and career reveals him quintessentially the man of his age and thus, in the full sense, the harbinger of our own.

Chapter I

The Early Years

Tissot's early life and milieu shaped his career in essential ways. Tissot himself often ascribed motivations for his medical and social thought to influences from his early life. His Swiss Calvinist environment marked him deeply, setting him apart from the other Encyclopedists, just as Rousseau's Genevan background marked him distinctively. Tissot attributed to his intrinsic culture a love of freedom and justice rooted in both the Swiss Waldstaetten of 1291 and the Genevan Reformers of 1536;[1] his call for social reform in the medical sphere was anchored in this dual legacy.

Tissot's views on freedom and justice from a twentieth-century perspective may seem limited. However, as one can read in Diderot's *Encyclopédie*,[2] the eighteenth-century perception of the political system of the Thirteen Swiss Cantons was one of admiration for the quasi-absence of shackles attached to the life of ordinary citizens and for their atmosphere of tolerance. Whether this view now seems an inflated claim for oligarchic Old Regime Switzerland does not invalidate Tissot's ties to a democratic heritage. Today the political and intellectual importance of the Swiss Confederation is blurred by her small population and the exiguous size of her territory.[3] Nevertheless, in the eighteenth century, well before the unification of Italy and Germany, this was not the case, for Switzerland's territory, population, and intellectual achievements compared with many of the states of Europe.[4] Geneva was then an independent republic, struggling to keep its independence and prominence in the face of the rising power of absolute states. The history of eighteenth-century Geneva is a complex mixture of glamour derived from banking and sciences and of a dark and troubled social fabric reflected in civil strife, foreign intervention, and exile.[5] The Pays de Vaud had been annexed by Bern in the early sixteenth century after a war of conquest against

Savoy, a sequel to the Burgundian Wars. The Reformation imposed from above, as well as disseminated from within by the preaching of men such as Farel and Viret,[6] sowed the seeds of a trend for compassion for the people that would have far-reaching consequences for Swiss attitudes toward education and the well-being of the population. This duality of the town (Geneva) and the country (Pays de Vaud), grounded in a deep Protestant faith, colored all of Tissot's life.

Samuel-Auguste-André-David Tissot was born on 20 March 1728 in the village of Grancy (Pays de Vaud), a healthy boy, as his father Pierre noted in his "livre de raison". The Tissots had been married for a little over a year, and this was their first-born. The couple would later have another son who would become an officer in the armies of Holland, and a daughter who would marry a minister named Pidou.

Pierre Tissot was a land surveyor commissary in Grancy. In his biography of Tissot,[7] Eynard tried to establish the Tissots as country squires; Doctor Tissot had attained such eminence in his career that it must have seemed irresistible to his nineteenth-century biographer to enhance his origins with a claim to nobility. A more sober assessment suggests that the Tissot family belonged to the educated professional segment of the rural population; and since then, scholars have recognized the important role the professions played in the modernization of the Ancien Régime. Pierre's brother, David Tissot was a Protestant minister in the nearby village of L'Isle. His wife was the daughter of a bourgeois of Geneva who had been an officer in the service of the Dutch Republic. This was, in the eighteenth century, a respectable way of earning a living in Geneva, as well as elsewhere in Switzerland, when small countries offered few opportunities on their own lands. In later years, Tissot, as physician, would deplore the custom, and denounced the lack of local employment in agriculture that forced young peasants to look for domestic or mercenary service.

Following the Protestant tradition of close family supervision of education, Pierre Tissot chose his brother David to act as a tutor for his son, when the lad was six years old. There at L'Isle, young Tissot developed his skills of observation for natural phenomena and human activities from the farm to the mansion. Tissot not only received from his pastor uncle his early training in writing, reading,

Latin, and all the "proper" subjects for a boy meant to attend the university, but he also lived and learned the religion which would inform his concern for others. That religion had its roots in the reading of the Bible and found its expression in the world through service for "the glory of God".[8] This attitude was deeply ingrained in Tissot through his early experiences of going with his uncle to visit the poor, the sick, and the afflicted. He observed the plight of peasants suffering from the effects of sickness, poor harvests, and most importantly the deadening weight tradition imposed on their lives. Whether in following the Almanac's injunctions ("a good day for bleeding or purging") or in discerning the etiology of cattle diseases (which had not advanced much beyond the witchcraft beliefs of the preceding century), these people remained trapped in the past.[9] In dealing with the Chandieus (the hereditary owner of the castle of L'Isle) Tissot learned his first political lesson about life under the government of Bern, but also a lesson in benevolent endeavor, and responsibility for those less powerful than oneself. When he wrote *Avis au peuple sur sa santé*, he recalled these formative years in the country among the peasants, but always from the perspective of the rural elite. At L'Isle, Tissot learned to enjoy a kind of life he would recommend to his patients. Young Tissot spent seven years in the company of his uncle, until the time came when his father and his uncle decided that he needed a larger horizon and a broader formal education. Their decision to send him to the Academy in Geneva seemed the obvious first step toward a career in medicine.

At Geneva, Tissot had his mother's relatives to welcome him and to supervise his education, behavior, and leisure activities. Moreover, the Academy was famous, not only for its preparation for the ministry but also for its teaching in philosophy as the eighteenth century understood it. This was the period of Bonnet, Calandrini, Cramer, Jalabert, Trembley, and others too numerous to mention. Their successors would include Saussure and Candolle.[10] At the Academy, Tissot was initiated into the intricacies of changing scientific methods which reflected the emergence of a natural science based more and more in observation and experimentation.

It might still be surprising in spite of the Genevan family connection to have Tissot pursuing his studies in Geneva rather than Lausanne. In the eighteenth century, however, the Lausanne

Academy, which had been founded in 1537, was mainly dedicated to the training of Protestant ministers and the Republic of Bern kept a close watch on the orthodoxy of its teaching. The choice of Geneva thus becomes clear: Tissot would be exposed there to the latest scientific achievements as well as to a political climate devoid of master/subject overtones.

At first the adolescent was not too keen on a new life in a city, especially a large one such as Geneva was at that time. But since he realized that this was the key to his career in medicine, which fulfilled his ideas of serving God and his fellow human beings, Tissot followed the advice of his elders and matriculated at the Academy on 15 May 1741.[11] Tissot was to lodge with Mr. Fougereux, the master of the fifth class.

The Academy, founded by Calvin in 1559, was housed in a building which stands today largely unchanged; it is still used as a College. The mind's eye can imagine thirteen year old Tissot getting acquainted with his new classmates under the elms in the courtyard, drinking water from the fountain in its center, attending class in the coolness of one of the first-floor rooms of the sixteenth-century clock-tower building, or rushing up the stairs of the south wing from which, some decades later, Bonaparte would harangue a not- too-happy citizenry. It took the boy some time to get used to his new pace of life and to take advantage of the teaching of his famous professors. But after a while he established himself among the first in his class. He valued the notes he took, neatly in Latin, on his courses sufficiently to keep them all his life; they are stored with his personal papers in the Lausanne public library where I found them.[12]

From his Geneva years, Tissot gained fond memories, good advice, and solid learning habits as he wrote years later to Zimmermann.[13] During this period another event marked him forever, namely his bout with smallpox in the summer of 1743 while on vacation in L'Isle. The experience did not mark him so much physically as intellectually, having a very deep effect on his outlook on medicine and medical treatment. The old physician who treated young Tissot prescribed the usual remedies, that is drugs intended to warm and sometimes even overheat the body to help the blood expel more easily the poison of smallpox through the skin. That the treatment was prescribed in spite of Sydenham's having denounced (in the seventeenth century) its pernicious results demonstrates how slowly any changes of therapeutics penetrated actual practice.[14] Fifteen year old Tissot, very sensitive to his body's reactions, quickly discovered that he felt much worse when he was given a *échauffans* like thériaque; he refused to take anymore of it or to be confined to a bed adorned with a down comforter in a room with closed windows (and in summer time to boot!) He recovered without too much physical damage, and subsequently used the experience to develop a successful treatment for smallpox based on cooling drinks and lots of fresh air. Tissot often recounted this youthful experience when writing about his new therapeutic views.[15]

In the early twentieth century, two strains of smallpox virus were identified: *variola major* and *minor*. One get generally infected by both at the same time. *Variola major* thrives at higher than normal body temperature and is the most deadly of the two; keeping a person warm increases its proliferation. *Variola minor*, which is inhibited by heat, gives as much protection against recurrent cases and is less prone to leave pronounced scars. Sydenham's and Tissot's cool treatment, inhibiting the most damaging, intuitively was correct and has been corroborated by these later discoveries.

In August 1745 at seventeen, Tissot received his master of arts degree from the Academy in Geneva; he then spent a few weeks at Grancy before embarking on the study of medicine. He chose the Faculty at Montpellier, an unusual choice for a student of the Pays de Vaud, at a time when most of the aspiring physicians of that land went to Basel for study and training. Basel hosted the only university of Ancien Régime Switzerland. It seems that Tissot was never attracted by Northern Countries and never learned German. For a mind like his, trained in the new scientific methods of observation, Montpellier was the perfect school, or so it seemed at a distance, especially since some tolerance for the Protestant religion lived on in the warm memory of its benefactor, Henry IV.

Certainly tolerance on religious matters was displayed with the foreign students attending the Medical School. But not quite the same tolerance was shown toward Protestant preachers; Bordeu, who studied medicine in Montpellier and graduated the year Tissot matriculated, recounted in letters to his father and brother how he witnessed the execution of a Protestant minister and how the

Protestant community kept watch all night over the hanged corpse
to prevent the medical students from stealing it for dissection
purposes.[16]

The State and the Church considered the Protestants as
outcasts, not to be buried in consecrated ground, since they had
refused the last rites. Protestants were to be buried like beasts, and
like beasts they could be used for dissection and medical learning.
The students were not as much concerned about the crime that had
led to the gibbet as they were concerned about learning. This
account reveals how avid the medical students at Montpellier were
for new learning and how eager they were to discover for themselves the anatomy of the body. The corpses of criminals were
often used for dissection; in some places, the authorities donated a
corpse a year to medical schools, and sometimes the students
helped themselves from the scaffold. Corpses would even rot
unburied when no family was around to care for the dead. The
authorities viewed this as deterrence and had no concern for the
health hazard so created. Furthermore, the incident reported by
Bordeu tells us that the dissection of dead patients was not yet
officially considered proper, or of any value for learning the
pathology of disease. A few years later, Tissot reported otherwise.

On 14 September 1745, Tissot left Grancy to travel southward to
Montpellier. He had time enough to reach his destination and get
himself organized before the opening of the "Grand Ordinaire"
(fall semester) on Saint Luke's Day (October 18). His father's
"livre de raison" mentioned that Tissot boarded with Sauvages, one
of the most distinguished teachers of the Faculty of Medicine.[17]
Sauvages, a botanist and physician, who introduced Linnean
nomenclature at Montpellier, wrote the first comprehensive treatise of nosology, a formidable attempt to classify diseases similarly
to Linnaeus' plant classification, using symptoms as the guiding
line. In *Nosologia methodica* (1763), Sauvages applied to medicine
the Baconian method of observation and correlation to help in
diagnoses. At first, it does not seem that student and professor
developed congenial ties. At the beginning of his stay, Tissot was
not too eager to study, as he conceded to Zimmermann.[18] Some
years later when Tissot was a doctor in Lausanne, he and Sauvages
maintained a correspondence that showed appreciation for each
other's work and accomplishments.[19]

Already in the Middle Ages the University of Montpellier had a distinguished reputation, yet the actual date of its founding is unknown. Its formal recognition dates back to a papal bull of 1220; and in 1289, it was confirmed as a university of three faculties: Law, Arts, and Medicine. The medieval Medical Faculty owed much of its fame to the infusion of Arab medical texts and to the scholarship of Jewish physicians. In the Renaissance, Rabelais was noted for teaching medicine from the original Greek medical books.[20] The Montpellier Medical School always projected an image of progressiveness, fostered in part by competition with the Paris Faculty and by a receptivity to outside stimulation and influence. Montpellier seemed not to have labored under the deadening weight of scholasticism that burdened other universities, but remained open to a keen sense of observation that permitted the Hippocratic heritage to flourish.

In the eighteenth century, the first historians of the University reported that the Montpellier Medical Faculty claimed first place for several innovations in dissection, anatomy, and botany.[21] Montpellier had permission (first granted in 1376 by the Duke of Anjou, Governor of Languedoc) to dissect the cadaver of one criminal every year; it boasted the first anatomy amphitheater, built around 1556 by the surgeon Rondelet,[22] while the Paris Faculty acquired its own only in 1604; the Montpellier Medical Library opened in 1536; its *Jardin des plantes*, was donated in 1597 by Henry IV as a balm to the city torn by religious wars; Paris had to wait until 1606 to get her own botanical garden. In clinical teaching, Montpellier led the way by requiring that no student could graduate without having spent a practicum of six months with a recognized doctor and having done rounds in the Hospitals of the Holy-Ghost or of Saint-Eloi, while the Paris Faculty let the surgeons ponder about the usefulness of hospital training for its students.[23] In the royal decree of 1707, Louis XIV officially endorsed the value for the medical students of acquiring practical knowledge in a hospital setting. In 1715 a chair of medical practice was established for the purpose of teaching students, as the royal decree said: "à consulter et à pratiquer". However, formal clinical teaching at the Saint-Eloi Hospital began only in 1760, with twenty students participating. The importance of clinical teaching in the training of a physician is usually attributed to the sagacity of Boerhaave or of François de la Boë, both of whom taught at Leyden. The Leydian model of a twelve-bed clinical ward (six-bed for men and six-bed for women) was adopted at Edinburgh and Vienna later in the eighteenth century.[24] Other chairs were established in the course of time. Around 1500, Louis XII formalized four chairs at the Faculty.   Two new chairs, in surgery/pharmacy and anatomy/botany were created by Henry IV at the same time that he established the *Jardin des plantes*;[25] two more chairs were granted by Louis XIV, one in chemistry in 1673 and in 1715 the other, already mentioned, in practical medicine.[26]

Tissot reported, in his correspondence with Zimmermann, that he daily visited the hospitals in the company of a Leyden-trained English doctor and that, as a *garçon-chirurgien*, he performed many autopsies on deceased patients from the wards. He commented that it was through this hospital training that he acquired the most useful medical knowledge, since he often found the lectures of the regular professors uninteresting and uninspiring.[27]

Tissot spent four years at Montpellier, somewhat longer than the ordinary three-year course of study. Each year was divided into two parts: the "Grand Ordinaire", from Saint Luke's Day (October 18) to Easter, and the "Petit Ordinaire", from Easter to Saint John's Day (June 21). A six-month period at the end of the course of study was added for the final examinations, so that the student received in short succession the bachelor, license, and doctoral degrees. Again, in his "livre de raison" Tissot's father gave some explanations for his son's delay. Three sheets covering the beginning of his son's stay at Montpellier are missing and in their stead is a note: "It is I who with good reasons cut out the three sheets missing here." A commentary inscribed by Colonel Tissot-Grenus added: "These were the expense accounts of my late brother, the Professor of Medicine, and the witness of his folly and prodigal spending at Montpellier."[28]   The father sought to destroy all traces of his son's youthful error: Tissot was seventeen when he went away to study in Montpellier; but the comments of the brother are more difficult to explain, except for spite, as the Colonel was known to be a lavish spender and was even reprimanded by the religious authorities for ostentatious entertainment.[29] Tissot himself admitted to the frivolity of his behavior when he first attended the University; he attributed his slip of conduct to the many attractions of the city coffeehouses and recognized that he did not spend enough time on the benches of the Faculty.[30] Yet, Tissot mended his ways and, as if to catch up for lost time, plunged himself in the study and practice of medicine, for a start during the terrible epidemic of smallpox that swept Montpellier in June 1746, and then in his studies where he soon earned the respect of his professors, beginning with Sauvages.

In 1748, upon the death of a Professor of Medicine named Fitzgerald,[31] Tissot was able to witness the elaborate process of choosing a new member of the Faculty: the legal notice of the vacancy and the opening of the competition for the post; the public disputes by the candidates on questions submitted by the professors; the public trial lectures; the vote by secret ballot; and finally the submission to the King of three names for his selection of an appointee. The whole process usually lasted over a year. A "Cérémonial" preserved at Montpellier relates the procedure and incidents of the nominations.[32] Observing the selection process for the successor to Fitzgerald was a lesson to Tissot on how to guard medicine from the intrusion of politics, a lesson he later used when, at the helm of the Lausanne Collège de Médicine, he had to fend off intrusions by their Excellencies of Bern. Amusingly, Tissot had no qualms about asserting that physicians ought to instruct governments on the best means to promote public health.[33]

The plan of study Tissot followed at Montpellier had not changed, at least in its formal setting, since the Ordinances of 1534, but in practice it was modernized at the will of the professors.[34] During the "Grand Ordinaire", courses in physiology, pathology, hygiene, and curative methods were given on a rotating basis by three of the professors. Anatomy was also taught during the fall semester. As long as the weather was warm, this course was devoted to the teaching of skeletal bones; as soon as the weather turned cold enough, dissection proper began. In the "Petit Ordinaire", the emphasis was on botany for one course, on drug preparation for another, and on demonstration of surgical techniques for the third. In 1698, demonstrations in chemistry were added to the "Petit Ordinaire" curriculum. Surgery and medicine at Montpellier do not appear to have exhibited the sharp difference and antagonism witnessed in Paris. At Montpellier it was even possible to earn an intermediary degree in surgical medicine between the bachelor and doctoral degrees. Tissot earned such a degree and always valued it, since it gave him dexterity for the autopsies he often performed on his deceased patients.

By 18 April 1749, Tissot was ready to defend his first thesis entitled: *Mania, Melancholia et Phrenitude*, and then one on *Hydrophobia* (rabies) for his bachelor's degree. He wrote to his uncle: "I proposed some new causes and remedies for this disease, not without encountering some resistance and difficulties from the professors ... thus they looked upon my thesis as a crime of 'lèse-Faculté'..." and this from a Faculty usually praised by historians of medicine for its openness to innovations. Tissot mentioned in the same letter that after thirteen more public examinations with one professor at a time and one private examination with all the professors, he was ready for the licensing examination and for the conferring of the doctoral degree which, he commented to his uncle: "were only ceremonies".[35]   At long last he became a medical doctor and was ready to go back to his family and country to practice his newly acquired knowledge.

Before closing this chapter on Tissot's formative years, I would like to discuss two health problems he encountered while in Montpellier. During his medical studies, Tissot caught the measles. In 1794 in a letter to Zimmermann, he reported this fact among others about his present health, without showing much concern over it, yet noting that since then he had kept a little dry cough.[36] This remark, a close reading of his manuscript on etisis, and a modern understanding of the nature of tuberculosis indicate that Tissot contracted tuberculosis in Montpellier, but only acknowledged the fact that he had the disease in the last five years of his life. This clue would explain many of the otherwise puzzling facets of Tissot's career. For example, his bursts of energy at writing books in a very short time and his periods of almost lethargy when he had no taste for anything intellectual, would fit the pattern of swinging moods that tuberculosis has been known to provoke by going alternately into remission and in active phase.

While away in Montpellier, Tissot had ardently wished to return home. It seems that, like many other eighteenth-century Swiss, he was easily homesick. Homesickness was, in fact, so common among the Swiss soldiers serving foreign powers that physicians were enticed to study it and tried to find its causes and remedies.[37]

"Nostalgia" as it was also called still intrigues twentieth-century physicians and tuberculosis has come to them as a possible explanation.[38] *Heimweh*, which has its entry under "Hemvé" in Diderot's *Encyclopédie*,[39] was then thought by some doctors to be caused by the quality of foreign air which was not as light and subtle as that of the Alps, while others looked at the difference in activity to explain it. *Heimweh* was so dreaded by the officers that they prohibited the singing of some songs, such as the *Ranz des vaches* (a shepherd's song), because the soldiers often deserted after hearing or singing it.[40] Even later in life, Tissot would suffer from *Heimweh* and cut short his sojourns first in Paris and then in Pavia.[41] It is quite possible that Tissot's moodiness was again a manifestation of his tuberculosis.

Tissot left Montpellier on 25 June 1749 and hastened home to Grancy where he found his mother seriously ill with dropsy. His father had hidden this condition so as not to worry his son to the point of his coming home before finishing all his examinations. Tissot tried completely different remedies from the usual ones which had failed so far to cure her and he had the happiness to see them work.[42] From the start, Tissot thus tried new cures where old ones had failed; his medicine would not be one of rhetoric and tradition, but one of observation, correlation, and experimentation. At Montpellier Tissot had learned to use observation in the best Hippocratic manner; he had been taught not to fall prey to prejudices whatever their nature: medical, social, or political. He had learned to trust his judgement, not his books alone; and he was ready to take his share of responsibilities.

Chapter II

The Physician of the Poor

Upon his return to the Pays de Vaud in the summer of 1749, Tissot practiced medicine in the small town of Morges and in the village of Grancy. Neither place was lacking in sick patients, but after the intellectual atmosphere of Sauvages' Montpellier, and the many opportunities his own position as "garçon-chirurgien" at the hospital had afforded him, Tissot found no great stimulation in the daily routine of caring for uncouth peasants. His childhood memories had made him yearn for the simplicity of country-living and for helping the companions of his early years, yet he thoroughly missed the challenge of academic life. Thus, he spent the winter of 1750-51 almost in retirement, pondering about what his real calling was. He dabbled at medical writing and contemplated going abroad for employment. He was pessimistic about his future, when in fact on the strength of his medical activity of the past two years, he was about to reach out for the career of his dreams. This chapter explains how Tissot, through chance and hard work, managed to escape from his rural predicament.

A few weeks after he had set up practice back home, a raging smallpox epidemic broke out. Tissot, drawing upon the experience he had acquired under similar circumstances in Montpellier, cared for many of the sick. He tried his method of cool treatment[1] which brought him some success and recoveries, but not enough to satisfy his ambition. He had witnessed too many deaths and too much permanent physical injury in the patients who recovered to be content with just a better cure.

Having heard of the inoculations Tronchin had performed in Amsterdam in 1748, Tissot decided to write to him in Geneva where Tronchin was residing in 1749.[2] The Genevan Doctor had already established a reputation, first as the cherished student of Boerhaave, then for his reintroduction of inoculation on the

Continent, and finally for his non-interventionist or expectant medicine and his emphasis on natural means of cure through diet and exercise. Tronchin's enduring fame rests on this last achievement. Tissot's initial request for advice on how to prevent outbreaks of smallpox through inoculation led to a warm correspondence and friendship between the two doctors. Tissot learned from his senior colleague not only about medical matters but also to be less flattering and subservient to his superiors.

Tissot suffered some kind of inferiority complex toward the urbanity of anyone more versed in city manners than he was. He had received a solid, if somewhat rough, education in the village of L'Isle. His first language was the *patois* spoken there, and he only learned French and Latin on almost equal footing, when his formal education began. Tissot had been exposed to two kinds of role models for a physician: the old-fashioned practitioner and the progressive-looking university professor. Neither was adequate for the town-doctor Tissot aspired to be, nor for the rising role of "directeur de conscience" which was beginning to rival that of the priest and minister, and which physicians increasingly were being called to play.

Tronchin exemplified the emerging enlightened physician who was at ease with rich and poor alike, and who followed the Hippocratic oath, sincere in his art of curing or, at least, of not harming. Here was a model Tissot could emulate. Tronchin, however, felt that Tissot was insulting his intelligence and his capabilities with his excessive modesty. He chided Tissot for his obsequious politeness, telling him to dispense with it or run the risk of being known only as a flatterer. Tissot heeded this counsel and learned to keep compliments at an appropriate level.[3]

After his direct contacts with Tronchin, Tissot devoted a large portion of the winter 1749-50 to studying the practice of inoculation and its literature, and later wrote several tracts and one book to promote or defend the method.[4] Following in Tronchin's steps, Tissot personally inoculated patients, not thinking of it as being beneath his dignity as a physician. Inoculations were often performed by surgeons who, in the eighteenth century, were considered inferiors to the university trained physicians. While Tronchin's activities were essentially focussed on the cities, Tissot introduced the practice of inoculation in the countryside, not only as a means to combat epidemics but also as a preventive measure to foil the spread of the disease.

After a few months of pondering about his future, Tissot decided in the spring of 1751 to move to Lausanne which was the seat of the Bernese Bailiff and of the Academy. He knew the importance of these two institutions, the political and the religious, to anyone who had ambition and yet was not too keen about expatriation.[5] He certainly had ambition and was a promising young physician, having graduated at the top of his class in Geneva as well as in Montpellier. The thought-provoking atmosphere of Sauvages' household had reinforced his taste for new medical ventures. And too, Tissot was some sort of child prodigy in his native village; he was determined to show his parents and friends back in Grancy what he could accomplish in Lausanne, drawing on the recommendation of the country-squires he had treated and on the strength of his enthusiasm for inoculation.

Moving to Lausanne was a brave effort to secure for himself a decent living in the Pays de Vaud, since the villages did not offer enough "paying" patients to sustain a beginner without supplementary income. Later in his career, Tissot often addressed the problem of insufficient health-care in the countryside because of the peasants' inability to pay a doctor adequately. Those who could pay, the well-to-do country squires, spent only the summer and fall on their estates; in winter and spring they lived in Lausanne in their *hôtels particuliers* of the "rue de Bourg" or the "quartier de la Cité". Moreover, the distances between their country estates and the next town were short enough that a city-doctor could, in acute need, be summoned from Lausanne, Nyon, Morges, or Yverdon within a reasonable amount of time, while the country surgeon administered basic treatments.

Medicine was also a personal calling for Tissot, and he did not hesitate to put forward new medical interpretations and cures. He had already done so in his medical theses, in the treatment of smallpox cases, in the cure of his mother's dropsy, and by the adoption of inoculation. Geneva and Montpellier had opened his mind to larger intellectual horizons; and the encounters he had there with foreigners had exposed him to a variety of competing views. On a smaller scale than Geneva or Montpellier, Lausanne offered Tissot the stimulus of its Academy, exchanges with foreign visitors, the proximity of the political authorities, and a population large enough to provide him with a living as a physician. A market-town, Lausanne maintained numerous contacts with the hinterlands. Tissot figured that a successful practice in Lausanne would allow him to keep contact with and help the peasants, and this without having to depend on their meager purses.

In recognition of the service he had rendered to the Pays de Vaud by introducing the practice of inoculation, Tissot was, in 1752, appointed by the Bernese authorities to the position of "médecin des pauvres" of Lausanne. At first Tissot shared the post with the aging Dr. d'Apples, who could no longer meet the demands alone. Lausanne had its full share of poor people and epidemics were frequent. Later Tissot took over entirely. Since the Middle Ages such regular paid positions had existed in several towns of the Pays de Vaud. The stipend was in kind (wine, wheat, wood) and in money paid by the civil authorities in proportion to the number of patients. Apothecaries and surgeons were also appointed for the service of the poor.[6] Similar positions existed in France and in the Germanies, where, for example, Johann-Peter Frank served as district physician in the Margraviate of Baden.[7]

In this practice, Tissot acquired invaluable knowledge of the most common diseases' treatment and he seized the opportunity to explore new remedies. Although twentieth-century sensibilities recoil from the idea of experimenting on the lowly, Tissot intended no disrespect by his innovative approach to curing. On the contrary, his search for less expensive remedies and his faith in the healing power of nature with a little help from the doctor, wholesome food, and rest were attitudes dictated by both the vitalist view he had acquired at Montpellier and his own pragmatism. It is, in fact, tempting to nominate Tissot as the model for Dupont de Nemours' observation in *Idées sur les secours à donner aux pauvres malades dans une grande ville*: "the position of physician of the poor should be given to a young man, well trained and full of promises. He will acquire a very valuable experience and develop into a first-rate physician and enhance his art."[8] In this tract, Dupont de Nemours was advocating optimum utilization of resources for the benefit of medical care.

Service to the poor made Tissot vividly aware of their plight in pre-industrial Lausanne. He had first hand experience of the vicious cycle of poverty and poor health. His published and manuscript works bespeak of how he tried throughout his career to break that cycle, sometimes with paternalistic overtones, sometimes with revolutionary accents. Tissot was always torn between the past and the future, which may be one of the reasons why he was so singularly attuned to the present.

This position offered Tissot a unique opportunity to develop his medical senses and intuition. He was able to accumulate experience quicker than most practitioners, collecting ample data on the success or failure of new as well as old treatments. The recurrence of diseases under the same circumstances drew his attention to the causes of diseases, not only to their symptoms. What he saw in his practice soon made him aware of the deficiency of the usual texts of medicine to accommodate his findings. Having a taste for writing on medical subjects, he soon embarked on a project to expand his Montpellier thesis on rabies; but, in the style of academic medicine, he felt compelled to buttress with copious quotations his own brief, yet innovative experience. Sauvages, to whom he had sent his manuscript, gently advised his former student first to see patients and then to write from true experience rather than bookish erudition.[9] Tissot heeded his professor's advice, saw numerous patients, and later, in his written works, drew extensively on his own experience.

The few years between Tissot's appointment to the position of physician to the poor and the publication of his first book remain somewhat obscure. Voltaire spent some months in Lausanne, and Tissot visited him occasionally, probably in the company of senior colleagues, welcoming the excuse to see the "fameux malade".[10] Tissot may also have tried to practice, with Gibbon (then residing in Lausanne), the English language he had learned while at the Academy in Geneva.[11] The Chandieus, who had known him as a child at L'Isle, regularly spent the winter months in Lausanne and often invited him.[12] Through the Chandieus, Tissot was introduced to salons in Lausanne. The city's location on several hills lent itself to separate neighborhoods based on political sympathies. The conservative aristocratic families lived mainly in the "Cité" near the residence of the Bailiff; many of their members were officers in the foreign service or tutors of German princes or Scottish gentry. The families of the professional lived near "Saint-

François" and the "rue de Bourg". The salons of the "Cité" were more politically oriented; those of the "rue de Bourg" were literary. With the Chandieus Tissot went to the "Cité"; later, after his marriage to Charlotte d'Apples, the daughter of a minister, he was a regular guest of the salons of the "rue de Bourg" as well.[13] In his adult life, Tissot seems to have enjoyed a hard day of work and a short evening of sparkling conversation. Most observers of these gatherings agreed that Tissot was more of a listener than a speaker. He was shy and reserved in demeanor which accounted in part for his success with the fair sex. An eligible bachelor, Tissot attracted the attention of young women.

In a letter dated 10 December 1754, he described to Zimmermann how his time was shared between "... Hippocrates, the Muses, and ladies, this charming school of grace."[14] To his friend, he justified his silence at parties, by explaining that when he had tried to overcome his shyness by witty remarks, he had been labelled a satirist. He admitted enjoying even more the popularity his silence brought than that of the period of his "bons mots".[15]

In the salons of the "rue de Bourg" Tissot met Suzanne Curchod, who was once Gibbon's sweetheart and who later became Mme Necker, wife to the banker and comptroller of finances to Louis XVI.[16] Suzanne was the daughter of a pastor who had settled in the village of Crassier. She was described as a beauty and a sparkling conversationalist. When in town, she was unquestionably the center of interest among the young set known as the "Société du Printemps". Everyone was fond of her and tried to comfort her when she became an orphan and when Gibbon did not keep his promise to marry her. Later, Tissot felt particularly close to her, since they shared the same experience of having grown up in a village and of having reached fame in their adulthood. Many letters from Suzanne and also from Jacques Necker to Tissot have survived and are witnesses to a long friendship that neither official honors nor fall from office would perturb: Tissot was to be Mme Necker's physician in her last illness.[17] When Gibbon broke his engagement to Suzanne, Tissot maintained his friendship with both parties. Indeed Gibbon and Tissot often appeared together at dinner parties at the Castle of the Bailiff or in the salons of the "Cité". They were friends throughout their lives, and together they continued their participation in the "Société du Printemps", even in the 1780s when they both were well-past their prime.

Tissot had the mumps in 1754 and, characteristically, he used his own case to promote his treatments.[18] His detailed description provides an important clue to some of his later preoccupations.[19] That year was memorable in Tissot's life, not only because of his self-study of the mumps, but also because his first book, *L'inoculation justifiée*, was published in 1754 also. Its success decisively raised Tissot from the obscure position of physician to the poor in a provincial town, to the role of a successful writer of popular medical tracts. Tissot is remembered most for the later role, and often, assessments about his achievements are limited to this aspect of his activities, thus obscuring the professional purpose of the work of his mature years, such as *Traité des nerfs et de leurs maladies* (1778-80) or *Essai sur les moyens de perfectionner les études de médecine* (1785).

Tissot became the new champion of inoculation, a role he certainly embraced primarily with the general good in mind. Yet, he was not completely unaware of the lift it gave to his reputation. *Inoculation justifiée* attracted the attention of many contemporaries and numerous long-lasting correspondences resulted. Haller and Tissot became correspondents, then friends, after Tissot sent Haller the first draft of the book.[20] La Condamine and Tissot exchanged letters for several years about the matter of inoculation and the controversy it was provoking on the European Continent.[21] Matthieu Maty, the London-based Huguenot physician and writer, wrote to Tissot informative letters on the practice of inoculation in England.[22] Through Maty, Tissot established contact with several English physicians, among them John Pringle, the brothers Hunter, George Baker, and James Kirkpatrick.[23] On 29 May 1760, Maty informed Tissot of his election to foreign correspondent of the Royal Society.[24] Dr. de Haen and Count Roncalli, two fierce opponents of inoculation, also exchanged letters with Tissot, letters that are a testimony to eighteenth-century politeness as well as to its practice of piercing irony.[25] The more than forty years of a fascinating correspondence between Tissot and Zimmermann began about the *Inoculation justifiée*. The very witty but often dark letters of Zimmermann reveal more of his personality than Tissot's, but nonetheless suggest that he appreciated his correspondent as a steady compassionate, trustworthy, and much admired colleague. Tissot's letters, which in spite of many wars have survived in Germany in a more complete entity than those of Zimmermann, tell of a constant friendship that, in my judgment, helped keep Zimmermann sane, and productive as a physician and writer, up to the storm of the French Revolution.[26]   These letters are an invaluable source for documenting Tissot's life; furthermore they provide insights into the inner-process of his medical consciousness and striving.

Pursuing his initial study of the existing literature on inoculation, Tissot discovered that the practice was promoted and explained in two types of books: those by English doctors, the most famous being Kirkpatrick's *Analysis of Inoculation* (1754), and those by French-speaking Protestants, of which the best known were by the Genevan physician Butini, *Traité de la petite vérole communiquée par l'inoculation* (1752), and by the clergyman Chais, *Discours apologétique sur la méthode de communiquer la petite vérole* (1754).[27] Twenty years earlier, Voltaire had written on inoculation in his *Onzième lettre philosophique* (*sur l'insertion de la petite vérole*), but Tissot viewed it more as a polemic work than a medical study.[28] Except for Voltaire's, these books addressed the problem of inoculation for a specialized audience. Tissot believed that a book for the general public was in order, and should be produced and disseminated quickly, so as to propagate the method of inoculation in Continental Europe.

Tissot's purpose in writing *Inoculation justifiée* was to enlighten the French-speaking public. He wrote fast, with no scholarly pretensions. The paucity of learned quotations confirms that he entertained no desire to impress scholarly circles. Indeed, he wrote to Haller that he worked: "without a sufficient library, hence it would be ridiculous to write for physicians, and this is not the aim of this pamphlet." The audience he had in mind was the general public and "women whom it is of the upmost importance to convince."[29]   With this remark, Tissot already exhibits a trend of the second generation of the Enlightenment, namely to call on women and their new role in domesticity to foster changes in the mentality of the general population. In this, the first letter of a long correspondence that lasted until Haller's death in 1777, Tissot wrote: "I believe inoculation useful. I sought to prove this usefulness with strong reasoning, solely built on good common sense and ordinary physics" (i.e. medicine). Tissot was to rely in all his subsequent books on this method. Haller replied, giving some advice about other authors who had written on inoculation, also instructing Tissot in the importance of precise spelling and grammar, warning him that such errors often open the door to petty quarrels.[30]

Inoculation justifiée was published shortly thereafter. The content covers the history of inoculation, a description of the procedure, and a cogently argued point-by-point review of the moral and physical objections. In fact, the 1760 article "Inoculation" in Diderot's *Encyclopédie*, written by Tronchin, amounts to a condensed version of Tissot's book.[31] It may be that Tronchin's signature was substituted for Tissot's, to give more prestige to the enterprise, since Tronchin was already famous for inoculating the children of the Duke of Orleans in 1756, whereas Tissot was a mere newcomer to the medical establishment. During the subsequent debate over inoculation, Tronchin praised Tissot's endeavors in favor of the practice, in particular *Lettre à M. de Haen en réponse à ses questions sur l'inoculation* (1759), writing to the Lausanne Doctor: "Jamais bonne cause ne fut mieux défendue."[32] After the *Encyclopédie*'s article, Tronchin never again officially contributed with his own pen to the defense of inoculation. Voltaire praised the book in a letter to Tissot: "Cet ouvrage est un service rendu à l'humanité."[33]

La Condamine the champion of inoculation at the Academie had encountered the practice during his 1735-43 expedition to South America, the purpose of which was to measure the length of one degree of the terrestrial arc at the Equator to settle the quarrel between Newtonians and Cartesians over the shape of the earth. In Paris, La Condamine's broad horizons had placed him at the hub of a network of correspondence that included many of the pro-inoculationists. As the battle over inoculation heated up, he was able to monitor and relay information to the protagonists favorable to inoculation. His letters to Tissot include not only data on the numbers of inoculations performed in different parts of Europe, but also valuable candid evaluations of the literature in the battle and of the authors themselves. He reassured Tissot that Count Roncalli was merely the ennobled son of a surgeon, with all the pretensions of his estate, whose written attacks "are sophisms bad enough to take care of themselves."[34] In the same letter, he is not much kinder to de Haen, another anti-inoculationist, who was however a reputable physician, a student of Boerhaave, professor of clinical medicine at Vienna.   La Condamine wrote that de Haen's *Réfutation de l'inoculation* "is a bundle of erroneous suppositions, false allegations, and sophisms." Turning his attention to the mathematical side of the quarrel, La Condamine offered an explanation of d'Alembert's attacks on the well-informed and carefully precise memoir of Bernoulli: "d'Alembert simply had just a petty habit of criticizing everything Bernoulli wrote." He added an even more devastating appreciation of d'Alembert's *Onzième opuscule mathématique*: "I know what is thought of the reasonings of M. d'Al. on this matter ... by the greatest geometricians of Europe, one among many says that if he had not seen the name of M. d'Al. at the head of this memoir ... he would not believe that it would be possible to demonstrate to its author that the three angles of a triangle are equivalent to two right angles."[35]

Nonetheless, beyond the wit and polemic so dear to eighteenth-century writers, the practice of inoculation was fostering deep questions on the ethics, purpose, and methods of medicine to prevent a disease through a controlled dose of infection by that disease. It was a gigantic departure from humoral medicine which held that disease resulted from an imbalance of humors. The proper balance of the humors was to be restored by drugs and interventions, such as emetics or bloodlettings. Inoculation was an active intervention, not performed to procure equilibrium, but purposely to induce an imbalance — a disease. The proponents of inoculation were conscious of the ground-breaking importance of their stand in favor of the practice. They sensed the deficiency of normal theories of medicine, whatever their tenets, to account for the success of inoculation. Yet, they had faith in it and the zeal of revolutionaries for it; they tried to promote it by the best means they knew. Most of the time, the operation was undertaken with careful control of the smallpox matter, of the patients, and their whereabouts; but, given the little that was known at the time concerning transmission of and immunization against disease, it constituted a leap of faith in experimental medicine on the part of the proponents. They acted almost as if their motto was: it has been tried; it worked; it should be adopted. They would not let themselves be bound to inaction by the lack of a traditional explanation or of a fitting place in a medical system.[36]

Tissot's *Inoculation justifiée* did fulfill its author's aim in informing the French-speaking public about the value of the practice, but it took years of argumentation and persuasion on his part to convince or silence the opponents of the method. In the course of the battle for inoculation, in particular over the value of a "preparation", Tissot acquired experience in the best manner to persuade the general public of the soundness of his advice. Tronchin, like the English inoculationists, favored a "preparation" of the person to be inoculated, which could differ widely from one practitioner to another.[37] For Tronchin, who was one of the first physicians to advocate a healthier way of life, "preparation" was mainly a question of hygiene, bathing and a bland diet. For some of the more energetic humoralists, it meant copious purging and bleeding; the frequently dangerous results of these acts fueled the objections of the opponents of inoculation. The rationale for the purging and bleeding was to weaken the body so as to lessen its reaction to the inoculated disease and thus to ensure a milder case. Tissot learned from the controversy that the public was ready for some sort of preventive medicine. Tissot perceived that diet and exercise could replace the emetic, the purge, and the lancet if the proper psychological attitudes were induced. Furthermore, diet and exercise were more safely administered by well-meaning relatives or neighbors than violent drugs. Since diet and exercise were to be explained to the public in terms of humoral medicine, which remained the predominant explanation of bodily functioning and mis-functioning among the lay population, Tissot thought that this linkage would permit shifting attitudes away from heroic cures toward regimen and the cultivation of a more hygienic way of life. He would develop these views in what I refer to as his Trilogy.[38]

In Tissot's view, *Inoculation justifiée* was a concise book, written in haste for the general public, not a work of erudite scholarship for his medical colleagues. With its publication Tissot became such a figure on the European scene that his uncle felt compelled to remind him that his worldly success should not provoke in him any affectations but rather should prompt him to deserve it by sustained work.[39] Tissot actively used his growing fame to promote inoculation. In fact, his own reputation paralleled the success of the method. The discovery of the "vaccine" by Jenner in 1796 displaced inoculation early in the nineteenth century.[40] So, not surprisingly, Tissot, who had been so akin to the eighteenth-century spirit, fell into oblivion in the next century. His medicine was perceived as inefficient at best and dangerous at worst. The same judgment was meted out to inoculation, without regard for the fact that where it had been widespread, vaccination was introduced with a minimum of reservation.

Inoculation justifiée's success incited Tissot to pursue writing on other medical subjects. The next chapter explores how the Lausanne Doctor personal and professional experiences determined the subjects he decided to treat and publish.

Chapter III

Early Medical Writings

From 1752 on, Tissot devoted most of his time to his position as physician of the Lausanne poor, yet he also hoped to further his career by medical writings. The epidemics (in particular those of bilious fever) which hit Lausanne taxed Tissot's energies.[1] By then, he had acquired a private practice, and his success with inoculation brought him many inquiries for information about the method as well as requests to perform it on specific patients.

This swirl of activities worried Tissot's friends and relatives. Dr. d'Apples thought that his young colleague was too lonely and, as a result, looked for more work and study to fill his hours. The old Doctor believed that providing Tissot with a family life would appease the tempest. Tissot himself sensed the void, writing to Zimmermann that he had "an innocent envy" of his correspondent's pleasant life, having under his roof a wife, a friend, and a lover all in the same person so that he did not need to attend parties to enjoy feminine company as he himself did.[2] Tissot's own parents might have felt the same way as Dr. d'Apples, but for another reason. They were concerned about their son's worldly success in the salons of Lausanne. What had happened in Montpellier, could happen also in Lausanne. Tissot might again devote too much time to pleasure and not enough to his medical career. So, it is easy to imagine Dr. d'Apples' role in arranging Tissot's marriage on 21 July 1755 to his niece Charlotte, the daughter of a minister and professor at the Academy. Together with her child (a girl) from a previous marriage, she had lived at her father's house, since 1754 when she had been granted a divorce, on the grounds of the loose life of her first husband.[3] Eynard wrote that her misfortune and her sweet disposition won Tissot's heart and that no hope of wealth influenced his choice.[4] I concur with Eynard that financial gain was not the main concern; the Tissots were to live on his medical practice earnings and his physician of the poor allowance. But, a love-match seems to fit better nineteenth-century assumptions than eighteenth-century conventions. Nonetheless, with his entrance into the d'Apples family, Tissot acquired connections and intellectual wealth to which he was certainly not indifferent.

For generations the d'Apples had been professors at the Academy, ministers, or physicians. In their house Tissot found a large, scholarly library which gave him many of the tools he had deplored lacking when he was writing *Inoculation justifiée*. Tissot was an avid reader; he is said to have had the habit of reading while having his hair set, even when dressing, although never at meals, something he classified as unhealthy.[5] Throughout his career Tissot bought books currently published, greatly expanding the d'Apples' library. A catalog of his library, anonymously established after his death, is deposited with his personal papers. Whoever began the cataloging on 10 June 1812 wrote that the library contained at least 14,000 volumes.[6] The catalog mentions more than 4,500 titles by at least 2,400 different authors. From the ancient classics in medicine (Hippocrates, Galen, the School of Salerno) and in literature (Homer, Tacitus, Virgil, Caesar, Lucretius) to the French Constitution of 1795, the library covered history, geography, travels, science and mathematics, religion and philosophy, economy (both public and private), agriculture, painting, music, and architecture; it counted some novels and plays, and numerous dictionaries, encyclopedias, transactions of various academies, and a collection of "éloges".[7]

Most of the books are from the second half of the eighteenth century; still entries from the seventeenth century account for about five percent of the total, and there are a few titles from the sixteenth century as well. The books were in several languages; just under one half of the titles were in French, over a third in Latin, about one-eighth in English and another 200 in Italian. Not too surprisingly, none were in German, since Tissot knew no German. This lacuna was not a serious problem for scientific and medical treatises because most German authors published theirs in Latin up to the nineteenth century.

Medicine is by far the most voluminous category in Tissot's library, accounting for about half the entries in the catalog. The medical collection ranges from ancient works to books published in the 1790s by Monro and Pott.[8] The volumes came from publishers in cities as distant as Philadelphia/Pennsylvania or Saint Petersburg/Russia. Their titles and dates closely follow Tissot's interests: English authors from the 1760s on and after 1780 many Italians.[9]

From the late 1770s and early 1780s, the library was enlarged by numerous treatises in botany, chemistry, physics, and mathematics, obviously intended to serve in the education of his nephew, as were the grammars and dictionaries of Latin and French acquired in the early 1770s.[10]

From the 1780s and 1790s, the catalog lists books on hospitals, prisons, medical police, and medical education. These books reflect the European-wide concern for better health-care.[11] In his writings on the reform of the hospital, Tissot was concerned with the quality of air and its renewal; he was well-informed on the subject, and it is no surprise, then, to find in his library not only the works of Lavoisier but also those of Priestley and of Scheele.[12] The diseases and health-care of women and children appear in the titles, and all the "classics" on these subjects are mentioned: Peu, Cadogan, Rousseau, Fourcroy,...[13] Surgery too had an important place since Tissot always cherished the surgeon diploma he had earned in Montpellier.

Tissot's library contained treatises on agriculture and, importantly, on physiocracy, such as the six volumes of *Physiocratie ou constitution naturelle* edited by Dupont de Nemours.[14] Books on the production, preservation, and trade of grain had their space on his shelves, and are reflected in his writings on ergoted rye, bad bread, and related problems.[15] These topics were close to Tissot's preoccupations with agricultural populations, that is their health which depended as much on proper medical care as on nutrition itself linked to their farming methods.[16] His concerns extended to the slaves with a book by Baytes [?] entitled *Directions to Those Who Hold Slaves* (Philadelphia, 1785). He owned two books by the American doctor Benjamin Rush, entitled *Research on the Influence of Physical Causes on Moral Faculties* (Philadelphia, 1786) and *Medical Observations* (Philadelphia, 1789), as well as copy of *Materia Medica Americana* (Erlangen, 1787).[17] Benjamin Franklin's works are listed, including a separate entry for *La science du bonhomme Richard*; and Dupont de Nemours' *Secours à donner aux pauvres malades dans les grandes villes* is entered with a publication date of 1786 in Philadelphia.[18]

More surprising is the number of entries dealing with Jewish history, institutions, and religion, as well as an exemplar of the Koran. These books probably were part of the original d'Apples' library.

Tissot also owned the classics on natural rights, such as Puffendorf and Burlamaqui, and the works of Locke and Hume, as well as books on the American Revolution and the questions it raised and/or answered.[19] Tissot kept up with philosophical and religious developments, as his owning of Paley's works suggest; and with revolutionary thought.[20] Copies of many proposals to the Assemblée Nationale are to be found in his library; they dealt with reforms of hospitals, medical schools, health care, children's clothing, and even the reform of public education by Talleyrand.[21] Tissot subscribed to the *Spectator* of London and to the *Mercure de France*. The catalog does not include Tissot's own books. However, one about his curative methods, *De methodo medenti Sydenhamii et Tissoti* (Breslau, 1764) written by the German physician Tralles, is listed.[22] The library was sold to an Englishman soon after the death of Tissot's nephew and disciple Marc d'Apples in 1840. The government of the Canton de Vaud judged that: "Old medical books were of no value, thus not worth the good money of the State."[23]

Tissot was fascinated with all aspects of life and all manner of scholarship. He was able to absorb others' work and to incorporate it in his writings to provide a general breadth and depth above that of the standard medical discourse of his day. He was scrupulous about citing his sources, the contemporary as well as the ancient, a practice that was not, at that time, the expected scholarly norm it has since become. Tissot's concern with proper citations might have reflected to some extent a modesty of character, but it certainly opened the door to later critics who branded him a popularizer or compiler, a judgment which completely missed Tissot's fine understanding of the mentality of his peers as well as the dimension of his learning.

The d'Apples-Tissot library was a gem which helped him earn the reputation he acquired in the 1760s. By then, he had learned to balance bookish erudition with personal experience. He read to expand and buttress his opinions, not to compile or plagiarize other authors. He had a distinctive talent for clear exposition and for synthesizing floating ideas in an attractive language which ensured success with his contemporaries. For Tissot, didactism was not merely a style, but also a personal impulse that pushed him to action. He saw the lack of medical knowledge of both physicians and general public hampering the progress and acceptance of the new discoveries and experiments in anatomy and physiology when it came to apply them to the field of practical medicine. He felt that prejudices and superstition stood in the way of accepting these new possibilities and perceived his task as that of developing a new interpretation of medicine for patient and physician alike.

In 1755, with almost a decade of medical experience and a fine library at his disposal, the newlywed Tissot was ready to embark on writing. Without delay, he collected data for his next book, in which he reported what he had observed and done during the 1755 summer epidemic of bilious fever.[24]

A daughter was born after a year of married life; the child died a few days after birth. Mrs. Tissot's health had suffered severely from the pregnancy and delivery. For months she was almost an invalid and she never carried to term another child. Tissot's relationship with her is ambiguous. He never gave examples from her health-records in his books, while he often used his mother's or his own diseases as case-studies. His letters to her are rather cold and business-like. She had a daughter, Suzanne Porta, by her first marriage, but he does not seem to have paid much attention to the child. Just a few conventional letters to her are left among his personal papers, whereas he conducted a warm correspondence with his wife's nephew, Marc d'Apples. Perhaps the girl was a sting to Tissot's male pride, a constant reminder of his failure to produce a strong child.

Little Suzanne's father, Marc-Antoine Porta (1724-1781), was an established jurist in Lausanne and became a bailival assessor in 1771; he was close to their Excellencies of Bern, which may explain why, after his marriage, Tissot looked more to the society of the "rue de Bourg" than to the "Cité" and to the company of wealthy foreigners rather than the Bailiff's. Tissot avoided comparison with Porta, known as "le licencieux" in the circles of the "rue de Bourg" and the Academy. On several occasions Tissot and Porta may have been in competition or could have interacted in a common project; judging by the record, Tissot each time chose the low profile. One such instance was the rebuilding of the Townhospital; Porta played a key role as supervisor of the lottery meant to raise the necessary funds for the new construction which however entailed no restructuring of the services.[25] Because of his position as physician of the poor, Tissot could not have been indifferent to the project; still he took no part in it. Twenty years later, the reorganization of the Lausanne Hospital caught his attention and interest; by then Porta was dead and Tissot was vice-president of the Collège de Médecine, a prominent official position from which he could speak.[26] Another occasion for conflict was the forced election of Porta to the Academy by the Bernese authorities, which nearly resulted in Tissot's resignation from that body.[27]

His marriage brought about what his parents and Dr. d'Apples had wished for; Tissot was concentrating on his career rather than on mundane distractions. His home library provided him an excuse for shortening his consulting hours as well as a haven for his medical writing. Shortly after his marriage, Tissot wrote to Zimmermann about his projected book on "habitual diseases", in which he planned to give an antidote to bleeding and purging against imaginary illnesses.[28] Zimmermann asked for a definition of habitual diseases. Tissot explained that he had begun the work by writing on nervous disorders which were linked to habits [lifestyle], since it was the subject that most appealed to him. He noted that he would perhaps limit his presentation to the latter and certainly would not discuss chronic complaints. In the same letter, Tissot mentioned that he had no regrets for the time spent on this work, as it was very useful in his practice. He was now convinced that a few simple principles accounted for the pathology of nervous diseases and that a small number of drugs, mostly dietetic, would cure them. The treatment, however, was long and tedious and few patients were willing to follow through for sufficient time to show improvement. As a result, nervous diseases were falsely labelled incurable. He added: "I have the rough draft of several other articles, but for now I will not polish them."[29]

In fact, Tissot did not finish and publish the part on nervous disorders until twenty years later.[30] He seemed to have become dissatisfied with what he already had written. Other projects captured his interest. Haller had asked him to supervise the publication in Lausanne of his *Physiology*. Tissot took the assignment seriously; he even wrote an introduction to *Physiology* that contains his only original contribution to the field, namely the non-sensitive and non-irritable nature of tendons.[31] When Haller also requested translations into Latin of medical observations by various authors that the Bernese Doctor was planning to have printed, Tissot, in a letter dated 12 September 1758, complained to Zimmermann that the task was tedious.

In a letter dated 21 June 1758, Tissot described to Zimmermann another subject that had engaged him. In his incipient *Traité de la nature*, he intended to answer the following question: "If the same principle which restores [health] ought to be that which preserves [health]. Then, which one is it?" Tissot elaborated on his mode of inquiry into the matter, and thus revealed how early he espoused the vitalist thoughts just developing at the Montpellier Medical School. He repeatedly named nature as the principle of restoration and preservation of health with which the physician has to collaborate. Unfortunately, Tissot never completed his projected *Traité de la nature*; he left only sparse notes. Instead, taking a clue from Haller's success in publishing medical observations, Tissot began writing of his own experiences in medicine.

During the raging epidemic of bilious fever that swept Lausanne in the summers of 1755 and 1756, Tissot tried a new cure that consisted of no bleeding, some mild purging, and a diet containing a lot of fresh fruit. He was rewarded with success and caught the attention of their Excellencies of Bern; they ordered that his prescriptions be printed in the form of a placard to be posted in every village in case of epidemic. When new outbreaks of the fever occurred in later years, the authorities indeed posted Tissot's prescriptions in every village to ensure its dissemination and application. Perhaps here is the seed of *Avis au peuple sur sa santé*; a poster meant to instruct on how to fight one disease was certainly useful, but a book instructing on how to care properly for many common diseases would be better. Moreover, when in 1758 Tissot published his account of the epidemic of 1755 under the title *Dissertatio de febricus biliosis, seu historia epidemica Lausannensis anni 1755*, he not only described what he had done, but also what he had seen in terms of suffering and lost lives due to the {mis}treatment by charlatans. In this case too, a poster was not enough to fight quackery, while a book might; furthermore a book would endure and always be available for reference, whereas a poster could all too easily be destroyed.

In *De febricus biliosis*, Tissot put into practice the advice of Sauvages to report and discuss only the cases he had treated: he marked his gratitude to his mentor by dedicating the work to him. *De febricus biliosis* saw several editions, the latest in 1813. It was translated into English, Italian, German and finally French in 1800.[32] Tissot appended to it a small tract entitled *Tentamen de morbis ex manustupratione ortis*, better known under the title *Onanisme*. On this work, which Tissot considerably expanded in the course of many editions, stands a large part of his enduring fame, so *Onanisme* will be the subject of the next chapter.

In writing *De febricus biliosis* in Latin, Tissot chose to address primarily the medical world, not the public at large as he had done with *Inoculation justifiée*. While the language medium is traditional, the content is not. Indeed, Tissot reported things as they were, with no adherence to any particular system of disease causation, and no speculation about causes he did not know. He remarked that the weather must have had some part in the epidemic, since the disease usually broke out in the spring after a warm wet winter. He described what he had observed in terms of symptoms, and what cured or helped the sick; even more importantly, he recounted minutely the measures that should prevent serious cases of the dread disease. For one, no bleeding; Tissot invoked the authority of Hippocrates to buttress his position against bleeding even as a preventive measure, and denounced Galen whose "principles are based more often on hypotheses rather than on medical observations".[33] Time and again, he pointed to prejudices held by the population about the treatment of bilious fever, such as the myths that raw fruit and fresh air are bad, while heavy and filling food are good. Tissot, recalling the experience he already had acquired at the Saint-Eloi Hospital in Montpellier, insisted on a proper diet of ripe fresh fruit, clear soup, and tart drink to flush out the putrid matter with the help of light purgatives. Tissot also described the physical feel of the belly of the sick, noting the hardening of the liver in a case of bilious fever.[34] Seen from the eighteenth-century medical context, this is a valuable account of Tissot's practice and how he reached diagnosis. Physical examination was rare at the time, if not unexistent, apart from the taking of the pulse and glancing at the aspect of bottled urine or at the blood's quality in the surgeon's basin. Considering that sickness was explained in terms of imbalance of humors, it is not surprising that traditional physicians were not curious about the state of internal organs, in health and/or disease.

While Tissot was treating the epidemic of bilious fever, he still was aware of the danger of smallpox, especially if an outbreak should follow on the current contagion. So he inoculated children as often as he could persuade parents to let him do so. At every opportunity, throughout the years, Tissot took up his pen in defense of inoculation to refute the accusations of de Haen or Roncalli on the dangers of the method or to plead with their Excellencies of Bern not to ban the practice in the cities.[35] To transmit his medical ideas to a wide audience, Tissot chose the vehicle of open letters addressed to doctors, which were printed and widely disseminated.[36] *Lettres* are of special interest to the history of medicine, for their organization of the material and extensive description of cases suggest a medicine grappling with a Baconian view of itself, reaching out for quantification as a way out of the stagnation of traditional medicine. *Lettres* offer an insight into Tissot's attempt to master a rapidly changing medicine and to effect a synthesis between the traditional medicine of humors and discourse and the new medicine of pathological causes and autopsy.

Especially in *Lettres*, Tissot recorded information on all kinds of diseases and cures, e.g. morbo nigro, dropsy, apoplexy, smallpox. Thus he hoped to find a trend in the repetition of symptoms and treatments which would permit him to formulate a new understanding of the process of healing and of the concept of health along the line of what he had described to Zimmermann about *Traité de la nature.* Yet, he was caught between tradition and enlightenment in the field of medical care, between precipitated heroic interventions and temperate action through change of regimen. In *Lettres*, Tissot interspersed old and new forms of investigations, so from a twentieth-century view, he seems to compromise, to temporize, like so many other authors of the Enlightenment. Very few were bold enough to defy the establishment in frontal attacks, as La Mettrie did.[37] Besides, *Lettres* are early works, written when Tissot was a promising beginner, searching for the best way to express what he saw as essential for bettering medicine.

Tissot, maturing in his art, realized that alleviating the symptoms of a disease was not the same as curing its causes, an opinion he shared with Haller: "I always have a bad opinion of treatments which are not based on the knowledge of causes."[38] Since causes were often hidden, Tissot came to realize that preventing diseases through proper hygiene was far more effective than speculating about their causes and cure. Tissot kept an interest in habitual diseases and their prevention and treatment by a healthy lifestyle. The next chapter devoted to *Onanisme* deals with what Tissot viewed as one particularly deleterious habit.

Chapter IV

Onanisme: Sin or Nervous Disease?

Tissot published a small work entitled *Tentamen de morbis ex manustupratione ortis*, better known under its French title *Onanisme*, as an appendix to *De febricus biliosis*. The unauthorized French translation of *Tentamen* which soon appeared in Paris was so poorly done that he decided to write a much expanded and revised French version. Shortly after its publication in 1760, *Onanisme* was translated into English, German, Italian, and Spanish; a Russian version came out in 1845. The last French edition appeared in 1991.[1]

From the time of its publication to the present day, *Onanisme* has been a cornerstone of Tissot's fame. In the eighteenth century the work attracted the attention of social reformers and physicians who were deploring the apparent depopulation of France in particular, and of Europe in general. Tissot chose its title from the English word onanism, coined after the name of Onan who spilled his semen on the ground to avoid siring descendents by the wife of his older brother (Genesis 38: 8-9). The word first appeared in Chambers' *Cyclopedia* (1721) which is listed in Tissot's library catalog. Contrary to what the etymology suggests, Tissot's book is not about the "funestes secrets" or the contraceptive technique of "coitus interrompus" which, in the eighteenth century, was spreading throughout the population. The "funestes secrets" so deplored by populationists and priests have no part in his preoccupations.[2] Rather, the subject of *Onanisme* is male masturbation, considered mainly as solitary enjoyment, and the deleterious effects on mental and physical health Tissot attributed to the practice. His view on the matter derived from the Calvinist tradition. Calvin held that sexual enjoyment is a means given by God to men and women to enjoy themselves and each other more deeply, and subsequently to favor procreation.[3] Tissot wrote that when a functional need existed, a pleasure to fulfill it also existed. He saw in masturbation the rejection of shared joy and fellowship for which God had created man and woman. The Catholic Church's teachings on the purpose of marriage and on the duty of the spouses to procreate were not foremost in Tissot's mind; neither were the Apostle Paul's admonitions to the Corinthians about conjugal rights and debts spouses ought to honor.[4] Tissot was mainly preoccupied with destructive selfishness, an egoism which robbed society of healthy persons.

Tissot wrote *Onanisme* and, for that matter, *Inoculation justifiée* as polemical and educational tracts to fight a scourge while enlightening the public on the potential of a different approach to medicine. Whether the scourge of onanism, considered from a twentieth-century context, is imaginary or real is beside the point. For Tissot and his contemporaries, masturbation was a real threat to the well-being of individuals and to the whole of society. However, the specificity of the French version offended Church and Censor and its printing was banned in France.[5]

Tissot wanted to explain the "habit" in medical terms, to transform the sinful perception of masturbation into that of a nervous disease which could be cured by medical methods (namely the "new medicine" methods of diet and exercise). More importantly, he wanted to prevent the "habit" not by means of restraint or guilty feelings, but by encouraging an active and purposeful life for everyone.[6] Therefore, he removed masturbation from the authority of the religious sphere that classified it as a sin and assigned its treatment to medical circles as a curable and preventable disease; a step which certainly added to the frustrations of a Church in retreat. *Onanisme* is the first instance in which Tissot was secularizing a problem, taking it away from clerical influences and turning it over to lay professionals. Here is one more marker on the road to the secularization of society of which Tissot was a proponent, one more manifestation of the "tournant des mentalités" in the 1760s.

However, this secularization turned out to be a mixed blessing (no pun intended) since the professionals of the Victorian era were as repressive to what they considered sexual deviants as had been the ecclesiastics of previous centuries. In our own time, Tissot is too often judged as repressive, because *Onanisme* served to buttress the Victorian vision of morality. His message about the danger of onanism, taken out of its true context, is therefore misunderstood. And because of the clarity of the description that still leaves some people uncomfortable, Tissot is occasionally depicted as verging on the obscene or the erotic. Thus, a French television broadcast on 8 January 1982 bore the title "Est-ce bien convenable?" and addressed the question of dissolute literature. This program was prompted by the sixty-fifth edition of *Onanisme* (1980) and the recent re-edition of *De la nymphomania* by Bienville (first edition 1771).[7] Tissot, who had condemned licentious books as part of the permissive attitude that fosters masturbation, would have been quite shocked to see *Onanisme* placed in the category of titillating literature.

Several authors have explored the motivation behind Tissot's writing of *Onanisme*, or, for that matter, behind any treatise discussing the ill effects of masturbation.[8] All interpretations of such writings intertwine control, economy, medicalization, repression, and the ubiquitous bourgeois ethos. Depending on the political leaning or the national origin of the commentator, one or another factor is stressed. Also part of the enduring success of *Onanisme* can perhaps be attributed to the taboos surrounding the subject and the curiosity it incites. Repression and curiosity are awesome stimulators; however, Tissot wrote out of a serious concern and emphatically sought to wrest young people away from a debilitating habit, which he believed furthered degeneracy and depopulation, a belief and concern he shared with many eighteenth-century conscientious citizens.[9] Yet, this does not tell the whole story behind the success of *Onanisme* nor the motivations that prompted the Lausanne Doctor to write it.

My aim is to situate this text in its context within Tissot's career, life, and eighteenth-century milieu, without making value judgements on its subject, or on who had, or is supposed to have had, the "habit". Circumstantial evidences would indicate that Tissot responded to personal marital problems when he wrote *Tentamen* and to career reasons when he translated and expanded it into a French version.

Looking at the years between the publication of *Inoculation justifiée* and *Onanisme*, Tissot's life presents several factors that may suggest marital problems. In 1754, Tissot had the mumps, and later wrote about, it without embarrassment in *Avis au peuple sur sa santé*, to encourage readers to follow his treatment of drinking only extract of balm with one quart of milk and eating some bread, which he claimed put him back on his feet in four days.[10] After the birth and death of his daughter in 1756, Tissot's married life was not easy, since this hardship had seriously altered his wife's health. Tissot disclosed to Zimmermann that he had little hope of ever fathering a child.[11] Mrs. Tissot, who was four years older than her husband, aged rapidly (as was common for women at the time) and was left in the shadow of a brilliant husband. Charlotte had such an unassuming comportment that she was easily overlooked; to wit Boisseau, in his "Notice sur l'auteur" of the 1826 edition of *De la santé des gens de lettres*, wrote: "He died celibate..."[12]

Of course by marrying in the d'Apples family, Tissot had acquired connections and status in the academic circles of Lausanne, a useful complement to his country-boy background. Still, it may be that he had been pressured into marriage by his family fearful that, in the relatively free environment of the Lausanne salons, he might return to the dissolute ways of his first year in Montpellier. On the surface, Tissot's marriage was one of convenience sealed in the traditional way of gaining access to desirable wealth and connections, here mostly of the intellectual sort. On a deeper level, Tissot might have entered matrimony to find steady companionship and shared love as he had written to his friend Zimmermann. The demands of tradition and the expectations of a novel sensibility toward love in matrimony weighed heavily on what Tissot sought in married life with a spouse who had been cheated in a previous union.

Charlotte's reserved demeanor could have stemmed from the fear of getting too emotionally involved in her new married life at the risk of being stung again by her second fashionable husband. She had ended her first marriage by filing for divorce on the ground of infidelity (a procedure allowed in Calvinist Lausanne); thus, she had consciously leaned toward the modern mentality of conjugal love and trust. Both spouses had aspirations for and expectations from the other. She wanted him to further his career in the best possible way with the help of the intellectual wealth found in the d'Apples connection and in matrimonial stability. He expected her to create a haven from the pressure of his medical practice without interfering in his work and leisure schedule.

Tissot's growing reputation as a champion of inoculation and as a successful practitioner opened wide the doors of society. He became a favorite of the well-to-do ladies, both as their physician and as their guest at parties. Numerous letters and short notes addressed to Tissot by women have been published.[13] These letters disclose another Tissot, the confessor, the indispensable friend, and a man, not merely the lofty physician chasing superstition and quackery, nor the taciturn guest, the "cold" person described by Gibbon.[14] That Tissot had temptation for extramarital encounters cannot be discounted. However, no proof or even hint of his succumbing to it are recorded.

Still, Nature had to be reckoned with and Tissot was tempted to look for solutions to his sexual fulfillment within the limits imposed by his marriage to an ailing wife and his fidelity to her. While at first, masturbation seemed an easy answer, it soon conflicted with Tissot's religious and medical beliefs. The state of knowledge concerning generation, as reproduction was then called, was such that Tissot like his contemporaries, under the influence of the Ancients (Pythagoras, Plato, Galen) linked brain and sperm matter. This medical view was shared by many (Frank for one) until the 1820s, when works on the nervous system's physiology put an end to it, at least in the enlightened part of the medical establishment.[15] But the idea has lingered in popular and pious circles down to our own times.[16] These protracted attitudes partially help to explain why *Onanisme* was often reprinted until 1905. Hence, for Tissot a waste of sperm was a waste of brain, and any kind of waste ran contrary to his Calvinist up-bringing. He came to realize that sexual satisfaction by masturbation was wasteful, perhaps even unnatural and thus pernicious when excessive; nevertheless he held the conventional idea that what was called nocturnal pollution was healthy in terms of humoral physiology since the body was rejecting its semen surplus, as long as that was not provoked by erotic thoughts and dreams.[17] In addition, Tissot's mumps case may have contributed to his inability to father a strong child that increased his feelings of sexual inadequacy. It is therefore reasonable to surmise that Tissot wrote his Latin tract, *Tentamen*, first to convince himself of the danger of onanism, then appended it to *De febricus* to test its validity. When it became a huge success, he developed a full-fledged study which reflected the worst aspects of the pomposity of a writer intoxicated by his own words and success.

Tissot did not invent onanism as an object of discourse; it was a concept and a practice much written and talked about in a pleasure seeking society which was also preoccupied with depopulation. Yet, he did focus attention on masturbation, as much to convince himself as others of the devastating effects of the habit. He was so persuasive that the author of the *Encyclopédie*'s article on "manstupration" cited Tissot's book as the basis of his article.[18] Later, *Onanisme* became the standard medical text for the fight against masturbation, and posterity assigned to Tissot the reputation of prosecutor of sexual freedom.

In the 1750s, Tissot was acquiring fame through his participation in the quarrel over inoculation; he needed a wider reputation to achieve the role of modernizer that he wanted to play in medicine. Because of trendy cultural pre-occupations in the 1760s, the topic of onanism offered him this fortuity which he was seized eagerly.[19] Later, when *Avis au peuple sur sa santé* attained an even greater success, Tissot could down play masturbation as a cause of many nervous ailments. By then he had outgrown the need to paint a bleak picture of the "habit". From the many letters he had received about onanism, he had learned to see its relative importance, with more equanimity, within the attainment of integral health and productive life.

Tissot's very large uncatalogued correspondence dating from 1763 to 1796 is revealing of his attitude.[20] He usually jotted down remarks about the diagnosis and treatment in the margin of the consultation letters he received. His secretary was to formulate a reply to the query on the basis of these notes that Tissot later signed.[21] On several letters addressing cases of onanism, Tissot wrote: "this is not the main cause of the disease, but an acrid bile is the culprit, the result of too much food and too little physical or mental exercise" and then prescribed: "a bland diet, no red meat, whey, brisk walk or, better, horseback riding." The advice of La Condamine may have had some bearing on this attitude. In a letter dated 2 June 1762, he wrote to Tissot: "I have heard much talk about your treatise on masturbation. This vice is no longer a problem at my age and I have never indulged in it. I would rather have you give a treatise on deafness. The organ of the ear is abandoned to its ill fate..."[22]

In the preface written for the 1774 edition of *Onanisme*, Tissot declared that he did not want anymore to be consulted for cases of onanism and that henceforth he would not respond to these letters: "this work is a general answer in which, with a little discernment, each one will find the most essential directives for one's case; in consulting one's personal physician one should be especially careful not to hide the cause of one's ailment."[23]

While before his correspondence had been mainly about matters of concern to physicians, now the general public was writing to him for advice on questions of everyday life, for better physical and mental health. *Onanisme* brought Tissot a different kind of fame. In the public eye he had become a leader. With the hindsight of two centuries, we can see here an example of the new secular mentality that was wont to replace the priest by the physician.

So far, I have discussed reasons linked to Tissot's personal circumstances to ascertain his motivations for writing *Onanisme*, but these alone are not sufficient to appraise fully why he wrote it, and certainly inadequate to explain the wide success of such a book. While his private needs served as catalyst to the work, Tissot was also aware of the current sensibilities that insured its public appeal. In writing *Onanisme*, Tissot was reacting to an old, yet increasing problem, homosexuality and to the appearance of the nuclear affectionate family.

Recent scholarship focussing on homosexuality led me to consider onanism within the context of the eighteenth-century gay subculture and of a changing mentality towards bi- and homosexuality acceptance. Attitudes toward these sexual orientations went from tolerance of particular aristocratic mores to abhorrence of effeminacy as degeneration and uselessness associated with aristocratic endeavors.[24]

Furthermore, the emphasis on Nature and the new image of the Natural that developed during the eighteenth century had a profound impact on the accepted views on women and their place in the family and society.[25] From a passive object, woman became an active subject engaged in forging the destiny of her family, the newly found affectionate nuclear family.

In Antiquity, specifically in pagan Rome, bi- and homo-sexuality were accepted or frowned upon not as deviant sexual practices, but as deviant male practice when a freeman placed himself in a passive sexual position.[26]   In Roman moral thought, it was acceptable for males to take their pleasure from slaves of either sexes or from young boys. Slaves were objects not supposed to have feelings of displeasure or pleasure; thus no harm was done by their sexual exploitation. The Romans assumed that the sexual immaturity of the boys so involved prevented them from feeling outraged. Here as in many other instances of eighteenth-century culture, it seems that the traditional understanding and morality of male nature owed to pagan Rome the idea that to be male was to be active, dominant, and possessive. It was manly to take actively one's pleasure. In contrast, it was despicable to give passively pleasure like a woman or a boy. In the same way, an active woman was unnatural and shameful in the usual way of seeing women as pathological and feeble creatures.[27] Then, the following questions are worth pondering. Was the traditional view holding or cracking apart under the assault of the new bourgeois mentality in family life and the respective role of man and woman within the newly defined privacy of the home? Specifically, is a clue to the success of *Onanisme* to be found in this new mentality?

In ancient Rome, as in eighteenth-century Europe, homosexuality was not only pederasty, it also involved adults of the same sex together. In the past, homosexuality was an open practice in aristocratic circles, but covert elsewhere in society. It seems that in the eighteenth century this attitude was changing, that a gay subculture was emerging outside of the court and the nobility, yet mimicking the aristocrats at least in manner of dress. This coming out of the closet was creating uneasiness, if not outright hatred in the population. Places to go to pick up a partner, gestures to signal one's preference were openly known. And one of the signs of identification among gays was masturbating in front of the potential compeer. In Paris, a special force of the police was devoted to fighting public homosexuality. The "mouches" patrolled the parks and arrested the offenders, often tricking them by not repulsing the first overture of exposure and masturbation. Sometimes, the crowd disclosed the fag, hissing him for his aristocratic attire out-of-place in worker-neighborhood.[28]

From the above accounts, it seems that homosexuality was either on the increase or more overt among the lower levels of society and was considered a public nuisance since it took place in the open, in the view of any passer-by looking or not for the "bonne aventure". Aristocratic homosexuality took place out of sight, if not out of the knowledge of the population. It was an accepted part of the manners of the nobility as were their extravagances of dress, food, and entertainment. It was a reflection of their soft, permissive conduct, of their luxury, which so far had not caused any major troubles in the minds or the customs of the people. Until then, nobody seemed to have been overwhelmingly concerned by the aristocracy's sexual behavior. However, when homosexuality became openly practiced by some in the general population, it was resented as a perversion; the effeminacy associated with it did not square with the prevalent manly attitudes of the people. Masturbation as a manifestation of homosexuality was singled out as the culprit of an effeminate degeneracy which led to depopulation. Ambivalent attitudes toward the aristocracy developed in the 1760s and paralleled the Enlightenment's questioning of the social status quo which allowed criticism of the nobility's mores to be almost openly ventured. Still, it was prudent not to call their habits sinful; to call the "habit" a sickness was a cleverer choice.

Tissot branded masturbating alone or in group a nervous disease, because he thought a link existed between sperm and brain matter, and also because he saw a kind of epilepsy in the physical manifestations of the male orgasm. Some causes of onanism were to be found in the easy lifestyle of the perpetrators, whose lack of purposeful activity led them into unnatural behavior and uncontrollable craving to relieve the boredom of their existence. Other causes were identified in licentious endeavors which excite the senses out of proportion. Along this line of reasoning, Tissot saw a revengeful nature striking back at the masturbator with the nervous disorder of onanism. The further away from nature a person was living, the more exposed {s}he was to falling prey to unnatural habits, and consequently to being sick of body or mind. Tissot more fully developed this theme in *Essai sur les maladies des gens du monde* which he published in 1770.

He wrote that onanism as a disease weakens the body because it overtaxes its functions in an unnatural manner, while natural pleasures are not tiring because reciprocal pleasure repairs the natural losses of love-making.[29] With this simple remark, he denounced the traditional attitude that only man is actively partici-pating and pleasure-taking in sexual intercourse and he proclaimed that woman too feels pleasure and participates in the act. Later, in his manuscript on the diseases of women, Tissot advised women to be active participants, to take charge of their health and their lives. He thus not only acknowledged, but also helped to propagate the new mentality that opened an active role in society to women. In fact, he had already done so when he wrote *Inoculation justifiée* specifically to persuade mothers of its usefulness. For Tissot, to be active is to be living as a human being, male or female, adult or child. Tissot objected to masturbation because it is a solitary enjoyment in which one takes pleasure without giving pleasure; it is a selfish out-of-control activity; and since pederasty and masturba-tion were often linked, he was also denouncing the homosexual who takes his pleasure from another denied "his" activity. There-fore one of the elements of Tissot's eighteenth-century success is that he understood the importance of addressing the two new topics of spreading homosexuality and assertive womanhood. In fact, under the cover of medicine, he treated these questions in the name of individual rights and worth.

Tissot also took to task the parents who exposed their children to corruption by relinquishing their educational duties to hastily chosen servants and/or tutors.[30] The "Grand Tour" had become an institution for the young well-to-do; going abroad with a tutor or a devoted friend was seen as an educative experience. Tissot threw some doubt on the wisdom of the enterprise and advocated that the best teachers were the parents, the mother for the tender age, the father for the growing child. In calling on the parents to educate their children, Tissot was actively promoting the family as the center of privacy, togetherness and love which hallmarked the modern nuclear family. His appeal went to the bourgeois who were the movers and the recipients of the new mentality. They were also the main book-buyers and they avidly bought each of Tissot's books.

For Tissot, masturbation had no place in the new order which was emerging. It was solitary enjoyment which ran contrary to the newly found shared joy of conjugal love. As a sign of homosexuality, onanism was a denial of the dignity and activity women and children deserved as well as an indictment of the effeminacy and non-productivity of the aristocrats. To all of the above, the emerging bourgeoisie heartily subscribed, hurrying to follow Tissot's lead.

As a sin, onanism had to be endured; as a disease, Tissot turned it into a curable condition. Once rid of the problem of masturbation and its attendant implications, individuals and society could proceed in private and public life to develop more harmonious relations and productive actions. Here was a prescription for progress, liberation, and fulfillment to be found in a rediscovered Nature and the gifts the Supreme Being had bestowed on everyone to enjoy. Here lies the key to Tissot's eighteenth-century success. Because of this overwhelming success, Tissot continued to be read and quoted in the nineteenth century, but his work was twisted to buttress a vision of sexuality foreign to his own. The message of joy was lost when the remedy was applied out of its original context. Tissot's advice was made to promote the repression of a sinful condition, not the treatment of a nervous disease. Guilt and secrecy prevailed once more.

Chapter V

Special Groups - Special Needs

In the closing decades of the Ancien Régime the individual, independently of a defined corporate body, was slowly becoming a center of interest. With this development came the advocacy of individual rights, which called into question the basis of organized society. Yet, it was soon discovered that human beings do not and cannot stand alone; they share common aspirations or common characteristics. Even in medicine, where the tenets of humoral medicine held that diseases came from unbalanced humors or from the peculiar constitution of the individual, recurrent symptoms under similar conditions in different persons led medical observers to look for classification of common diseases or for correlation between habits and health. The most famous of these pioneers was the Montpellier physician Sauvages. Tissot expanded his mentor's quest from disease to health, from grouping diseases to grouping individuals with special health needs or distinct habits, ultimately advocating the right to health as part of an individual's rights.

A major part of Tissot's medical writings are devoted to the health of individuals and of specific groups of people: three published books and at least two other manuscripts.[1] *Avis au peuple sur sa santé* (1761), *De la santé des gens de lettres* (1768), and *Essai sur les maladies des gens du monde* (1770)) exemplify Tissot's early preoccupations with educating the lay public about the possibilities of regimen and simple treatments to prevent or cure most diseases. The aim of the Trilogy matched that of the *Encyclopédie* with its emphasis on self-help and education to fight abuses of any sort, to offer the means to escape routine and stagnation so as to embark on a road of progress and happiness, which the Encyclopedists were quick to point out, could not be attained without health. In the Trilogy Tissot tried to provide a different solution to the problem of eliminating quackery than the numerous edicts, which in the name of professionalizing medicine, were repressing the activities of the empirics. To demask quackery, Tissot had to enlighten the population on the real value of a well-understood medicine. He wanted to instruct ordinary persons on how to avoid bad medicine and costly treatments by the perennial use of private hygiene. He aimed at enlarging the number of people who could benefit from the proper understanding of regimen.[2]

During the 1780s and 1790s, Tissot's own experience and the rising medicalization of society motivated him to aim at reforming medical institutions. In 1785, he published *Essai sur les moyens de perfectionner les études de médecine*.[3] In manuscript lecture notes he expanded, the advice on the health-care of children and women included in the Trilogy and adapted it to the specific use of physicians. By then, the focus of who deserved medical care and who should provide it had also changed in society at large, thus Tissot's emphasis on an academically trained physician treating women and children of the bourgeoisie reflected current trends. Why Tissot never published these manuscripts is somewhat puzzling. Perhaps he applied to himself what he had said in *De la santé des gens de lettres* about the wisdom of locking up in drawers one's old age works to preserve one's reputation.[4] Yet, without the mature years' manuscripts the full scope of Tissot's medical philosophy cannot be apprehended.

Together with *Onanisme* the books of the Trilogy have been the most studied of Tissot's works and the appraisal of his contribution to medicine is usually derived from them. Since scholarly attention has narrowly focussed on single books, always interpreted within a rigid context: sexual repression for *Onanisme*; popularization of medicine for *Avis au peuple sur sa santé*; literary criticism for *De la santé des gens de lettres*; or a medical thesis for *Traité des nerfs*, Tissot has generally been viewed as a mere popularizer of current ideas about individual health and as a proponent of medicalization.[5] These studies are valuable tools, but none integrates the progression of Tissot's thought from *Avis au peuple sur sa santé* to *De la santé des gens de lettres*, and finally to *Essai sur les maladies des gens du monde*: a progression already reflected in the choice of titles.[6]

Tissot's thought concerning healthier ways of life represents more than popularization and medicalization. His division of the population according to their occupation is distinctly novel and broader than Ramazzini's.[7] It signals the breaking down of old patterns, a marked stepping away from traditional views of society. As was the case for *classes stériles* and *classes productives* of the Physiocrats, Tissot's groupings represent new forms of classification that cut across the formal structures of the Ancien Régime. To recognize *gens de lettres* as a group is indeed to acknowledge the emergence of a new social entity, one very close to a bourgeoisie of talent. To write a book especially for a new emerging class is explicitly to endorse modernity. Tissot in his successive treatises addressed the needs of the ascendent bourgeoisie, in particular their participation in, and their expectations from, the care dispensed by their family doctors. He wanted to provide a new orientation to the quest for health, one based on a true interpretation of ancient medicine and a correctly understood human physiology. He believed that this project would result in new truths and new achievements in medicine. He envisaged new roles for both physician and patient.

Understanding Tissot's Calvinist background is essential for interpreting his endeavors. Calvin as a social and economic thinker has often been neglected in favor of Calvin the religious reformer, the theocratic theologian, and the advocate of predestination. A more balanced view has been proposed by Biéler.[8] Consequently, the social component of Tissot's medical career should not be interpreted without reference to the social thought of Calvin, nor be considered fragmentarily. For Tissot, to write medical treatises in French for the people was an eighteenth-century equivalent to the sixteenth-century translating of the Bible in the vernacular, in order to render the content intelligible to ordinary persons.

Tissot's attitude toward medical thought and practice can best be captured by an analogy: he would do to ancient medical writings what the Humanists had done to the Bible, to restore it to its pristine truth with the help of modern knowledge. The Reformed tradition had also emphasized the "reading" of the Book of Nature as a way to glorify God.[9] This emphasis on "reading", Hooykaas argued in his *Religion and the Rise of Modern Science*, had far-reaching consequences for the Scientific Revolution.[10] Tissot transposed this concept (reading of the Book of Nature) into the reading of the "book of the body" for the mutual enhancement of medicine and individual health, as well as a proper step towards the glorification of God. He would instruct the general public to read the medical signs of the body, to gain personal understanding of health, very much as the Reformers had insisted on the indispensability for every Christian to read the Bible in order to reach personal faith. In the same vein, Tissot would train a new kind of physician who would replace the Catholic "directeur de conscience" with an adviser for physical as well as mental health, and who would work in close partnership with his advisee. This last step constitutes a major assault on ecclesiastical supremacy in everyday life, transferring leadership to the laity. It is directly in line with the general spirit of the *Encyclopédie*, a spirit, no one could deny, had the power to revolutionize common practice. In Montpellier, Tissot had been closely exposed to the intrusion of the Catholic Church into health and personal matters. There, he had encountered the Royal Edict which prevented the physician from returning to the bedside of a dangerously ill person who refused to see the priest.[11] Therefore, Tissot published the Trilogy to teach the population to read the medical language of the body and circumvent the lack of medical help.

Tissot aimed at being the new Hippocrates of a new medicine which had begun with Harvey's discovery of the circulation of the blood.[12] In his view, this medicine must be practiced by a new brand of physicians adapted to a new culture, child of the Enlightenment epitomized in the *Encyclopédie*. He was deeply aware of the change in mentality that the Reformation had initiated and that the Enlightenment was bringing to fruition. That Tissot only partly fulfilled his goal in his published works does not invalidate it, especially since the manuscripts spelled out his intent clearly. He wanted to shake off fatalism, superstition, pretense, and inertia in medicine, as his Reformation predecessors had tried to expel these prejudices from religious life, and as many of his contemporaries of the Enlightenment were striving to oust them from the social and political realm. He also tried to guard himself from denouncing only "traditional" superstitions in medicine and not to fall prey to new ones in the form of faddish cures or panacea, such as opium or quinine had become for many eighteenth-century physicians.[13] In retrospect, Tissot's project seems out-of-proportion with the usual portrait given in recent studies, the vulgarizer of medicine, the provincial doctor who could not speak with the authority he would have derived from a Chair in a prestigious university.[14] Yet, a comprehensive study of his published and manuscript works on individual health reveals a far more complex and forceful image of the man: the image not only of a reformer but of a revolutionary of medicine.

When, in 1761, Tissot undertook to write *Avis au peuple*, he crossed, consciously or not, an important threshold: medicine was to become the concern of everyone, sick and healthy, rich and poor, rulers and governed. With this book Tissot was fulfilling his childhood ambition of helping the country folk with whom he grew up to attain better health. Tissot's path to this first goal may seem like a long detour; fresh from medical school he could have gone directly (and did for a couple of years) to the village, served there, and... starved. However, adulthood had made him both more ambitious and more discerning in his medical career. He knew that a direct course of action would help just one village for a short time, whereas a clearly written, succinct book about the most common acute diseases was certainly a more valuable tool for reaching out to the corners of the Pays de Vaud than the solitary labors of a country physician. A book in a household would always be immediately available for reference when needed, if only to help administer proper emergency care, while a physician was summoned ... and often delayed by the poor conditions of the roads. He could write a book in a few months, but, under the best of conditions, it would take years and the creation of a special school to train enough able country-surgeons to staff the entire Pays de Vaud. In *Avis*, Tissot set out to put on paper concise information on how to recognize and treat common diseases; when to call for the help of a medical practitioner; and what to report in order to get the best diagnosis and remedies for the case.[15] Tissot hoped to help his country-fellows to cope better with the hazards of their lives. He wanted to give them a sensible, reasonable, and inexpensive way to better their lot. A few years later, Tissot addressed the problem of training medical personnel especially for serving in the villages of the Pays de Vaud.[16]

Initially Tissot wrote *Avis au peuple* specifically for the villagers of the Pays de Vaud. He was quite surprised when it caught attention abroad and even more so when medical reviewers attacked him for writing, in the Hippocratic tradition, for the population of a specific area with its peculiar climate and customs influencing its diseases. A measure of the success of *Avis au peuple* is that within five years of its publication it came out in seven different translations and French editions. It was translated ultimately into at least fifteen languages and was reprinted many times in the nineteenth century.[17]

With the success of *Avis*, the number of requests for consultations Tissot received grew tremendously; patients' letters and carriages headed to Lausanne with the hope of reaching the Swiss Aesculapius. Tissot earned the friendship and the congratulations of famous and common readers alike; a money reward from Geneva; and several offers of official positions.[18] Senac, the aging doctor of Louis XV, tried to lure him to Paris, stressing the glittering success the capital could offer him.[19] Tissot was certainly ambitious, but unlike Tronchin, who would stay in Paris, he thought that Lausanne was convenient enough and that fame was not worth the pains of *Heimweh*.[20] Tronchin had good reasons for leaving Geneva, in particular its political situation, which was very ticklish with continual tensions between oligarchy and citizenry. This is not to imply that the political situation in Lausanne was without clouds; far from it. But the two doctors stood in very different positions relative to their governments: Tronchin was a member of the oligarchic circle of the Republic of Geneva; Tissot was not even a bourgeois of Lausanne, itself only a subject town of the Republic of Bern. In 1763, in recognition of his services in numerous epidemics and of his successes in attracting wealthy foreigners to sojourn in the town, Tissot received the Lausanne bourgeoisie, free of the customary fees. This was no meager gift: it normally cost about 4,000 florins per head of family to acquire bourgeoisie rights in Lausanne. Bestowing this status on Tissot was a gesture designed to make him feel more at home in Lausanne and to preempt his considering a move to a larger stage such as Senac was suggesting. In fact, throughout his life, Tissot received honors and gifts from his government only when the question of his leaving arose! Tronchin did not tolerate having no say in the medical affairs of his city; Tissot was more patient and hoped to be able to work within the system.

The publication of *Avis au peuple* prompted Rousseau to establish contact with Tissot. Jean-Jacques' distrust of medicine is too well known to need recounting here; he was attracted to Tissot's kind personality and compassion for everyone, regardless of their wealth. *Avis*, in its natural approach to health care, its emphasis on simple cures and inexpensive drugs, and most importantly its sustained stress on education and self-help, could only appeal to Rousseau. Tissot could find echoes of his own feelings in Jean-Jacques' works; he defended him ardently to Haller, rejecting the accusations of impiety that *Profession du vicaire savoyard* had created. Tissot noted that Rousseau had raised no new objection to Christianity, that the existence of God, the spirituality and immortality of the soul were not denied; and that he had only been so clumsy as to irritate Christians and Philosophes alike.[21] Tissot was appalled by the general condemnation of Rousseau, while Voltaire could go almost undisturbed. To Zimmermann, Tissot exploded: "What! One has against the Law, tolerated, cajoled, courted, and praised a man, whose works are less interesting and more dangerous, in which evil is only compensated by the exquisite and not by the righteous, whose example increases luxury, worsens morals; and one rejects a wise man whose presence could diminish evil, one has savored evil and one now rejects the counter-poison."[22] Tissot had learned to despise Voltaire for the harassments to which he descended in order to get his way and for using his ill-health to capture attention. Like others, he also suspected that Voltaire had provoked some of Rousseau's troubles with the Genevan oligarchy. Their relations remained on an even keel until Rousseau's death, an accomplishment not many could claim. Rousseau wrote to Tissot in the summer of 1766, after Tissot had gone to Môtiers at his urging to care for a young woman sick after childbirth: "You are placing me in a dilemma, I must believe in medicine or in miracles, after having written against both."[23] Tissot hoped to help him in his moral and physical sufferings; he also wished that Rousseau's stay in England would be beneficial to both ailments. Unfortunately the visit was a poor experience. In spite of his affection and admiration for Rousseau, Tissot could not help him.[24]

Tissot's reputation was such that he received several invitations from foreign governments to become part of their medical estab-

lishment. At first, he was not too keen about leaving his country
and turned down the offers suggesting his friend Zimmermann as
an alternate.[25] However in 1765, he was tempted by the invitation
to join the court of Poland as First Physician to the King.[26] Their
Excellencies learned of the project, and fearing the loss of a valuable doctor, offered Tissot the title of professor of medicine at the
Lausanne Academy. The Academy had no medical Faculty, so the
chair was honorary and carried no teaching duties; Tissot was only
expected to give an inaugural address. The Bernese went so far as
to add an extraordinary gift of money for their new Professor; but
with characteristic haughtiness in their letter of appreciation they
informed Tissot that, upon his yearly solicitation, they might renew
the gesture. Tissot wrote to Haller that he was above begging: the
money he earned would be through his work as a physician, not
through letters of supplication.[27]

The Polish incident was closed. The honorary position at the
Lausanne Academy would soon give Tissot a chance to state
publicly his views on preventive medicine, but in the long run, the
ambiguity of the situation made him yearn for a true teaching position at a medical school. Because Tissot had seen the effects of a
poor understanding of the rules of personal hygiene in many
patients (rich or poor), he took the occasion of his inaugural
lecture at the Lausanne Academy on 9 April 1766 to deliver a
lesson *De valetudine litteratorum*, on the topic of the health of
intellectuals as linked to hygiene. When Tissot published it, he
prudently dedicated the Latin edition (1766) to the King of Poland
and the French version entitled *De la santé des gens de lettres*
(1768) to their Excellencies of Bern.[28] With *De la santé*, Tissot
was sharpening his concern for groups of people rather than single
individuals. He was moving closer to the definition of a social
concept of health. Later, in *Essai sur les maladies des gens du
monde* (1770), he stated his social concerns more clearly. His
experience as physician of the poor had shown him the limit of the
Bernese authorities' benevolence. His practice with wealthy clients
had made him painfully aware of the futility and the arrogance of
their demands. Tissot the revolutionary was slowly emerging from
the chrysalis of Tissot the reformer.

Tissot also recognized that he could accomplish more from his
base in Lausanne than if he was a court or state physician outside

of his familiar surroundings. In Lausanne, people came to consult him or wrote to him for advice; they depended on him. Tissot appreciated the freedom of action he gained from being called upon rather than called in. The same motivation that made him write *Avis au peuple*, namely the recognition that he could not serve everywhere at once, and that a book widely distributed could serve as a surrogate physician, enticed him to take the pen again this time to admonish wealthy people. He hoped that such a book, written from a neutral and essentially powerless city by an independent physician, could be accepted in all quarters by everyone without jealousy or hurt pride. The success of the book would then allow him more financial and intellectual independence to pursue his task, free from the chicaneries of precedence and pecuniary reward. So Tissot kept rejecting offers to leave Lausanne to preserve his freedom of action, and because his aging parents required his medical help; his own health as well was deteriorating.[29]

In the same year (1761) that *Avis au peuple sur sa santé* was published, Auenbrugger's *Inventum Novum ex percussione thoracis humani* and Morgagni's *De sedibus et causis morborum per anatomen indagatis* (held to mark the birth of modern anatomical pathology) came out of the printershop.[30] These three books met different medical receptions, but all three had a definite impact on the way medicine was to evolve in the nineteenth century. Auenbrugger's book, a radical departure from accepted medical practice which used hardly any physical examination, emphasized chest's percussion to reach a diagnosis. It was received with caution, when not simply ignored. In March 1761, Tissot wrote to Zimmermann that he had read it with pleasure; nevertheless, in a later edition of *Avis*, when he described the method, he wrote that he was not entirely confident of its validity for a sure diagnosis.[31] He seems to have had some trouble exploiting the full potential of Auenbrugger's method. Nonetheless, he used it and later taught it in his clinics at Pavia, since he was a convinced partisan of a complete physical examination before prognosis or diagnosis.[32] Morgagni's treatise laid the foundation for a systematic use of correlating symptoms during disease with findings at the *post mortem*. From the beginning of his career Tissot had performed, as often as he could, autopsies on patients he had lost, sometimes even offering money to entice relatives to give their permission.[33]   In 1779, Tissot supervised a new edition of Morgagni's treatise for which he provided a Latin introduction.[34]   When he became professor of clinical medicine, his students routinely performed autopsies of the deceased patients they had treated in his Pavia clinical wards. To Tissot these autopsies were an integral part of medical training. *Avis au peuple* emphasized expectant medicine, regimen, and simple treatment, with the view of making the sick partners in their own health care.

Physical examination, autopsy, and expectant medicine would be some of the principal tenets of nineteenth-century medicine and are credited with much of the progress made in curing since then. Auenbrugger and Morgagni have kept their place of honor in the medical history written in whiggish style, while Tissot lost his. His books were written in the vernacular and for a large audience and today are considered mere popularizations; Auenbrugger's and Morgagni's written in the style of Ancien Régime's science, in Latin, and for physicians, are still viewed as scholarship *par excellence*.

The choice of title, in particular the word "avis", while reflecting the emerging mentality of improvement by education, also implied a possibility of choice: one can accept or reject advice, using one's own judgment to check its validity and then decide to follow up or not.   It became the stamp of a certain kind of spirit, one which appealed to the reader's intelligence and capacity for judgment. After the 1760s this use of the word spread fast, due partly to the considerable success of Tissot's own *Avis*, seed and fruit of the "tournant des mentalités".[35]   More generally, the use of the word "avis" became a declaration of the author's intent to enlighten the population and move them to action.

For many eighteenth-century thinkers, including Tissot, who extended the implications of the Scientific Revolution to the study of human beings and society, human or social nature appeared less as an unalterable condition to be suffered and more as raw material apt to improve.   Driven by curiosity and by a will "to subdue the earth", the Philosophes' thoughts later matured to challenge the status quo, which has been characterized by Peter Gay as "the recovery of nerve" that prompted modernization.[36]   The new mentality was beginning to loosen the grasp of fatalism and indolence which had beset the minds of the people. There was a new confidence in the ability to develop talents and to modify environments. A faith in progress was beginning to filter through.

Agriculture was changing, new and better crops and ways of cultivation were being developed. New crops in the form of clover and other forage plants, which returned nitrogen to the soil, were planted instead of leaving the land fallow. This fodder was fed to cattle with better results than had been obtained by turning them loose on fallow pasture. A by-product of the better fed cattle was more manure which, in turn, increased the yield of the field fertilized with it. Turnips (a source of vitamin C) and potatoes slowly took their place on the tables of the poor. Iron plows replaced old wooden plows, and often horses instead of oxen were harnessed to the implement, allowing farmers to plow deeper in the arable earth. As a result, more abundant crops were harvested, better cattle were raised, and the specter of endemic famine became less threatening.[37] These agricultural changes had first occurred in the Low-Countries in the late seventeenth century, from where they had been imported into England at the beginning of the eighteenth, then later into France and Switzerland.[38]

Their Excellencies of Bern were among the first in Switzerland to encourage new ventures in agriculture. For example, early in the eighteenth century the Bernese introduced, in the Pays d'Enhaut, the cultivation of potatoes. Because the harvest of a given potato plot feeds more people than that of a wheat of the same size, it was possible to turn formerly cultivated fields into pasture for dairy cattle. As a result cheese production increased, yielding two benefits: more protein for the local population and a new commodity for export.[39] The increased supply of food, even if not quite in plentiful quantity, played an important role in the improvement of both the health and the wealth of the people.[40] For the Physiocrats, pre-eminently among other writers, better agricultural practices were the means to stamp out famine and poverty and to bring about wealth and plenty. Several of Tissot's landowner patients, who subscribed to physiocratic thought, were experimenting with or implementing new crops.

In the realm of medicine, mentalities were changing too. Previous reverence for the achievements and teachings of Ancient Medicine was questioned, even if the superficial discourse still exhibited the old rhetoric of humoralism. This questioning was brought about by recent discoveries of new drugs (Peruvian bark) or novel intervention (inoculation) to cure or prevent diseases, and by applying the scientific spirit of observation and experiment to medicine.[41] Increasingly, physiology and pathology were subjects of scholarly inquiries; this research yielded new understandings of health and disease. Consequently, new concepts of treatments and new hopes of improved health developed, which reflected the new discoveries and attendant theories.[42] This questioning of Ancient Medicine must also be linked to the outbreaks of new diseases (syphilis); to the increased deadliness of others (measles, scarlet fever), which Ancient Medicine was powerless to cure; and to the disappearance of still other diseases (leprosy, black death), which had not recurred for decades by the second half of the eighteenth century. The questions to be addressed were different and they called for different solutions.[43]

Tissot shared that hope and this questioning. He saw the value of the new medicine for a healthier life. He first turned his attention to what he thought was the most deprived and most valuable part of the population: the people of the countryside. He wrote in the preface to *Avis au peuple*: "While we take care of its [the population's] most dazzling portion in the cities, its most numerous and useful part wretchedly perishes in the countryside."[44] This interest in the health of the people was not unique to Tissot.[45] The wealth represented by a healthy and numerous people was acknowledged by both mercantilist and nascent capitalist theories. The profit earned by strong farmers and artisans as well as the power wielded through tough soldiers was part, but not all, of the populationist discourse. A healthy and growing population was also thought to be the reflection of the value of political institutions.[46] The eighteenth-century government's interest in the health of the people can be, and has been, differently interpreted mainly on account of the scholar's political and intellectual leanings. From crass exploitation to sublime humanitarianism, every shade of interpretation can be found in the past and present literature. However, what is of interest here is the emergence of a new sensibility. Tissot realized the gain a healthy people would bring to his country; however, his main motivation was to stop and perhaps reverse a general weakening of health which he thought brought depopulation. He abhorred both unnecessary suffering of the body and useless wasting of monetary resources.

Tissot wanted to give the people the means to acquire or retain good health through changed mental attitudes toward the values of their own bodies, and to teach them how to spend their cash resources for better health care. At the same time, he wanted to help the well-meaning elite of the land to bring enlightened medicine to their folk. Tissot believed in the value of example. He hoped that the local elite in villages that were removed from medical care, would first try on themselves the precepts he had expounded in the *Avis*. Their personal success would then give them authority to guide their people in the treatment of diseases.

The hopes for a better life Tissot had benevolently raised throughout *Avis au peuple* bred both revolution and disdain; **revolution**, through his advocacy of a comprehensive public health to alleviate the misery of the population and his placing squarely in the hands of the political authorities the responsibility of the welfare of the people; and **disdain**, from the medical establishment that dismissed as dangerous the idea of thrusting into untrained hands the means to diagnose and cure diseases. Nonetheless, the success of *Avis au peuple* stimulated others to write self-help medical books with a particular audience in mind. Buchan's *Domestic Medicine* (1769) was directed at the urban British middle-class, while some decades later Gunn in Tennessee, borrowing Buchan's title, wrote for the frontier population of America.[47]

Nineteenth-century history harshly criticized Tissot's attempt in *Avis* to bring medicine to the countryside: the enterprise was judged fraught with danger, or useless and wasteful at best. Today, however, his intention in *Avis* must be recognized as a marker on the road to a social conception of health. Last century medicine aspired to be scientifically sanctioned, and it saw in Tissot only a well-intentioned but pedantic, old-fashioned doctor. As a first approximation, this view is confirmed by a superficial reading of his works, but a deeper investigation of his motivations and purpose reveals a reformist — almost a revolutionary — committed to deliver proper medical care to the population at large.

Tissot hoped to shake the apathy of the people and the complacency of the elite, forcing individuals to take responsibility for their own health. Certainly, a current of opinion about the importance

of preserving one's health through regimen existed in the Encyclopedist Era.   With its source in Ancient Greece, preventive
medicine remained a concern of the privileged classes and was
largely an endeavor of the bourgeoisie, as William Coleman has
pointed out so well.[48] Tissot's originality lay in his systematic effort
to bring to all levels of society the knowledge necessary to preserve
good health without disposing of a fortune. He also drew attention
to health problems that were common to many individuals and
addressed them globally in a unifying fashion. Tissot insisted on
the urgency of change by arguing that the problem was not individualistic or fragmentary, but general within the population. He
pointed to some groups, holding them accountable for the
unhealthy state of others. It was bad enough in his view that
because of ignorance sets of individuals suffered ill health, as he
had emphasized in *Avis au peuple* and in *De la santé*. It became
intolerable for him that the excesses of one group should aggravate
the poor health and sufferings of another, thereby contributing to a
general weakening of the population. He summoned enough
boldness to denounce in *Sur les maladies* this social and medical
deficiency of the Old Regime: "Whenever the peasant is forced to
run some errands, it is only because he has to serve the fashion-
ables and then become the victim of their fitful style of life."[49]

Tissot was part of the concerted effort to turn around the tide of
depopulation and degeneracy that was forecasted (incorrectly it
has since been shown) by social and medical theorists of the
eighteenth century.[50]   *Avis* provided the embryo of a social
program of medical care for counteracting the scourge of the
quack on the life of the peasant. *Avis* was addressed first to the
ministers and the school teachers of the villages, i.e. the most lowly
(or democratic) of the representatives of authority, and only
secondarily to the aristocratic and wealthy inhabitants of the
countryside, the autocratic elements of authority. Tissot wanted
the powers-that-be to participate in the health care of their
charges, to provide instruments and money to ministers and school
teachers to enable them to distribute medical help more wisely. He
advised the country clergy and the school teachers to improve their
medical skills by studying his *Avis*, or by making place for medical
subjects in the curriculum of their formative years.[51] His ultimate
aim was to provide the villagers with properly trained medical

personnel. Tissot saw his own book as a palliative, even though he knew that peasants in the countryside would sometimes find *Avis* hard to afford or to read on their own. Yet he wrote: "I am not doubting that amongst the yeomen, several of whom, full of sense, judgment, and good will, shall read with pleasure this book and eagerly spread its maxims."[52]   Tissot would not let himself be discouraged by the magnitude of the task. Around him enough good will was shown by the well-to-do in their charitable concerns that Tissot thought he could enlist them also in his project: "With the help of few questions to relatives, or a visit to the sick, the gentry will estimate the kind of disease and by proper management will prevent a lot of calamities."[53]   He hoped to motivate the people to acquire better health; he wanted to render them conscious of their own value, in the same way they already knew the value of their cattle and took good care of them. He noted: "However as soon as he, his wife or children are concerned, he goes without help, or makes do with anything handy, no matter how harmful."[54] To achieve his goal, Tissot realized that he also had to raise the elite's consciousness of their responsibility for the improvement of both health-care and agriculture.

In 1760, when Tissot was writing *Avis*, he was close to the people; and he knew from his frequent visits to the adjacent country estates of his gentry patients, the role they could play in his social health-care program: "True charity feels that, lacking knowledge, it can harm, and this fear restrains it, but it eagerly grasps any hints that can help."[55] Madame de Corcelles in a letter to a friend confirmed this: "Louison [her maid], suddenly seized by a high fever as if cast on her, is spitting blood; ... To get a physician in the middle of the night and the Jorat, judge it? I throw myself in *Avis au peuple* ... I followed everything and so well served my dear sick that she is saved thank Heaven ... This *Avis au peuple* is really a masterwork,"[56] Tissot also recognized the difficulty of changing customary ways: "If the people could only reason, it would be easy to undeceive them, but those that lead them ought to reason for them."[57] He was a reformer who wanted to improve the lot of the countryfolk through simple ways, with simple drugs and diet. He wished to inform them of the danger of neglect of their health as well as of the perils of overtrust in the itinerant quack's skills, of whom he wrote: "Ignorant, impudent liar and rogue, he will always seduce the uncouth and gullible people unable to judge of anything."[58]   He wanted to rid the people of costly prejudice and superstition which were taking a heavy toll on their lives: "The third reason of depopulation is the way in which the people are cared for while sick ... I have witnessed minor diseases turned deadly because of their treatments."[59]

In the early 1760s, Tissot saw the people as children who, although clever, lacked the knowledge to make informed decisions in health matter. He tried to provide them with correct information about curing diseases. He wanted to counteract their beliefs in the mysterious, complicated, and costly practices of the charlatans: "A surer remedy would be to convince the people, a thing easily done, that it will cost them less to be well cared for than to be bullied."[60]

In the late 1760s, when Tissot had become a fashionable doctor, when he had seen the high society of Europe flock to his door, sick of over-indulgence and boredom, he embraced a romantic vision of the peasant and of natural life. He then wrote in *Sur les maladies*: "Should one ask who has the best conditions for a healthy life, everyone will answer without hesitations, the peasant, who has many advantages over the craftsman ... the further away from the peasant's style of life, the worst one's health, yet our present day peasants are less healthy than their ancestors or even than some savage tribes who, to this day, do not know many diseases and die mostly of accidents or old age ... our peasants don't uniquely live from farming; some have been domestic servants, others soldiers, who weakened their health in these occupations and infected their villages with city customs ... bourgeois are still further away ... and lastly are the well-to-do ... who have no calling and fill their days with pleasure; but since natural and true pleasures are only associated with occupation and needs, they have had to turn to artificial pleasures..."[61] To emphasize the essential difference between the healthy natural life of the peasant and the cluttered artificial life of the gentry, Tissot compared the conduct of the gentry to that of a hypochondriac whom nothing can satisfy nor cure. In the same stroke, he also denounced the corrupting effect that domestic and military services had on the peasants. Tissot never lost an occasion to attack dependency of any kind, that of the nobility upon the king as well as that of the peasantry upon the wealthy. In *Avis au peuple*, he saw ignorance hurting the people; in *Sur les maladies*, Tissot denounced self-conceit and uselessness. The decade of the 1760s had been a hot-bed of political and social thought; the spirit of the *Encyclopédie* was coming of age. The under-pinning was nature and the various themes of natural rights. Tissot transferred the theme of natural rights to the realm of a practical physiology: when the "natural rights" of the body were respected by its owner, the result was health; when artificial habits governed the life of a person, the "natural rights" of the body were violated, nature was brutalized, and ill health followed. Tissot had already touched upon that theme in *Onanisme*. As time passed between the publication of *Avis au peuple* and the writing of *Sur les maladies*, he became more concerned with nature and its role in Neo-Hippocratic medicine. His drive for medical care and a healthier way of life also embodied a deeper yearning for a different kind of social relations.

Under the pretext of promoting health, Tissot attacked superstition in *Avis au peuple*, bad habits in *De la santé*, and pretension in *Sur les maladies*. In each treatise he called for a rejection of fetters, for an emancipation from routine, for a realization of the full possibility and true worth of human life. Indeed, Tissot admonished the peasant: "Shake off your fatalism"; the scholar: "The world is larger than your room"; and finally the aristocrat: "Jettison your dependence on patronage and pretension." For each group, he wanted an expanded horizon, a fuller life reached through nature, for nature casts out the useless. The message of contempt for the parasites of society was made clearer in each succeeding book. In *Avis* Tissot took to task the quack who speaks in florid terms, promises the impossible, pockets the money of the credulous, and escapes with a slight-of-hand.[62] *De la santé* was intended, as was *Avis au peuple*, for a class of individuals for whom Tissot felt empathy and at the same time impatience for their lack of awareness to the value of their natural bodies. Both groups ignored the call of nature and mismanaged their resources. This mismanagement of nature was the real culprit, and Tissot wanted his fellow intellectuals to comprehend the value of healthy bodies for balanced minds. He challenged them to measure honestly their intellectual achievements against the pain inflicted on their bodies by negligence of nature and over-preoccupation with their learned research: "Is pride in one's accomplishments worth the price of poor health and ultimately incapacity to work?" Then he declared: "One is too learned when one is so at the expenses of one's health; what is the use of knowledge without happiness?"[63] Only persons with healthy bodies and balanced minds can enjoy a productive life, a life which does not abuse the talents they received from the Supreme Being, a life of which they will see the end without fear, for they have lived a purposeful life (rather than a parasitical one) directed by their conscience.[64]

The title, *Essai sur les maladies des gens du monde*, reveals Tissot's position toward the wealthy, since it substituted "maladie" for "santé" used in the preceding titles. Health may be restored by the natural means of diet, exercise, and simple treatment. Disease denotes a serious condition, often immune to cure by nature; the sternness of his judgment is reinforced by the fact that medical possibilities outside of natural ways were questioned and doubted by eighteenth-century Neo-Hippocratism culminating in the nihilist medicine of the early nineteenth century.[65] For Tissot sickly persons depend on others, a state not far from parasitism.

Sur les maladies makes for pleasant reading with its romantic and slightly irreverent tone; one of its English translators dubbed it a "medical novel".[66] At first it brings a smile for its quaintness: "The aristocrat ought not to favor hours which are those of the wicked wanting to be ignored."[67]   But the smile turns to amazement at Tissot's daring; between the lines lurked a Tissot who was lashing out at the system of privileges. Openly he wrote of health, but behind his rhetoric about natural life and the effects that the Galenic non-naturals have on the health of the peasant and of the aristocrat, Tissot was denouncing an unnatural state of affairs not only confined to the human body but also present in the body politic. "Indolence feeds on itself ... ultimately one finds only painful situations ... where needs have no end and happiness has no beginning."[68]   In his view, this state was so unnatural that it brought disease to the individual and blemishes to the wealthy class, making them incapable of leadership and pre-disposing them to beget feeble children unable to uphold their social positions: such a condition could not last without calamitous outcome.

Sur les maladies had two editions within a year, and then took its place among the several complete works printed later. The success was modest compared to that of *Avis au peuple* (at least 46 editions) or even of *De la santé* which had three editions in 1768 and twenty-one more to our day. *Sur les maladies* was translated into English, German, Italian, and Spanish, whereas *De la santé* had also been translated into Greek, and Polish, while *Avis au peuple* had appeared in fifteen different languages.[69]

Within ten years Tissot had shifted his attention from the country-folk, first to the intelligentsia, and lastly to the courtiers. Each time he saw over-work or over-activity as a hindrance to good health. Tissot defined good health by a state of equilibrium in the body: "when all functions occur regularly, easily, and without any awkward feelings."[70] In that sense Tissot was a humoralist physician; he followed the age-old definition of balance of humors as the way to good health. But he departed from the older ideas of cure when he rejected bleeding, purging, vomiting, and heroic drugs as the primary agents of recovery; instead, he promoted an expectant medicine that relied on the force of nature to effect recovery with minimal help from the art. Hence the stronger and closer to natural life the body was, the better the chance of recovery appeared, since the force of nature was not enfeebled. Obviously, the chances were with the active peasant, not the idle aristocrat.

Tissot had the foresight to mark the dangers of over-exertion for the sake of production, but he did not extol laziness: "usefulness and happiness cannot be separated and it is difficult to have one without the other."[71] In *De la santé* he often referred to the craftsman spending long hours at his bench; he wrote of the small reward for long days of work, of the toll that such practice exacted from health.[72] His contacts with Britain made him aware of the coming of industrialization, of the accelerating pace of production, of the pressure to perform and its detrimental effects on health. This awareness led him to define the country as the haven of a natural mode of life in opposition to the bustle of the urban environment with its noisy workshops. Tissot participated in the vision of a romanticized countryside fallen victim to the empty agitation and pretense of the city.[73] Even worse, in Tissot's view, was the game of patronage played at court which was taking its participants away from their true place in society, their role as leaders.[74] At court, the aristocrats bartered their responsibility for a golden cage; or as Madame Necker put it: "...in a word what one calls duties leave no time for duty."[75] They were enslaved by an illusion which destroyed their health and their will to fulfill their proper calling: "Ambition striving for honor, praises, and wealth, and driven by luxury, agitates ceaselessly the soul of the fashionable, this is enough to destroy his health and to expose him to frequent setbacks."[76] Nonetheless he warned his readers not simply to ape the peasant way of life, for each group had its own proper regimen; nor to become so enslaved to their "health" habits that any small disturbance would be incapacitating.[77]

Tissot wanted his readers to ponder the meaning of their lives and callings, to set in proper proportion their well-being, their ambition, and their way of life: "It is only by keeping the right simplicity that one can enjoy constant pleasure..."[78] He meant his Trilogy to be the starting point of this reflection and the key for everyone to attain good health and full enjoyment of life.[79] This beginning should, he thought, be complemented by a reform of medical education and of hospitals and by a comprehensive policy of public health. Here lies the hinge in Tissot's thinking, the articulation between a partial solution at the individual's level and the general solution found in the concept of public health. Here is the key also to his unpublished writings on medical police.[80]

Tissot's contemporaries certainly perceived this social and political criticism and they chose discreetly to ignore *Sur les maladies* and to lavish praise on *Avis au peuple* which described health to be regained and not disease to be fought. *Avis au peuple* gave the enlightened elite a role as leaders in the movement for a healthier life, whereas *Sur les maladies* demeaned them as sickly and useless creatures. Only an exemplar of *Avis au peuple* found its way into Queen Marie-Antoinette's library.

Tronchin, who was an advocate of a more natural way of life and who also encouraged dieting, exercising, and bathing as treatments, seems to have enjoyed better success with the aristocracy. An aristocrat himself, he could cajole his gentry patients into following his advice by the trappings in which he wrapped it. He designed a standing desk to diminish the bad effects of too much sitting and too much intellectual work. He established the fashion for flat shoes and shorter dress to enable his well-to-do female patients to go for brisk walks unrestrained by high heels and yards of fabric. Cleverly, he prescribed his pills not for their effect (they were often placebos) but for the schedule they imposed, e.g. to take certain remedies upon rising at 7 am; one-half hour before a light lunch; or at retiring at 9 pm.[81] They had complementary roles. Tissot developed theories and wrote books about the natural way to health; Tronchin prescribed by letter and consultation. Today, the Genevan Doctor is well remembered and celebrated for his witty prescriptions: "Monsieur de Voltaire has been living, since he arrived in Paris on the capital of his strength; his friends ought to wish that he would live only on the income", while Tissot is neglected, in part because of his "pompous style".[82]

De la santé and *Sur les maladies* were reprinted together in 1859, but only the first work was judged worth reviewing by Daremberg in 1865.[83] Or would the second book again be apt to awaken susceptibilities in the high circles of the Second Empire and thus should better be left to the private appraisal of its readers? After this 1859 edition, only *De la santé* was reprinted in 1981 and again in 1991. Is *Sur les maladies* too *passé* to arouse interest or just too radical to fit the conventional image Tissot has been assigned in recent scholarship? The subtle revolutionary tone of *Sur les maladies* failed Tissot's intent; in the past it offended many, in the present it disturbs established ideas. Tissot anticipated that only a revolution in mores would transform the ways of the aristocrats and save them from extinction. He meant *Sur les maladies* as a warning signal of immediate danger to the well-to-do: if heeded, catastrophe could be averted; if not society would continue without them. For Tissot, society had no need for feeble and frivolous members. While this was understood at the time, it was ignored like many other attempts at reform.[84] The revolutionary implications of *Sur les maladies* were vindicated by history, even if they are glossed over by historians.

Witnesses from Tissot's own time, Daremberg's review, and Azouvi's preface to the 1981 edition disclose the reactions to *De la santé* at intervals of about a hundred-year each. *De la santé* first appeared in Lausanne under the title *Sermo inauguralis de valetudine litteratorum* (1766), followed quickly by an unauthorized French translation published in Paris (1767). As with *Onanisme*, Tissot was less than happy with the Parisian translation; he embarked on his own, in spite of the fact that he was beginning to hate the tedious task of translating and revising his past works. He wrote to Zimmermann that he had to do it since he hated even more to see his books taken as "passport" for the ideas of their translators.[85] Tissot's expanded French version came out in 1768. Numerous letters attested to the success scholars had in restoring their health, and then maintaining it by following Tissot's prescriptions. Bonnet wrote Tissot thanking him for "the important help given to this small part of humankind who enlightens the other while destroying itself."[86]

Daremberg saw no interest in the reprinting of Tissot's books, except that this edition offered an elegant volume to the discriminating collector.   For Daremberg, hygiene and lifestyle had changed so much over the last century that he wondered about the soundness of this commercial venture.   He failed to perceive the role Tissot had played in the changes; he saw *De la santé* as a narrow enterprise; he disagreed with Tissot's definition of "gens de lettres" as inevitably sedentary beings; he argued that to reduce intellectuals to the diet Tissot proposed is worse than the ill-effects it is supposed to prevent; he disagreed with him about the danger of tobacco making it a question of fashion rather than health.[87] Daremberg did not like *De la santé*; he found it *passé*. How could it have been otherwise?   It was a book written for a past age. Daremberg was still too close to the Ancien Régime, the French Revolution and their mode of thought. He had to distance himself by demonstrating the shallowness of Tissot's observations; Daremberg called them anecdotes since he found them wanting in scientific rigor; he praised the greater value of more recent works in the same field.[88] In spite of Daremberg's proclamation that medicine had drastically changed because it was now anchored on solid observation, the new experimental medicine of Claude Bernard would soon make Daremberg's faith in certain medical ideas almost as old-fashioned as Tissot's.[89] Daremberg looked at Tissot's book through narrow nineteenth-century spectacles and faulted it for failing to address the mental health of the banker or the bureaucrat of the Second Empire, whom he believed to fall within Tissot's category of literary men, since they hardly moved from their desks. Daremberg missed completely Tissot's point of educating eighteenth-century literary persons rather than physicians. Judging Tissot's book as a treatise of medicine for nineteenth-century doctors, indeed Daremberg found it wanting.

Medicine and the method of history have so radically changed that Azouvi can appreciate *De la santé* for what it was meant to be: an aid to better health for a group of individuals sharing some common habits. He places this work in the current of Rousseauist views which held civilization and culture to be breeders of degeneracy and disease; and he points out Tissot's intention to denounce bodily inaction as the seed of nervous disease: the hypochondria of the literary and the hysteria of the idle. Azouvi locates Tissot in his proper context as witness and prophet of his time. Today, Tissot's *De la santé* is part of our intellectual heritage.

While the Trilogy, written in 1760s, was well known, Tissot's writings of the 1780s and 1790s remained largely private. Nonetheless, these later manuscripts complete the earlier works, since some of them expand on topics treated briefly in the Trilogy.[90] His unpublished writings also disclose new currents in the general re-thinking of medical care. Therefore, studying how and why Tissot took up again the subjects of the health-care of women and of rearing children can throw light on his philosophy of medicine, and on his place in the drive for professionalizing medicine.

In spite of a wide interest in the history of childhood,[91] historians of medicine have usually traveled lightly over the roads of the medical world of children before the nineteenth century, except perhaps to signal the efforts of Rousseau and some of his contemporaries.[92] But this scant interest does not give an accurate picture of what was really happening in the field of children medicine. In the second half of the eighteenth century, physicians and lay persons demonstrated a fast growing concern for the medical welfare of children; this effort ought to be incorporated in the studies of the transformation of childhood.[93]

The roots of many endeavors of the Enlightenment can be traced through the Renaissance to Antiquity; the eighteenth-century concern for children is no exception. Furthermore, the interest in Nature fostered by the Scientific Revolution in conjunction with mercantilist theories made the study of population an intriguing and possibly rewarding enterprise. The new fascination with statistics led to a fresh evaluation of the calamitous effect of the prevailing conditions of the recent past on the survival of children. While the mere collection of facts and figures cannot suffice to change a mentality, the availability of data encouraged serious study, as in the works of Halley and Petty on the Bills of Mortality of London.[94] What had previously been vague impressions and suppositions on depopulation and death rate emerged as glaring facts from the statistical study of mortality tables.[95] A cry of alarm was first sounded by political economists; some physicians (in particular those of the Montpellier School) challenged by these findings, took up the gauntlet and questioned their medical tradition: the Galenic which held that infants' characteristics were hot and humid, hence their temperament was most prone to diseases if not intrinsically sick; the mechanistic which held that toddlers had a soft fiber, a constitution very conducive to illnesses; and finally the Hippocratic which advised avoiding hopeless cases. With such traditions, it is not surprising that the health and care of children was not the foremost pursuit of medicine in spite of Hippocrates' writings on the pre- and post-natal care of mother and infant.[96]

Physicians looked afresh to natural phenomena and their Aristotelian explanations through final causes as natural means to solve the ills of civilization. Smallpox, for example, had been a ravager of children and in spite of its danger, the method of inoculation was a solid preventive measure, usually applied early in life. Since inoculation was a natural way, why not seek other natural ways to improve children's chances of survival, remarked the would-be "paediatricians".[97] For now, the concern of educators and physicians shifted to the very young child. Previously, interest in the education or the value of children had been delayed until they reached the approximate age of seven, also considered the age of reason, when they had outgrown the precarious stage of infancy (in rough terms, only half of the newborns would live that long and a quarter of them would have died in the course of their first year).

Another aspect of the new mentality toward childhood can be found in the attempts by parents to limit their fecundity to better the chances of survival of their already born children.[98] This desire of the adults to diminish vital waste can be linked to their consciousness about the value of their own health. The physicians who were party to this medicalization of the world of the adults were also part of the new medical awareness of the needs of children. Thus, Tissot, who had played an unequivocal role in the promotion of healthy habits in adult life, also paid careful attention to the needs of childhood. To a 1768 query of Zimmermann about how to establish a successful practice, Tissot answered that "the cures which accredit most swiftly a physician are those of women and children,..."[99]

Yet, according to the historian of pediatrics Ulmann: "the authors of the works published at that time [eighteenth century] on the subject of the medicine of children pretended to treat anew a neglected topic while in fact they repeated under their own names theories developed by their predecessors; still this does not mean that all originality is absent of this literature."[100]

Tissot's manuscript, *De l'éducation physique et des maladies des petits enfants*, dates from the late 1780s (the latest quotations are from books published in 1784), when Tissot had direct, everyday experience with a child, his grand-nephew Auguste d'Apples, whose family shared a house with the Tissots. The manuscript was written over a period of years, with corrections added on the original as well as on a copy. Tissot probably abandoned the work at the death of Auguste d'Apples in 1790 and may have taken it up again five or six years later, not long before his own death in 1797. His handwriting is much weaker in the corrections than in the original version. Tissot gave a clue for the dating when he praised Etmüller's treatise entitled *Valetudiarum infantibile* (Leipzig, 1675), writing: "it is impossible to say it better than Etmüller did one hundred and ten years ago."[101]

In the eighteenth century physical education covered a much broader domain than it does today. It was much more than exercise and gymnastics; it was a whole way of life spent in accord with hygienic rules based on the Galenic non-naturals. In *Sur les maladies* even more than in *Avis au peuple*, Tissot had placed hope in a different upbringing of children as a cure for the ills of that part of society and had indicated, in fact, that the improvement of society depended on a better physical education of all children. In *De la santé*, Tissot departed from the strictly medical sphere to give his views on the formal instruction of children and on how best to integrate it with a healthy life.

If Ulmann's remark is well taken, what is compilation and what is original in Tissot's thought about the rearing and care of children? What is clearly new in Tissot is the psychological dimension of his advice, and his appeal to the latest advances in physiology to justify this advice. The child is no longer seen as a miniature adult nor as an insensitive creature incapable of feelings, wants, or deep long-lasting hurts.

When, in the Trilogy, Tissot wrote about the health and rearing of children, he was advising parents or non-medical persons. He was then addressing general questions of nutrition and clothing, much in the fashion of the books Ballexserd or Des Essartz had published in the 1760s. However, in *Des petits enfants*, Tissot was unequivocally writing for the medical profession, as he was in some others of his manuscripts dating from the same epoch (*De la médecine civile* and *Traité des maladies des femmes*[102]), since he declared that when writing for a physician, one ought to examine the material fully and very attentively.[103] These works reflected his mature judgment on the role of medical and political authorities in the improvement of the welfare of society. They might have been written as lecture notes at a time when Tissot hoped to see a faculty of medicine added to the Lausanne Academy. Also, the newly formed Collège de Médecine with Tissot at the helm wished to train more medical staff for the Pays de Vaud or at least to offer them continuing education.[104]   These manuscripts written in French dealt with general practice and were directed to physicians eager to learn about the newest advances in their art, yet unable to spend the time and money to pursue such investigations on their own; for this reason, the manuscripts contained few references to ancient authors and many to Tissot's own experience. They were meant as guides on the path to the new role the physician had to play in the mental, physical, and public health of the medicalized world of the nascent bourgeoisie.

Des petits enfants could fall into the category of compilation which is how Ulmann dismissed most of the efforts at a so-called renewed pediatrics. But with this work, Tissot attempted the task of persuading, of the soundness of his advice, physicians accus-tomed to take their clues from such established authorities as Hippocrates, Galen, Sydenham, or Boerhaave. So he offered them such references but also buttressed his arguments by invoking recent works mainly by British doctors such as Buchan, Cadogan, or Hunter, and by referring to nearly current issues of learned journals.[105] Furthermore, he always justified his prescription by an anatomical or physiological explanation. For instance, Haller's irritability was called upon to explain many observations of the functioning of the body. So Tissot attributed many accidents of the first few days to the irritability of the infant's senses exacerbated by the changes in environment, nutrition, and even the knotting of the umbilical cord, which provoked convulsions and vomiting.[106] Tissot also used his own observations and what he called final causes to persuade his readers of the validity of his remarks. For Tissot, final causes were operations performed by nature in the course of life without any help, because they had to take place. In that sense he was an Aristotelian who contemplated the beauty of finality and of teleology, and whose admiration for God's Creation and Wisdom was thus increased. Yet, he was also a pragmatic who showed reservation in the indiscriminate emphasis on final causes to let nature run its own course unaided. The best example is his treatment of the knotting of the umbilical cord. By sheer prudence, Tissot advised that the umbilical cord always be knotted; the fact that animals do not nor the observation that some children do not suffer from its omission were not to be taken as proofs of its inutility. Tissot had seen infants die of a hemorrhage from the umbilicus, but at the same time he strongly warned physicians and judges not to condemn as murderer the mother, who giving birth unattended, did not tie her newborn's cord and had the child die from umbilicus hemorrhage. Ignorance or trust in nature, not malice, should be considered the culprit, and the mother should have the benefit of the doubt.[107] Tissot, with this remark, was not only prompting caution in forensic medicine and juridical decisions; he was also advocating the presence at birth of a physician or trained midwife to insure the proper treatment of the newborn, in fact justifying the medicalization of birthing.

Tissot was well aware that he was not the first nor the only one to write in favor of mothers nursing their babies or of ample unrestrained clothing for infants.[108] He cited Buffon as being among the first to have done so. He candidly admitted who influenced him the most and why: "Mr. Locke, man of infinite genius, great observator, very skilled physician, is properly the first who treated this topic [nutrition], on which he said excellent things and I recommend the reading of his work to all the fathers and all the physicians."[109] Traditionally, if not reluctantly accepted, the role of mother had been to take care of the very young child, while the father's role was understood as coming later with formal education, when the child (the son particularly) was seven years old.[110]   In recommending to fathers to instruct themselves in infant-rearing Tissot might have had two purposes in mind; the first one, to advise fathers on the proper way to care for small children (after all their wives might die in childbirth), enabling them to teach the care-giver sound practice of child-rearing; the second one, under the cover of enlightening fathers about child-rearing, to prepare them to accept and share their wives' new practices on the subject.[111] The former was traditional advice; the latter was modern in its intent to give women a leading role.

Tissot applauded Locke's recommendation of cold bathing and plenty of fresh air to develop strong bodies; this advice was certainly congenial to Tissot's prescription of cooling remedies and pure air in the case of disease.[112]   With Rousseau, in contrast, Tissot is rather stern; he had more admiration for the novelist than the moralist: "*Emile*, published five years after the treatises of Brouzet and Des Essartz, treated of the same subject; while it was written with a great deal of warmth and was more widely read by women and men alike, *Emile* spread their doctrines and made them more acceptable; yet, its reading shows immediately that he [Rousseau] had not seen children nor had the necessary principles to deal in a reliable way with this matter and that in criticizing often Locke, he only belabored or exaggerated Locke's precepts."[113] With this comment, Tissot betrayed a slight flutter of jealousy: Rousseau's Emile was not to see a physician; he needed only a preceptor to teach him the proper rules of hygiene to be kept healthy.   The   pedagogue   was   displacing   the   pediatrician. Eighteenth-century physicians were in a transient position; they had replaced the priest in many functions, and they were the coun-selors and confidants of their secularized bourgeois clientele. Jeal-ous of their new role in preventive medicine and in the ruling of people's lives, they did not want to be ousted from that position by a tutor. Especially since in *Onanisme*, Tissot had already been wary of preceptors and had encouraged parents to supervise personally their children's education. This wounded professional pride is quite openly displayed in Tissot's reference to two books by physicians who gave the same advice as Rousseau did, and yet were ignored by the general public. No one today would quarrel with the statement that with *Emile*, Rousseau was the "porte-parole" of his age, even if some of his opinions are somewhat excessive. But for Tissot, who was trying to exemplify in his medical practice and writings the new role of physician, it was apparently not possible to stay impartial.[114]

Since Tissot was writing for physicians, he explained in great detail the differences in physiology and morbidity between children and adults. He did not think that childhood was synonymous with illness because of its constitution, but that childhood presented a delicate dynamical balance always evolving stage by stage into the adult equilibrium and that each step was a potential danger-spot in which things could go wrong and disease set in.[115] The core of the work covers the child, and all of his or her needs, from the time of birth to the age of the eruption of the last tooth. He was as concerned by the emotional state of young children as by their physical well-being. He advised speaking and handling infants gently. Parents should look for causes of their cries, and not simply feed or rock them to quiet the screams. He had very harsh words for the practice of rocking "it is like intoxication and brings imbecility" and babies were to be fed only if they avidly sucked a finger.[116]

Tissot's manuscript also displayed, compared to other contemporary works, an unusual sensitivity to the social and economic influences on the rearing of children. He dismissed the belief that country children were stronger than urban children and advocated the necessity of proper clothing for everyone. Tissot argued, seemingly contradicting what he had written in *Sur les maladies*, that the children of the people encountered more adverse circumstances to their well-being than those born to wealthy parents. He noted however: "it is true that when they enjoy the same degree of good health, the children of the people are ahead of the privileged in every thing that depends on physical skills, which are strengths sooner developed out of the needs of everyday life in the children who are not always helped nor even anticipated in all their needs."[117] Self-reliance and autonomy were necessary to an harmonious development, while dependence on outside help stunt the process. Tissot had not varied in his appraisal of the wealthy's lifestyle: it was far from being the most conducive to good health. On the next page, he stated: "Footwear belongs to any kind of weather, to all countries, and to every estate, only poverty taught to do without it."[118] He also insisted that a child's temper should be watched, so as not to spoil it or break it; parents had the duty to develop it to its full potential.

Like his contemporaries who wrote on infant care, Tissot devoted a good deal of attention to breast feeding. Yet one aspect of the process is almost neglected in his manuscript: weaning. Tissot, contrary to Ballexserd, did not discuss the problem of the "sevreuse". Tissot simply advocated a gradual weaning starting at about six months, at which time the child should be offered other foods, such as fruits, to complement the mother's milk; then progressively others should be added bit by bit to accustom the child to digesting different foods.[119] Tissot has a long section on pap as substitute or complement for milk, and on the best method to feed a child artificially. Tissot noted that most of the common paps looked more like paste than food, and are useless because indigestible by the infant. He blamed many accidents occurring to babies on the unhygienic practice of using one's finger to feed the pap; instead he advocated using clean cowmilk boiled with some water and fed to the child in a clean cup, never with a rag soaked with it.[120] Tissot was aware of the atrocious toll that the lack of proper nutrition was extracting from the foundlings. He hoped that his advice about artificial feeding for a child reared at home would be put to good use in hospitals, together with his admonitions about the cleanliness of bedding, diapers, and infants. He insisted on simplicity of surroundings and clothing for children, easier to keep clean than elaborate one.[121]

Tissot included sections on when to begin to feed the newborn and on how to choose a wet-nurse. Wet-nursing was at the core of the debate on reforming motherhood. The problem loomed large on Tissot's mind; he was to discuss again the choice, the suitabilility, and the regulation of wet-nurses in *Traité des maladies des femmes* and in *De la médecine civile*.[122] Tissot was against having an adult suck the mother's breast to activate the production of milk or chew first the solid food of the baby: the child was the one to do it; he noted that he disagreed with Ballexserd on this question.[123] At each step in life, Tissot wanted children to accomplish things on their own, or as if on their own, while being encouraged into new discoveries by their parents.[124] Experiences bring judgment;

Tissot's reading of *Emile* (in spite of the criticism) had not entirely been lost.

Turning to the choice of a wet-nurse, Tissot assumed that the nurse would be living at the newborn's home rather than having the infant taken to the wet-nurse's house in the country. Tissot was writing for the late eighteenth-century bourgeois who were accustomed to keeping babies at home. The nobility still sent theirs away, as they considered children a hindrance to their social life. The artisans for whom the mother's earnings were essential to the family budget sent their offsprings for about two years to peasants' households to be nursed and cared for.[125] Tissot advised against hiring a wet-nurse whose child was too young (less than three months); he then wrote down the diet the wet-nurse should follow to make her milk compatible to her suckling's age. In his judgment, a mother, who would from crass interest deprive her own baby, would make a very poor wet-nurse; yet he warned parents to consider and respect both health and feelings of the wet-nurse transported to a foreign environment, away from her child and husband. When the infant was sick, the doctor should also call on her: "The health of the child is one with that of the wet-nurse..."[126]

As usual when he was dealing with diet and exercise, Tissot used the Galenic non-naturals to review the proper regimen for the wet-nurse; at the entry "passions" he wrote: "under this heading one should comment upon the consequences of the 'commerce' between the wet-nurse and her husband, on one hand: pregnancy, on the other hand: the effect on the milk."[127] As far as pregnancy was concerned, he thought that a nursing woman could not conceive as easily as one who was not. This was standard thinking in the eighteenth century and it is still thought true today since nursing often inhibits ovulation at least for some time. It was also common wisdom to say that intercourse altered the quality of the milk, and it was very severely forbidden to the French royal nurses.[128] Tissot departed from this common belief; he thought that the frustrated desires had worse effects on the quality of the milk than their actual fulfillment. He seriously took into account the feelings of women in sexual matters in regard to their well-being and elaborated on the subject in *Traité des maladies des femmes*. He quoted van Swieten to buttress his argument, but van

Swieten's words were not as unambiguously strong as his. Tissot may have found in the writings of the sixteenth-century physician Joubert support for this unusual thought about the "passions" of wet-nurses.[129] Joubert wrote bluntly about the harmful effects of frustrated desires for a nursing woman and her suckling and added that he was not in the habit of giving advice to others that he did not follow himself: an adage Tissot shared with Joubert.[130] In *Des petits enfants*, he wanted to foster modernity by many references to recent books and, particularly, to current issues of the new professional journals. This is probably why he did not cite Joubert, a physician of the old medicine, who was not considered a "classic" as Galen or Avicenna were; such a reference would have defeated his purpose; still, he needed one to buttress his idea, so he used van Swieten, a respected, deceased eighteenth-century physician.

Tissot recommended that the wet-nurse should not sleep in the same room as the baby and absolutely never in the same bed. He was adamant about this last point which he justified with the aid of the Galenic non-naturals (air and rest). Heavy on Tissot's mind was the risk of "overlay" an all too common accident, sometimes also a convenient one to get rid of unwanted babies.[131]

In the last and most technical part of the manuscript devoted to dentition, Tissot presented a general medical history of teeth and teething, and a thorough review of the prognosis and treatment of ailments related to them, since he thought that only the proper and complete knowledge of a subject equipped the physician to deal with it. Here again, he distrusted final causes: "Although cutting a tooth is natural, one should not believe the process painless, thus neglecting it."[132] Teething loomed large in the concerns of those writing on children's health.[133] It was supposed to create all kinds of problems, ranging from rash and fever to convulsions and death. Tissot observed: "I have enough material to prove that from one hundred children who are well-formed and well-cared for, no more than one will die from teething ... and that only one out ten of the well-cared for are sick enough with teething to give any worry to their parents."[134] He was using the novel field of statistics to buttress his principal line of argument: prevention was the best cure, prevention in the form of the right physical and hygienic upbringing. Tissot recommended soothing the gums by chewing or gentle rubbing, or, if the pain became really serious, relieving it by a small incision in the gums where the tooth should come out as was widely done in England under the authority of Hunter. This operation should be done by a properly trained surgeon with a lancet and not with a fingernail. Tissot was adamant: blood-letting was no remedy for children, although leeches placed behind the ears, as he had seen practiced in Montpellier and had tried himself several times, could help to diminish inflammation.[135] In the last sentence of the manuscript, Tissot repeated his advice of never neglecting the slightest deterioration in the health of a child, as it could lead to weakness and languor for life.

Tissot's advice on child-rearing conformed to the view of his time, with one significant exception: the question of the feelings of infants, their mother or wet-nurse. Tissot always aimed at their happiness through caring for their material as well as emotional comfort. He could not repeat often enough that a frustrated baby in swaddling clothes would develop into a sullen peevish adult, but he was no advocate of permissiveness either.[136] Some other points are worth mentioning. In *Des petits enfants*, Tissot offered a more detailed treatment of the first age of childhood than Ballexserd, whose treatise covered upbringing, from birth through fifteen years old in a small volume of 238 pages in octavo. Incidentally, Rousseau accused Ballexserd of plagiarism, but the charges cannot withstand the scrutiny of impartial eyes.[137] Venel's book addressed the health of girls and he devoted a large part of it to the value of exercise and the abuse of corsets. Venel's main point was that girls, like boys, should have an active life since charm and health result from naturally elegant, strong bodies. He worked on the premise that only healthy women will give birth to healthy children, and only healthy girls can turn into healthy women. Venel was a model of the new male midwife; he was the founder of the first midwifery school and obstetric hospital in Switzerland. He showed primarily a populationist intent rather than a advocacy of individual happiness and fulfillment. Tissot was to address in *Traité des maladies des femmes* the specific happiness of women as women, not only as future wives or mothers.

All the eighteenth-century authors who wrote on the upbringing of children, albeit some (Helvetius) more openly than others, expounded the view that children are the hope of nations.[138] Through its children, especially those receiving a proper physical and intellectual education from their enlightened parents, a nation will build a future of growing attainment.[139] The foundlings were not left out of the concern of the reform-minded writers. Raulin had very strong words about the ties between their well-being and the political authorities' enlightenment.[140] The program of the Encyclopedists started with youth, unspoiled and open to learning. A new wave of children, brought up differently than their parents, ought to fulfill the dreams of a new society through evolution or revolution; indeed, the line of demarcation is a thin one. Tissot's manuscript, *Des petits enfants*, demonstrates his commitment to the new mentality.

While he was writing on the health of children, Tissot also wrote on that of women in the longest of his unpublished manuscripts.[141] Tissot loved what he referred to as his "travail de cabinet" (writing); but he worked with bursts of energy, then let himself be side-tracked by his practice, another project, or entered periods of lethargy due to his own failing health (all characteristic of tuberculosis). So he became overconfident in his capacity to complete the treatises he was working on simultaneously, misled as he was by his ability to have done so twenty years earlier when he had worked on *De la santé*, *Sur les maladies*, and *Traité des nerfs* as well as on revisions of *Avis au peuple* and *Onanisme*. Finally, he also showed signs of growing bored with the hassle of publishing. After Zimmermann's death on 7 October 1795, Tissot undertook at the request of his widow to write his "éloge". In barely more than a year, Tissot wrote and published a book entitled *Vie de Zimmermann*, and probably neglected his other works to complete this book on his friend.[142] By February of 1797, when Tissot worked again on *Des maladies des femmes* (as some additions indicate), he had only a few months to live and never finished the revisions.

Des maladies des femmes provide another valuable key to understanding Tissot's medical philosophy. Here, even more than in *Traité des nerfs*, he drew for his medical practice the full consequences of his humoralism adapted to the theories of irritability and fiber. *Des maladies des femmes* shows him at the peak of the mastery of his own medical thought as well as of his partaking to the latest medical trends. In particular he argued his views on women in close connection with the vitalist thought of the Montpellier School as exemplified in the work of Roussel.[143] Tissot does not explicitly refer to Roussel, which is in line with the eighteenth-century custom of not specifically citing what is supposed to be well-known (especially when the author was still alive), for fear of insulting the scholarship of the reader. Since he carefully identified his sources outside of contemporary French writings which might be less familiar to his prospective readers, Tissot may indeed have omitted to cite Roussel's only because he assumed that the work was widely known. In *Des maladies des femmes*, Tissot used more materials from recent professional journals than in any other of his works. The *Philosophical Transactions*, the *Essays of Edinburgh*, the *Annales de chirurgie*, or the *Comptes-rendus de la Société royale de médecine* are frequently quoted, even more often than medical books. His choice of words also reveals a clear spirit of modernization. Twice he used the word antiseptic, which was first used in the English language in 1751 or in the French idiom in 1763, then by Priestley in 1774.[144] His reference to the concept that pus' discharge is not always a positive sign, but should frequently be combatted with antiseptic fomentations is even more important as evidence of a new reflection on humoral medicine than his use of the word antiseptic. *Des maladies des femmes* provides a coherent exposition of the accepted physiology and anatomy of women, on which Tissot based his knowledge of feminine nature. He added his own experience with his female patients to arrive at a special understanding of feminity and to draw new conclusions for the treatment of diseases related to the reproductive system. The table of contents demonstrates the scope of the project.[145]

Tissot opened with a review of the different nature and organization of man and woman, mainly to demonstrate that women's "fiber" was softer than that of men. He explained the difference by final causes: women are meant to bear children, in pregnancy and delivery their bodies are exposed to tremendous changes. A strong fiber would counteract these changes, whereas a soft fiber would easily give way to an enlarged uterus or the push of a child's head. Tissot perceived this as an advantage in childbearing, but as hindrance to very good health. He argued that a soft fiber does not allow the functions of the body to take place as well as they should to assure optimum health. It predisposes to congestion and obstruction as well as to accumulating fat; the nervous system is more susceptible to disturbances in a body of soft fibers; so Tissot concluded that women are more prone to mobility of the nervous type which he explained as an over-reaction of the nerves to bodily disturbances such as bad digestion. He also attributed to women's soft fiber his observation that in general more men than women will die of acute diseases and more women than men of chronic diseases.[146] On several occasions he gave a precise description of the size and position of the uterus to enable the consulting physician to determine by means of manual examination the proper causes of the different complaints or troubles, for example the lack of menstruation.

Tissot wrote *Des maladies des femmes* especially for the physicians who treated women of the bourgeoisie. This choice of audience explains why he insisted that the lack of physical education and the kind of life led by wealthy women were exaggerating the softness of their fiber to the point of impairing the functions the soft fiber was meant to favor. He charged both doctors and women with the responsibility for improving the health of the female sex: the physician had to explain to his patient her particular needs and weaknesses; the woman had to watch her bodily reactions to external factors and report her symptoms accurately to her physician, and she had to heed her doctor's counsel.

According to Tissot, the physician should give a three-part consultation before attempting diagnosis and prognosis, and finally prescribing a treatment: 1) historical in which the patient recalled all the details of the disease and its treatment from its onset up to the present day; 2) physical in which the doctor, through careful palpation, checked the state of his patient's body; and 3) psychological in which he judged and weighed his findings against the motivations underlying the chosen descriptions of ills and symptoms. Tissot had in mind specific cases in which a patient might want to mislead her physician concerning the real nature of her complaints, so as to receive the wrong prescription for her state but the right one for her purpose: a woman who hid her pregnancy claiming a loss of menses without acknowledging the possible cause, thus hoping to receive an abortive drug; or a women truly suffering from a suppression who claimed to be younger than she really was just in order to regain her periods as a sign of youth. Tissot took seriously the Hippocratic Oath of not giving an abortive substance to a pregnant woman, yet he showed concern for the ill effects of the missing menses: "the disturbance of such an important function is in general always harmful, many adverse results stem from women's ill-advised conduct during their periods, endangering their health, that of their future children as well as their happiness and that of their entourage; each women should observe what is damaging to her and renounce it forever."[147]

Tissot, like many of his contemporaries, explained the normal and necessary discharge of menstruation through a plethora created when no pregnancy took place since no foetus needed the menstrual blood as nourishment before nutrition through the placenta and umbilical cord was established. In the humoral system, plethora of any of the humors was a potential source of disorder. But at the same time the suspension of menstruation could also mean that the body was not producing this normal plethora due to a weakness which had to be identified. So Tissot advised searching seriously and conscientiously for the cause of the suspension before blindly forcing a resolution: "medicine does not know yet of any substance that certainly determines the periods and that is without a doubt a wise occurrence."[148] In his view, all the supposedly specifics *emménagogues* were dangerous because they were hot, acrid, and irritant. The physician, Tissot noted, should always balance the present discomfort against the risk of the treatment and not yield to fashion: "it is one of those cases in which many physicians practice medicine from public demand without observing that they dispense bad medicine..."[149] He further added that a treatment which had no effects for several weeks should be discontinued and replaced by milder drugs, exercise, diet, cleanliness... and trust in nature. Once the physician has discovered the real cause of the suspension, the proper treatment for correcting this fundamental condition must be prescribed, even if the physician has to disguise it, to please the women or her relatives, as a remedy to reactivate the menses. Tissot noted that, in Edinburgh, electricity was used to restore periods, on the premise that electricity increased the rapidity of the circulation of the blood and the fluidity of the humors, hence induced the plethora which was a condition favorable to menstruation; but he did not recommend it, since he considered electricity as an "heroic" drug.[150]

Since menstruation was judged to be so critical a time, Tissot devoted a whole chapter to what should be done when sickness struck during the menstrual discharge.   Here again he was dispelling misconceptions and customs, especially that of refraining if not outwardly abstaining from administering any drug or treatment during this time.   He recognized that this custom was so well anchored that sometimes the fear of taking remedies destroyed all the good that might be expected from the treatment.

Tissot addressed the question of breast-feeding and its consequences for the health of the new mother.   He had a very long chapter on the risk of improper care during lactation as well as on its artificial suppression.   *Lait épanché* (milk re-absorbed by the mother's body) was believed to create all kinds of health problems. Tissot agreed with this view up to the point where he objected that it was too often an easy solution for the physician to blame *lait épanché* for any complaints, any time in the life of a woman who once bore a child.[151] He advised doctors to prevent congestion of the breast and to instruct the nursing mother in the symptoms to watch; he assumed that mothers were nursing their babies and instructed their physicians accordingly.   In *Des maladies des femmes* Tissot sharply criticized the practice of wet-nursing.   Yet, he admitted that sometimes there were valid reasons for the mother not to breast-feed her baby.   He described how to avoid a bad wet-nurse, especially one with venereal diseases.   Tissot concluded that the best way to avoid all the dangers of wet-nursing was to manage without it.[152] He then moved to the use of animal's milk in feeding babies.   Here as in *Des petits enfants*, he wrote that the best choice is boiled cowmilk diluted with some water to use first as a supplement to, later as a substitute for the mother's milk. Tissot also tried to dispel the idea that any milk was bad for an infant and that only artificial feeding with a pap of grain and beer was a guarantee of success.   The idea behind this regimen was that with the milk the infant also absorbed the character's traits of the human or animal female.   Tissot dismissed this theory which had been published anonymously in 1738: "fifty years ago", and added that La Mettrie attributed it to the Abbé Moreau de St. Elie.[153]

In his chapter on "pâles couleurs" or chlorosis, Tissot described a situation of languor in adolescence in which the complexion has a greenish color.[154] He wrote that in the prevalent view this disease was related to the lack of menses at the so-called normal age for the discharge to appear. He took a different position, noting that while girls were primarily subject to this disease, boys were not exempt from it; he thus saw it as a problem related to physical education and to the ways in which wealthy girls were brought up. In an addition to the copied version, he remarked: "the pale colors are much less common since physical education has become better." A few pages further the clean copy reads: "I am not afraid to say that one does not find now a tenth of the *oppilations* [pale colors with loss of the menses] than one had in the past."[155] Nonetheless, chlorosis took almost epidemic proportion in the nineteenth century.[156]

A. Clair Siddall, in a well-documented article, argued for an iatro-etiology of the disease, since the prevalent cure was bloodletting.[157] Siddall also based his argument on the increased consultation of doctors by nineteenth-century wealthy persons. His point was that more girls suffered from the disease because more of them were brought to a physician for a mild condition which was rendered worse when treated by bloodletting; in the case of chlorosis the medicalization of society was a mixed blessing.[158] By contrast, Tissot did not bleed for chlorosis, he prescribed exercise and diet to which he added an iron based medicament.

In *Avis au peuple*, Tissot had already treated the case of chlorosis and had prescribed a drug for the use of country girls suffering from pale colors.[159] Those girls were not sick from a lack of exercise, but from poor nutrition. The prescription was for a preparation of iron; however Tissot cautioned that this drug was too strong for well-to-do girls and gave an adequate formula for them, which also contained iron.[160] Here he spoke as the humoralist who warned of the need to adapt the remedy to the temperament and condition of the patient. Yet, Tissot placed his highest hopes for the success of the cure in exercise and activity, the best way to animate the functions and to distract from the sadness that often accompanied pale colors. He also wrote that many persons considered marriage a cure for chlorosis; he advised against it, except when the languor resulted from not having the object of one's love. Otherwise, marriage was merely one more burden piled on an already weak constitution.[161] With the treatment of pale colors, Tissot insisted once more on the value of natural cures as well as on the worth of looking into the psychological features behind diseases.

In *Des maladies des femmes*, Tissot displayed concern and respect for the special needs and personality of women.   He instructed physicians to prescribe solely treatments female patients would accept and to attempt only the examinations to which a modest woman would consent.[162]   He based his therapies on women's active participation, assigning the responsibility for cure to their initiative, first by seeking consultation early, second by changing their way of life in responding actively to the age-old prejudice of soft and weak female bodies. Tissot wanted physicians to understand the positive values and the respective roles of nature and final causes, and therefore to recognize their own prejudices and cultural biases.[163]   Tissot defined the particular problem of woman's health as two-fold: physiological and cultural. Physicians and women had to understand this duality and hence had to aim at the best possible health-care for the happiness of women, preeminently as individuals, not only as providers of citizens.

Tissot certainly was a promoter of medicalization and an advocate for a larger role for the physician in the planning of people's lives. However, he saw this role of "directeur de conscience" as a partnership between patient and doctor. Consequently, he wrote first for the people, teaching them the value of enlightened medicine; then he turned to special groups of individuals rendering them aware of the nature of their physiological needs; and finally he charged physicians with building the bridge to an educated partnership in health and the concommittant pursuit of happiness.

Chapter VI

Success and Illness

By the 1760s Tissot had definitively become a leading medical writer. His Trilogy had brought him fame with the lay public. His defense of inoculation had spawned a mixture of vicious attacks by detractors of the practice and praises by its advocates. In the 1770s he kept publishing revised editions of his books, while writing new medical treatises and attending to a growing private practice. All of these activities, even the fights, furthered his medical career, but at the same time, he paid with illness for his success.

In marriage Tissot had hoped to find at home what he had been looking for at the numerous parties and dinners he had attended as a bachelor: the supportive and challenging feminine companionship of a lively speaker embedded in a good listener. Charlotte d'Apples was neither. Tissot was too preoccupied with advancing his career to spend the necessary time to build the relationship further than the bedroom. The death of his infant daughter and the resulting ill health of his wife took even that away. Tissot retreated more than ever to his dear "cabinet" and wrote almost with a vengeance, making extensive use of the fine library in his father-in-law's house. After a few years and a few books Tissot, the overworked physician of the poor, became an oversought doctor for the fashionable.[1]

The round of parties engaged him again, while his medical practice absorbed more of his time. His health faltered; in his letters to Zimmermann, Tissot complained repeatedly of head-colds, nagging coughs, eye problems, and indigestion. When he also lost sleep, Tissot blamed the social demands of his wealthy patients eager to entertain and dine their doctor. In fact, Tissot was over-extending himself in his medical practice and writings, without paying enough attention to the "little dry cough" he had kept since his measles case while a student in Montpellier. Tissot insisted on blaming food indulgences and social whirls for his poor health. He was diagnosing in himself the causes of disease he denounced in his wealthy patients. He not only had to cure them, but himself too, for he had fallen prey to the contagion of their disorders. At this point, Tissot never thought to correlate the sequels of his measles case with his repetitive bouts of fever. Nonetheless, the symptoms described to Zimmermann indicate that already in the 1760s Tissot was suffering from tuberculosis, a fact he acknowledged only in the 1790s.[2]

Tissot was not ready to recognize how his own style of life was endangering his health, nor was he ready to take the necessary steps to cure himself. For him, building a career and pursuing medical success was more important than enjoying the company of his wife and step-daughter. In writing, he could denounce the solitary pleasure of onanism for the sake of the affectionate family new mentality, but in real life, Tissot could not recognize the results of his own selfish actions. The appeal of the world was too strong, the "médecin galant" epithet which he had ascribed to himself in a letter to Zimmermann about his inclinations before his marriage was back, haunting his family.[3] They assumed that he needed a child to retain him at home, or out of his study, as the only way to improve his health; unfortunately his wife had miscarriage after miscarriage, and Tissot lost hope of ever having a son.[4] In an effort to lure Tissot away from mundane pursuits and back into a more sedate bourgeois lifestyle, his sister-in-law, on the verge of death, urged him and his wife to adopt her last son, aged two. In 1762, young Marc d'Apples came to live with the Tissots. At first the arrival of the child did not change much in Tissot's customary ways. It was 26 April 1763 before he mentioned the boy to Zimmermann, although he had written approximately every month during the past year. The letters were full of news about Rousseau and reactions to *Emile* or about Suzanne Curchod "too beautiful and too learned for me to dare to pretend to be her friend. I am neither young enough nor ignorant enough for her to turn me into a schoolboy,..."[5]

Slowly, however, Marc was becoming part of his uncle's life in ways Tissot would never have suspected a child could. Remembering the fond time passed with his own uncle, he took an earnest interest in the boy's welfare and education. Marc brought joyful activity in the house which drew Tissot out of his study; he discovered the pleasure of family life and began to appreciate the ever quiet presence of his wife. He became devoted to Marc. In fact, some decisions Tissot made about his own career were motivated by what he perceived was in the best interest of his nephew as well as by circumstances in Marc's life which redirected Tissot's medical interests to include the reform of medical education, public hygiene, and health-care for women and infants.[6]

Tissot's reputation as a medical writer was attracting many wealthy or notorious patients to Lausanne; the Prince Louis Eugene of Wurtemberg was one of the most devoted. While by now Tissot was rarely attacked for his defense of inoculation, medical reviewers did fault him for writing *Avis au peuple* for a specific country with peculiar climate and customs and for trusting the delicate task of caring for the sick in the hands of non-medical persons. He was chagrined by the critics because he had no other ambition than to help the population of the Pays de Vaud. Tissot admitted the impossibility of writing for everyone everywhere, as he also recognized the implausibility of a universal remedy.[7] For Tissot, anyone claiming to have or to know of a universal remedy was a quack, deceiving the population. In his view, the causes of diseases were multifarious and many of them still unknown; multiple causes could not be cured by a single remedy no matter how complex the prescription. The duty of the physician was to look for the particular disease, then to prescribe a specific treatment meant to cure its cause and not merely to mitigate its symptoms. Being interested in determining the causes of diseases in order to devise better cures, Tissot concluded that finding the reasons for good health was of prime importance. Consequently, he showed interest in physiological theories and research. He himself did some experimentation along the lines of Haller's work and demonstrated the insensitivity of sinew. His main interest, however, always lay in pathology which he thought was a less controversial subject.

In the 1760s, because of their physiological research, Tissot and Haller were accused by de Haen of irreligiosity.[8] Previously, de Haen had viciously attacked Tissot on the practice of inoculation, even bringing insinuations of witchcraft to buttress his arguments. De Haen, running out of steam in his fight against inoculation, shifted his ground of assault to different areas of medicine: first to the description and definition of pleuresy, second to the theory of irritability and its supposedly inherent atheism. De Haen was introducing the concept of materialism (which he scorned) and the attendant problem of the inter-connections between mind and body into medical quarrels. In the eighteenth century, materialism was a serious issue which could be somewhat openly discussed as a "scientific approach" to an understanding of life. Still, La Mettrie, as one proponent of materialism, had to flee France and seek refuge at the court of Frederick the Great; he had died there a few years before de Haen's attacks.[9] Buffon, Diderot, and other Encyclopedists had to speak in half-words so as not to displease the powerful Sorbonne.[10] De Haen was a fiercely devout Catholic Dutchman established at the Habsburg court in Vienna. His contention can be better understood when one recalls the torments of religious wars and the bitter struggle to gain freedom from the Spanish Habsburg's dominion the Netherlands had suffered in the sixteenth and seventeenth centuries. The complete independence of the Dutch Republic (the northern, mainly Protestant, part of the country) was finally recognized in 1648 at the Treaty of Westphalia.

Religious skepticism was more a threat to the Catholic version of Christianity than to the Reformed. Protestantism had always advocated looking for one's own set of answers in the Bible.[11] By the eighteenth century, the emphasis on individual determination of Biblical meaning had led to various interpretations of God's role in the Creation and in everyday life. These variations were not always pleasing to the Protestant clergy, especially when proclaimed high and loud by d'Alembert in the *Encyclopédie* article "Genève" in which some Genevan pastors were suspected of deism.[12] Nevertheless, the concept of a rational God creating a world that the human mind could comprehend and master was congenial to the enlightened mentality. Therefore, the Protestant members of the Enlightenment had little trouble in reconciling their religion with reason; the same was not true of the Catholics, many of whom turned to deism or materialism to reconcile their enlightened reasonings with their religious beliefs.

Tissot reacting to de Haen's allegations of impiety wrote: "If the discovery of irritability can produce some moral effect on a righteous spirit, it is to make him admire its Author whose immortal wisdom brought about through such a simple way the most beautiful phenomenon of the nature of man alive."[13] De Haen had misread the Protestant mentality, which aims at understanding the world as a means to glorify the Creator and not to reject God.[14] But Tissot's disgust at de Haen's method of mixing religious and scientific issues gave him one more reason to turn to the social aspect of medicine rather than to its theoretical understanding. The social dimension of medicine was also controversial, but on a political plane. Tissot tried to stay above quarrels, often at the price of not publishing his thoughts. For him, medicine was a social calling, prompted by religion, to relieve the suffering of all, thus it was necessary to instruct the political authorities on the best way to procure good health through reasonable care for the population entrusted to them.[15] Tissot felt that any form of government could be rendered aware of medical problems and conscious of its duty to alleviate them.

In spite of the theoretical bent that still marks all of Tissot's books, he was a practical man, always looking for the most direct way to achieve his purpose. He had no time for sophistry, so he dropped his interest in a field that brought him this type of chicanery and instead devoted his efforts to practical medicine. Among Tissot's published works, *Traité des nerfs et de leurs maladies* (1770-1780) perfectly illustrates this shift of emphasis.[16] In *Traité des nerfs* he could be as theoretical as he wished, using irritability and psychosomatic interpretation to his heart's content. Nonetheless, his aim was always a practical one, namely to understand the nature of nervous diseases and to be able to cure them. The unpublished *De la médecine civile* was the direct product of his socio-medical concerns and of the role he thought the state should play in public health.[17]

The Philosophes' emphasis on education and reason revived in many Protestants the spirit of the Reformation with its appeal to dispel superstition and ignorance. Steps toward improving general education and social conditions were taken in several of the Swiss cantons.[18] Driven by the same impetus, Tissot turned his attention to the reorganization of the health service for the poor and to the education of medical personnel and wrote *Mémoire sur les moyens de procurer au peuple les secours les plus utiles dans les maladies*.[19] His efforts were fruitless, due to a combination of foot-dragging on the part of the Bernese authorities, who were never enthusiastic about innovations introduced by their subjects, and to the suscepti- bilities of the different councils of Lausanne which were very jealous of what little was left of their prerogatives. They were therefore unwilling to listen when Tissot proposed creating an entirely new school for the training of midwives and surgeons. He decided to wait for another occasion to implement his reforms, since he knew of the difficulties Haller was encountering. The opportunity came in the 1765 when their Excellencies of Bern requested that Tissot draw up a plan for the upgrading of health services in their lands. He adapted his former *Mémoire* and submit- ted *Plan d'instruction pour des médecins de village*.[20] Strangely enough since Bern had initiated the project, Tissot's proposal to train medical personnel in a hospital-setting came to next to noth- ing, even though the Bernese had in the past rewarded his success at fighting epidemics with a gold medal and membership in their Société économique.[21] If their Excellencies had been fishing for compliments, they received some in Tissot's proposal, which recog- nized in the Inselspital in Bern the best place to establish a school for country surgeons. But this plea for a new school could also be interpreted as a criticism of their prized hospital and was resented as such.

Others recognized the potential that Tissot could bring to their state. Not far from Bern, Solothurn (one of the thirteen cantons of Old Regime Switzerland) offered him the post of State Physician. He refused, on account of not mastering German, the language in Solothurn. He recommended Zimmermann for the position; in the end, Solothurn chose a Jesuit medic.[22] From abroad, Dr. Wolff, physician to the Prince Czartorysky, contacted Tissot on behalf of the newly elected King of Poland who was looking for a suitable candidate for the position of first physician.[23]

The offer, however, presented a dilemma. For Tissot, Catholic Poland would be a country of mixed opportunity. As the King's physician, he would have the power to implement some of his dearest projects; but the same position would also bring jealousy and intrigues, especially since he was a Protestant. Tissot did not want to encounter animosity and opposition to his views for reasons mainly dictated by bigotry.[24] He could not blatantly refuse; an honorable excuse had to be found. To decline the offer, he pleaded his responsibility to his aging parents and the long hazardous travel. Stanislas-Augustus, who wanted to bring enlightened absolutism to his strife-torn country, reassuringly wrote to Tissot of the warmest possible welcome at his court; the King had read the religious concern between Tissot's lines.[25]

Tissot pondered the question for more than a year. On the one hand, the Polish position offered the chance to see his views on preventive medicine implemented; on the other, it offered the risk of *Heimweh* and chicanery. Tissot wrote to Haller asking for his help in disentangling the pros and cons of the situation.[26] Haller, who knew the advantages and inconveniences of an official position in a foreign country (he had been professor of medicine at Goettingen and first physician to the Elector of Hanover) and of trying to be a reformer under their Excellencies of Bern, found it very difficult to give an impartial answer. In fact, Haller found the decision so difficult that he spoke of Tissot's Polish project to some influential members of the Senate of Bern and transmitted to Tissot their dismay at the prospect of his expatriation.[27] Tissot had not expected his friend to give an official turn to his request for advice and gently scolded Haller on the matter. Tissot had wanted impartial advice and was still naive about how to handle the oligarchy of Bern, whereas Haller knew, all too well, what motivated them. For once, their Excellencies reacted quickly; three days after Haller's letter, Tissot was called to the Castle by the Bernese Bailiff and handed his letter of appointment as professor of medicine at the Lausanne Academy.[28] The Town-Council of Two Hundred was also debating what (title, money) to offer him in order to prevent his accepting the last offer of Stanislas-Augustus (housing and board, carriage and horses, a yearly pension of 1000 gold ducats, and 400 ducats to defray travel cost).[29]

The appointment, dated 30 January 1766, gave Tissot the right of deliberation and suffrage in the Academy Council. The Academy had no medical faculty and was very sensitive to infringements on its prerogative. The Council grudgingly accepted the *de facto* academic appointment. Tissot was overwhelmed by the unprecedented solicitude Bern had shown him. He again refused the offer of the Polish King, when, in fact, he had decided to try the post for a few years. At this point in his career and with the added responsibility of his nephew's adoption, Tissot thought that he could ill afford to hurt the pride of their Excellencies by declining the professorship they had bestowed on him.

Tissot's timorous attitude can be explained by the fear of *Heimweh* and by a sober appraisal of the power he could actually wield in Poland, a nation known to be subject to cabals and favoritism.[30] Once out of favor with the King, he would be nothing, and even when in favor he would have to cope with the usual jealousy that plagued any foreigner in a position of power. Where could he turn if things went wrong in Poland, after having angered their Excellencies of Bern by refusing their professorship and departing from Lausanne? Childhood stories engraved on his mind the lesson of his Helvete ancestors, who having burned their fields before leaving their homeland, were forced by Julius-Caesar to return to its self-inflicted bareness. He lacked sufficient confidence in his reputation to run the risk.

Tissot was right as later events proved. Others tried their luck in Poland and ran afoul of the internecine quarrels for which it was notorious.[31] Stanislas-Augustus himself encountered difficulties with his program of reforms, which, after factions had invited foreign intervention, ended with his abdication and the dismemberment of his Kingdom in 1795. In accepting Tissot's refusal, the King wrote in his own hand that he was very pleased to have been instrumental in advancing Tissot's career since the professorship nomination was, in fact, a counter-offer to his own.[32]

Their Excellencies of Bern, cashing in on their favor, requested extended duties from their newly appointed professor. Tissot had to travel by horseback near and far to organize the fight against epidemics, since Lausanne or the Pays de Vaud were rarely spared a yearly return of bilious fever. While he was generally successful at saving lives when the fever was raging, he was not satisfied, because as soon as he returned to Lausanne, the quacks took over again, since few qualified medical practitioners were available in the countryside. Tissot thought that preventive measures of proper diet and hygiene should also be implemented. For their Excellencies, treating epidemic fevers was one thing, preventing them was another. The Bernese were ready to improve transportation or agriculture if that meant money returning to their treasury. Money spent for improvements not directly taxable did not interest them. Even with Haller in their midst, the Bernese saw no point in preventive medical expenditures.[33]

Dashing to the four corners of the Pays de Vaud, Tissot was exposed to infection and exhaustion. He actually was sick for weeks at a time, hardly able to answer the many consults he received, even less to see patients in Lausanne. He needed rest, not more distraction. To get away from the pressure, Tissot bought a house, Montrion, just outside Lausanne, where Voltaire had previously resided. The pleasure of country living and the escape from callers restored some strength to Tissot. He explained to Zimmermann that he walked to his lodging in Lausanne every afternoon and that this exercise helped him digest and sleep better.[34]

Tissot had barely settled in his new lifestyle when he received another offer from a foreign court. Dr. Werlhoff, first physician to the Elector of Hanover, died in 1767. His position was offered to Tissot. The Elector and King of England George III wanted a well-known physician for his Hanoverian Court. Tissot had many contacts with British physicians, including Pringle with whom he corresponded on medical matters and about the possible recall of Haller at the University of Goettingen.[35] Tissot was tempted to accept the position. Hanover was not as far as Warsaw, religious differences were down to a variation on the Reformation theme, and Haller spoke highly of the intellectual atmosphere of the Electorate.

Tissot's mother having recently died, and his brother, an officer in the Dutch Republic armies, being now stationed in India, Tissot thought that his father should not be left alone. Furthermore, recalling that he had earlier written to Haller: "Where would I be more free than in Lausanne?" Tissot suggested his friend Zimmermann who was eager to get out of his hometown of Brugg which he found too restraining.[36] Zimmermann was appointed to the post; he did not, however, receive the compensation and benefits offered to Tissot. Rather Zimmermann was hired with the same conditions as the late Dr. Werlhoff, which amounted to about one third less.[37] Later Zimmermann bitterly lamented the move, and Tissot regretted his part in the appointment.[38]

The next year, through the good offices of the Prince of Wurtemberg, Tissot was contacted by the Court of Vienna for the

possible inoculation of the Imperial children. Smallpox was such a
robber of lives at the Hofburg that Joseph II had lost his two wives
and his only daughter to the scourge. Maria-Theresa was not
against the practice of inoculation and showed interest in Tissot.
Haller forewarned Tissot of the risks of encountering once more
the wrath and acid pen of de Haen, as well as the displeasure of the
Hanoverian Court should he decide to stay, adding that court's
intrigues and servitude were never compensated by wealth or
honor.[39] It was true that Tronchin had succeeded in overcoming
all obstacles when he inoculated the children of the Duke of
Orleans, but Tronchin had at the Court of Versailles or in Paris no
enemy such as Tissot had in de Haen. It was clearly less dangerous
to treat the Duke of Orleans' children than those of Maria-Theresa
herself. In fact, de Haen went so far as to suggest that it would be
impious to let an alien heretic introduce a foreign substance into
the bodies of the Archdukes! Tissot declined the Viennese offer
but accepted one from the Senate of the Republic of Venice to
advise them on inoculation. Again Tissot chose to write rather
than to travel for the cause he cherished. Anyway, the princes who
wanted to have their children inoculated by Tissot came to
Lausanne for the purpose, as witnessed by many letters of appreciation and thanks.[40]

Tissot, who in refusing the offer of the King of Poland and of the
Elector of Hanover, had invoked the excuse of aging parents
needing his care, lost his uncle, his mother, and his father within a
few years. His father passed away on 4 September 1768. It is difficult not to see a coincidence in the fact that on October 1st, the
Council of the Sixty of Lausanne called Tissot to fill a vacancy and
waived on his behalf the restriction of at least ten years of bourgeoisie tenure to hold office in the Council.[41] Lausanne had been
quick to recognize that with the death of his father, Tissot had one
less tie in the Pays de Vaud. The Council of Sixty had also acted on
the premise that Tissot's fame was attracting many people to
Lausanne, bringing revenues not only to the doctor but to the town
merchants and innkeepers as well, and even to the bourgeois
families who rented parts of their houses to wealthy foreigners.[42]
In spite of Tissot's repeated refusals of outside offers, influential
personalities were still trying to attract him to their particular
projects.

One such project was the founding in Paris of a model hospital where the best physicians, surgeons, and pharmacists would practice and teach. The project was the brain-child of Chamousset who had convinced Choiseul, then War Minister, of the feasibility of the project and of the fame it would bring to the Kingdom.[43] During his adult life, Chamousset tried to help the underprivileged, but he unfortunately attracted more mockery than respect for his philanthropic enterprises. The Count and Countess of Golowkin, wealthy patients of Tissot while in Lausanne, had suggested Tissot's name when the search for a suitable director was open.[44] Chamousset approached Tissot in an undated letter, probably written late in 1770, since Tissot mentioned to Zimmermann that he had been pressed for the past two months to accept a very lucrative position.[45]

Hospital building was flourishing in the eighteenth century. Hospitals served several purposes, such as removing old-age paupers and young orphans from the streets, procuring health care for the sick as well as medical experience and knowledge for the students and professors of medicine and surgery. For Chamousset the last purpose was the most important. In his letter to Tissot, he described what he hoped to achieve with this new institution for medical research and curing. Chamousset proposed keeping an exact account of each disease, with symptoms, diagnosis, remedy, and results of the cases. Then any other information obtained about the same disease was to be added to the report collected at the hospital. All similar cases were to be filed in a single box to be deposited in the private library of the hospital. When enough information had been gathered to arrive at a sound judgment of diagnosis, prognosis, treatment, and success, the outcome was to be made available to all hospitals in the hope that they would reciprocate. Chamousset was, in fact, describing the Baconian scientific method applied to medicine which Tissot would use later when teaching clinical medicine at Pavia.[46]

Tissot's answer is lost. He seldom kept copies of his answers, but usually jotted down, on the letter itself, a few indications of his intentions to be developed in his response. Unfortunately, the letter from Chamousset carries no notes nor comments. Tissot was not inclined to go to Paris to take up a position as Choiseul's "protégé". First, Tissot was not in the habit of being anyone's "protégé", and, second, he felt a special loyalty to Geneva, his mother's birthplace. At the time, Geneva was hard-pressed by the politics of Choiseul who was trying to choke Genevan business by promoting the growth of another town, Versoix.[47] Their Excellencies of Bern, as allies of Geneva, were not happy about Choiseul's dealings at Versoix which threatened their own lucrative trade along Lake Geneva. Nor were they pleased with the social agitation in Geneva. They, in fact, tried to enroll Tissot in a diplomatic mission to Paris. The correspondence between Tissot and Haller is full of allusions to the worries of their Excellencies over the Franco-Genevan imbroglio and to their steps to preserve their own interests with both parties. The Bernese thought to entrust Tissot with a money offer to Choiseul's sister who was in turn expected to discourage her brother from the Versoix enterprise.[48]

Tissot seemed the perfect candidate for the mission. Chamousset's standing offer suggested that he was respected by Choiseul and would make his presence in Paris appear natural. His relations with the Neckers would introduce him in financial and political circles; and Tronchin was his friend. Since Tissot declined to take part in the scheme, we can only speculate whether or not his intervention would have made any difference in the final settlement. Soon anyway, Choiseul fell from power and was exiled to his estate on 24 December 1770. Both the project of Versoix as a watchmaking rival to Geneva and the model hospital dreamed by Chamousset were abandoned. In April 1771, Tissot wrote to Zimmermann: "I did not tell you more about the Paris vocation because I gave it up a few days after writing to you about it."[49]

Tissot, repeatedly sick from overwork and exposure to epidemics in Lausanne, first tried to recover his health by spending more time at his country home. He had hoped that fresh air and quiet hours with his family would improve his digestion and help him recover sleep. When this proved not sufficient to restore his health, he acceded to his family's pleas and went away for a trip and a cure at Spa. Tissot often suggested travelling as a way to improve one's health away from everyday obligations and pressures. He left alone on 18 May 1772 and returned on August 11, spending about five weeks in Spa.[50] While in Spa, Tissot tried to behave as much as possible as a patient. He took the waters, went for long horseback rides, participated in the social life so far as to play the game of dropping calling cards on the newcomers to the resort. He avoided the parties and set fixed hours during which he was a physician. And he missed his family, especially his nephew Marc. The outgoing journey by way of Basel, Mannheim, and Aachen proved to be much more tiring that what Tissot had anticipated. Delays caused by bad weather or lack of horses at relay stations hampered the travelers' progress and made a regular schedule next to impossible. The return trip via Brussels and Lyons was even worse because of the heat of summer. The experience turned out not to be one of healing, but one of harassment by wealthy patients who solicited Tissot to spend a few hours at their homes in the course of his travels and entrapped him for days at a time.[51] On his way home Tissot visited an abbey of Bernardins near Say-sur-Saône; he noted the huge building and the immense endowment used only for the upkeep of a few persons while so much poverty was present in the neighborhood.[52] Tissot would return to the problem of the best use of resources when he wrote on the reform of the hospital or on public hygiene.[53] He finally arrived in Lausanne, only to take to his bed for several weeks. All the good he had hoped to get from the trip and the benefit he received from taking the waters were lost. For eight days he suffered from the most violent fever and from continual headaches. He treated himself with lukewarm baths, fruit juices, whey, the whole cooling regimen... and occasional bloodletting.[54] He recovered, but felt very weak for many more days; by October, he was finally feeling better than he had been in years.

Tissot was ready to give his time, energy, and medical knowledge without thinking of fatigue or gain when he felt it was a question of health, but would not tolerate arrogance or whimsy. The Duchess of Courtland spent the winter of 1770-1771 in Lausanne and regularly consulted Tissot. When she felt cured, (many thought her restored health was a miracle), she left Lausanne and entrusted a messenger to take some money and a tobacco box to her doctor to show appreciation for his care. When he opened the snuff-box, Tissot found some tobacco residue in it; obviously the gift had been used before; he then closed the box and returned it to the messenger without a word. Later, when asked how he liked the snuff-box, he wrote back to the inquirer: "I am not in the habit of using secondhand furnishings; a worn object is a gift from master to servant and not one from a prince to an individual who has had the advantage of rendering him a few services."[55] Tissot's attitude may reflect more than the susceptibilities of a single man: it exemplifies the drive for professionalization of the late eighteenth-century physicians. In a society that was turning ever more to money for all its transactions and was affirming the value of individual, the physicians were fighting to gain independent status, to be recognized on their own merit, to be paid fees for service performed. Tissot repeatedly shunned court or great household appointments, which in the past had been the crowning of a medical career, since for him to be a physician so attached was to be reduced to the status of a servant. The Tissot/Zimmermann correspondence of the 1770s abounds in references to how a physician should earn his living and to the proper relations between patient and physician. In fact the two questions were linked. In Antiquity, physicians treated their free and slave patients differently. To the free they gave advice; with them they discussed every aspect and anything pertaining to their recovery of good health and its maintenance. It was an expensive and time-consuming relation few could afford. In contrast, the doctors of the slaves never spoke to their patients; they examined them in silence and then prescribed a treatment without giving explanations. These encounters were short and minimal in time as well as in cost. The dual behavior endured with slight variations. As long as society was clearly divided into rich and poor, this system did not need much adapting. By the eighteenth century, however, a third group had appeared: the bourgeoisie. Much argumentation has been lavished on the role and importance of the rise of the bourgeoisie; a review of the arguments would lead too far afield. The important fact is that eighteenth-century physicians responded to the phenomenon by adjusting their practice. For the use of the bourgeoisie, Tissot published books meant at explaining the tenets of good health, therefore disseminating them further than could a dialog between physician and patient. He also wrote for the benefit of his colleagues about medical education and the proper duty of a physician of the bourgeoisie.[56]

Still, the problem of professionalization ran deeper than educating physicians and patients. It was a general question of patronage versus independent status not only for the physicians, but also for writers, musicians, painters, artists, and independent professionals. In their letters, Tissot and Zimmermann slowly developed new understandings of professionalization. They discussed how physicians had been and still were pensioneers of the State caring for paupers, or dependents of a nobleman's good will for a New Year gift in return for twelve months of scrupulous attention, or hired hands attending to the health's needs of private households; and how doctors were succeeding in becoming independent from patronage. They dealt with the question of emolument and how the voluntary gifts of jewelry, medals, snuff-boxes that noble patients had bestowed on their physicians were to be replaced with hard cash computed on a fee-for-services basis. Also discussed was the question of whether physicians were to call on their patients at home or whether they were to be consulted in their own houses; should the place of consultation be different for rich and poor? Tissot and Zimmermann realized the transitory nature of their situation. Changes did not happen without tensions and doubts in theirs as well as other minds. Their professional desires were clashing with traditional ways. This was especially true for Zimmermann who, in 1768, had accepted the position of court physician in Hanover; with it came a handsome pension and the possibility of a brilliant private practice. In the courtly atmosphere of Hanover, Zimmermann could not escape dependency on princely patronage. On the surface, he seemed to cherish his ennoblement by Catherine the Great, his consulting for Frederick II, his caring of George III's sons, but he confessed to Tissot that he always resented being on call as a servant, especially since it was through these kingly relationships that he was known and consulted by the upward and status-conscious bourgeoisie of Hanover. He came to envy Tissot who could refuse any and all offers to become court-physician because he did not need any patronage beyond his reputation. Tissot had won professional independence by hard work in unprestigious Lausanne. The resolution of the conflict between past and future medicine never came to fruition in Zimmermann's practice; it might be one of the sources of his foundering into manic depression. In contrast, Tissot, successfully wedding traditional and modern medicine, attained a prominent position as an independent practitioner.

Another aspect of Tissot's fight for professional independent status can be found in the 1769 incident between their Excellencies of Bern and the Lausanne Academy, on the right of suffrage of a *de facto* appointed honorary professor.[57] Tissot was upset by the intransigent attitude of Bern on behalf of the lawyer Marc-Antoine Porta, a man the Academy had found unfit to seat because of his scandalous life. Tissot would have resigned his own honorary chair had it not been for the soothing intervention of Haller. Tissot did not want to share the same title as a licentious man who, incidentally, had been his wife's first husband. Haller wrote: "One must forgive many things to one's fatherland."[58] Yet, the converse was not to be expected. Bern would not forgive the Lausanne Academicians nor in fact anyone else. To wit, while Voltaire was residing in the Pays de Vaud, a Bernese Bailiff gave him this friendly advice: "You have maligned the dear God, the dear God will forgive you, however don't even try to speak ill of their Excellencies of Bern, for they will never forgive you."[59] Tissot would have to forgive many times, as Haller had done and had encouraged him to do. He never openly complained of the heavy hand of the Bear of Bern but continued to hope that with time "it" would see the light of modernity. "One must be useful to be rewarded" Haller wrote him referring as much to their Excellencies' line of conduct as to his own faith.[60] Tissot's intent was likewise to serve God, not to earn money and honor for vanity's sake: this should throw some light on his indifference to ostentatious positions and eagerness for useful endeavors.[61]

Yet, Tissot had first to face his own ill health which forced him to curtail his activities. He was gravely sick in November and December 1773, with fever, pains in the left eye and such a weak stomach that he could not even take any medicine. He was unable to move or to speak, although he kept all his faculties.[62] In June 1774, he took another trip to get away from the demands of his wealthy patients and from the burden of revising his books. This time he went to Plombières, a much shorter journey than the preceding one to Spa. His wife accompanied him and acted as the guardian of his rest and peace, fending off the requests of the ladies avid to consult the famous Swiss Aesculapius. Tissot was convalescent for almost a year, while his wife carefully ensured that he observed for himself what he had prescribed to others, that is moderate physical exercise, few hours of intellectual activity, and enough sleep.

In spite of his illnesses Tissot saw his influence broaden during the 1770s through the numerous revisions and translations of *Avis au peuple* and *Onanisme*. He wrote to Zimmermann that he was including a long chapter on regimen in *Onanisme*, as such a book was read while those on regimen won't![63] All the while, he was working cautiously on his monumental *Traité des nerfs*. His first intention had been to write on "vapeurs"; however after the *Onanisme*'s condemnation by the French censorship, Tissot became wary of dealing directly with the repercussions of sexuality and approached the subject from a more theoretical point of view.[64]

Tissot was not satisfied by publishing only for the general public. He wanted not only to educate patients, but also to train his own medical disciples. His professorship at the Lausanne Academy was honorific and, except for the inaugural lecture, offered him no opportunity to teach. A few years earlier, Bern had initiated a revision of the role of the Academy and Tissot had hoped to see it enlarged with a Medical Faculty, but nothing materialized. Having taken seriously his nephew's education, Tissot discovered the joy of teaching, of passing on one's experience and knowledge. However, much as Marc was willing to listen to his uncle, this was not enough for Tissot who wanted to reach a larger audience of physicians.

This period of semi-retirement forced by convalescence allowed Tissot to reflect on his accomplishments and to redirect them to deeper levels, to that of the structure of the medical establishment. He had been out of medical school for about twenty-five years, and now with Marc showing an interest in the profession, Tissot wanted to have an active role. He was eager to adapt medical literature and teaching to the new demands of an increasingly critical attitude toward traditional explanations of the functioning of the body as well as to the new social pressures for preserving life. Romantic dreams of natural man living in harmony with his surroundings, be they human, animal, or vegetal, were developing into thoughts of a better life through a better understanding of life itself. The Encyclopedists, like Tissot who can be counted as a distant member of their circle, were much concerned with how to improve living conditions and health throughout society in order to achieve a fuller and happier life. Tissot had already sensed this new dimension in human potential. He had specifically written *Avis au peuple* to broaden the category of those who could have access to decent medical care. Now he had to define better what was meant by "decent" medical care.

Although Tissot was committed to the humoral system of medicine, his medical framework was not so rigid as to preclude his absorbing new physiological discoveries. His strong attachment to humoral medicine helps to explain his ability to reach and influence his contemporaries as well as his rapid fall into obscurity after his death. He brought humoral medicine to the limits of its possibilities, leaving behind the abuses of heroic treatments and bringing in the expectant attitudes of the Neo-Hippocratics. Since Tissot considered the causes of diseases more important than their symptoms, he always preferred the deep slow effects of mild, carefully chosen drugs and of proper regimen to the quick-acting intervention of the emetic or the mercurial. Yet, the use of bloodletting in Tissot's medical practice presents a complex picture. He bled less often than his contemporaries did and never for preventive measures, although when he did, he prescribed drawing large amounts of blood. He recommended bloodletting only in the case of a high fever (when plenty of cool drink, fresh air, and rest had failed) resulting from an acute inflammatory situation that he saw as an obviously plethoric condition, or when fearing miscarriages. In honest humoralist fashion Tissot evolved his medical philosophy from a balanced compromise of humoral and Neo-Hippocratic medicine with a touch of iatro-mechanism as well as some vitalism in order to open medical treatment to innovative possibilities.

The Doges of Venice, who had consulted Tissot on inoculation, must have been pleased with his advice since in early April 1775 they offered him a professorship at their distinguished University of Padua where Vesalius, Acquapente, Ramazzini, and Morgagni had taught and Harvey had studied.[65] Tissot pondered his answer for weeks. Lieuthaud, the first physician of Louis XV, had written to Tissot praising *Traité de l'épilepsie*: "in a word, since long ago I consider you the foremost physician of Europe. You deserve to be on a larger stage."[66] The Venetian offer could provide that larger stage. Tissot had so far resisted the appeal of prestige; this time it was harder for him to turn away from such a call. Considering that the offer was for six years, Tissot felt that he could arrange for his return to Lausanne afterwards; in the meantime his nephew would complete his bachelor of arts degree and medical doctorate under the best conditions. Tissot turned the pros and cons of accepting the appointment over and over in his head. Finally, on 20 May 1775, he accepted, only to recall the letter; and on the 23rd, he sent a categorical refusal.[67] He explained to Haller that once again he had followed the rule of not looking for greener pastures when one is very well settled.[68] Tissot was afraid of *Heimweh*; he needed still the reassurance of familiar surroundings to give the best of himself, and he knew all too well how his dear friend in Hanover was paying with continual depression and ill health for his restlessness at Brugg. He did not want to risk the same fate. In 1775, Lausanne was still enough for him.

That same summer, Zimmermann came to visit him. This was the first and last meeting of the long-time penpals. Tissot hoped that their few weeks together would help his friend overcome his pessimistic outlook on life, but to no avail. Zimmermann could not understand how Tissot could stand to live in such a small place with such capricious weather! They parted still in good terms, yet they enjoyed each other's company more through letters than in person. In his letters, Zimmermann was sparkling; in life, he was tiring. Tissot himself was finely spirited in writing but bashful and cold in society. Because of his rural youth, he always felt clumsy. His contemporaries reported that Tissot enjoyed parties from a spectator's point of view, he rarely engaged in conversation, dancing, or card playing on his own initiative. Nonetheless, Tissot had recommended to litterati to get out of their studies for a few hours of evening rest in pleasing company and gingerly followed his own advice.

Two summers passed and Tissot received another visitor who, with his modesty and good taste, was to play a salient role in Tissot's life.[69] This traveler who came not to be cured but to observe, was the Emperor Joseph II travelling under the name of Count Falkenstein; he went to see Haller in Bern but not Voltaire at Ferney.[70] That reason alone could have sufficed to make Tissot love him. Tissot had grown very tired of Voltaire and of his arrogance, and he felt closer to Haller who never abused his seniority and high reputation. Voltaire was dejected and felt slighted when he realized Joseph II would not visit him.

Haller, who was sick during the summer of 1777, died on December 12. The letters exchanged that autumn give many details about Haller's illness and Tissot's prescriptions and reassurances. During his last months Haller was preoccupied to the point of torment by his physiological experiments on animals and the suffering he had inflicted on them. At last, he found peace in the realization that the God from Whom he feared judgment was a just God Who did understand his medical intentions and Who did forgive the repented sinner. Haller's death was an immense loss to Tissot as well as a call to fill the void, to affirm his position, to seek larger horizons, to train disciples.

The newly organized Société royale de médecine elected Tissot as one of its first foreign corresponding members. In fact, in a letter from Paris dated 11 December 1777, Vicq d'Azyr informed Tissot of the project and requested the honor of adding his name to the list of their members.[71] The formal charter of the Société came in August 1778, confirming the Royal Decree of 1776, and officially sanctioning the seances which had been held in Paris for over two years. These meetings had stirred up the jealousy of the Paris Faculty of Medicine and the two bodies engaged in a power-struggle.[72] The aim of the Société was to by-pass the inertia of the medical Faculty, to serve as a consultative board to the royal ministers on questions of public health and hygiene, and to try to collect medical data to determine better the etiology of epidemic diseases.[73] The work of the Société royale de médecine lay very close to Tissot's own preoccupations, and he found in his new membership one more reason to wish to spend some time in Paris. Tronchin had been in Paris for many years and had written Tissot of his success there. By now the Neckers were also well established in the capital, and it was rumored that Tissot would be chosen to head the hospital founded in 1778 by Mme Necker.

So, under the pretext of his nephew's education, Tissot travelled to Paris. Both left in September 1779 and spent about ten months there.[74] Mrs. Tissot stayed behind in Lausanne, and his letters to her offer some information on his life and experiences, although these messages are frustratingly incomplete: Tissot informed his wife of his projected whereabouts and activities but gave no account of the events themselves.[75] Thus, he wrote that he would "dine the following Tuesday at the Neckers", while his next letter did not even mention whether the dinner took place. His letters provide no evidence on whom he saw or what subjects he discussed, no glimpse of his Parisian life. He was less parsimonious with details when it came to describing architecture, painting, music, or the cost of living. What were the reasons behind this silence? Perhaps he thought that she was not interested in the spirited conversation of the Neckers' circle. The worldly anecdotes of the Lausanne high society mention only him, never his wife.[76] Or, perhaps, he was unwilling to commit to paper the topics discussed at these gatherings for fear of the censorship's use of his reports.

Tissot did not like the hectic pace of life that eager patients and social whirls made him live in Paris. He felt homesick and fell ill while there. He wanted to return to Lausanne; at the same time he wished his nephew to pursue his studies in Paris, but could not consider leaving him behind. With the return of spring, Tissot's health improved, and he was better able to assess the situation. He decided to stay a few more months. His nephew, who had followed the lectures of Vicq d'Azyr among others, was offered by Buffon his own key to the "Jardin du Roy" and the possibility of studying botany there in very favorable conditions during June and July 1780.[77] Such an opportunity was not to be missed, and Tissot also figured out that with the return of summer his wealthy patients would leave for their country estates, allowing him more time for his own medical interests and studies of the medical establishments of the capital.

However, after this couple of months devoted to botany, Tissot decided to return to Lausanne. The directorship of the Necker Hospital had not materialized; it had been offered to a younger physician from Geneva named Gallatin.[78] It is possible that Tissot did not pursue the offer after a few months in Paris on account of his dislike of the hustle and bustle of life there. Nevertheless, the Parisian experience proved very useful to Tissot. He had been able to watch closely how medicine was taught and how hospitals were run; he certainly met Tenon and Lavoisier while in Paris and subsequently drew upon their works when he wrote on hospital reform.[79] He attended meetings of the Société royale de médecine and what he heard discussed and reported during these meetings reinforced his opinion of the urgency of medical reforms. Later, as Vice-President of the Lausanne Collège de Médecine, he tried to emulate on a much smaller scale the work of the Société. The Société dealt with abuses of medical practice, granting of drug's privileges, diffusion of preventive measures and with collecting material and information to define a theory of disease propagation and prevention; it also engaged in rationalizing the Kingdom's medical resources toward more judicious uses, particularly true for hospitals.

The sojourn in Paris made Tissot even more aware of his position in this revitalizing current of the medical establishment, a position he had already sensed in the numerous articles he had been asked to write for the *Grande Encyclopédie de Paris*.[80] While in Paris, Tissot had attended some lectures with Marc; their content convinced him that he too had something to teach in medicine. He returned to Lausanne determined this time to look for an opportunity to teach and to guide his nephew in further medical studies. At long last, he had managed to dominate his illnesses and to gather the necessary energy to complete the writing of *Traité des nerfs*. With the publication of *Traité des nerfs* in 1778 and 1780, Tissot gathered more successes; he reached a rank of authority in the medical profession itself. The years of reflection were over, Tissot was ready to embark on a new course of which, in a sense, *Traité des nerfs* was the prelude.[81]

Chapter VII

Individual Versus Societal Ills

For almost twenty years, Tissot slowly nurtured his works on nervous diseases. At first, he projected a book in the form of letters; perhaps he was influenced by Rousseau's success with *Nouvelle Héloïse* or Fontenelle's *Entretiens sur la pluralité des mondes* (a model for the popular scientific expositions of the Enlightenment).[1] A few remnants of the early project which he had described to Zimmermann are left among Tissot's personal papers.[2] When in the late 1770s Tissot published his finally completed six volumes *Traité des nerfs et de leurs maladies*, he had, however, changed his targeted audience from the general public to the medical profession and shifted genre from friendly letters to serious descriptions of the nervous system's anatomy and physiology, and discussions of pathological cases and their medical care. One theme had, nevertheless, remained constant throughout the gestation: the link between psyche and soma. Tissot, as a true disciple of Sauvages, always emphasized the reciprocal influence of physical and moral causes; thus he correlated nervous ailments and psychic disorders.

In Tissot's mind, *Onanisme* was a prologue to his larger work on nerves. Its success encouraged him to pursue writing for the lay public. Tissot refrained from publishing his letters on vapors and hysteria on account of the troubles he had with the censorship about *Onanisme*; however, he went public with his works on the health of individuals,[3] meanwhile accumulating materials for *Traité des nerfs*. As his career progressed, Tissot realized that specialized professional writing might be less likely a target of censorship and that physicians, too, were seeking his expertise.

Traité des nerfs was an ambitious project. Tissot had planned thirty-four chapters. As he was more often sick than well during the twenty years of its drafting, he had to scale it down and be content to publish only the parts he had completed by 1780. He had also lost enthusiasm for an enterprise which had dragged on far too long. To Zimmermann, he even confided: "Had I known all the troubles it would give me and how small the satisfaction would be; I would never have embarked upon its writing."[4] In the early 1780s, Tissot's interests in medicine were shifting once more; his accepting Joseph II's call to be professor of practical medicine at the University of Pavia was one manifestation of this new orientation.[5]

In 1770 their Excellencies of Bern had granted to Tissot a publication privilege of ten years for *Traité des nerfs*. He applied for a second ten-year privilege, which was granted in 1778, on the ground that his poor health had prevented him from completing the writing and from supervising the editing of the multi-volume work as first planned.[6]

The first volume of *Traité des nerfs* had appeared in 1770 under the title *Traité de l'épilepsie*. It was supposed to be chapter XX of the work. The next four volumes, chapters I to XII, came out between 1778 and 1780. Already in the early 1770s Chapters I to V on the anatomy of the nervous system had been printed as one volume which, however, was not put on the market. Chapter VI on the physiology of the nervous system occupied another volume. Volumes three and four comprised chapters VII to XII which dealt with the physical and moral causes of nervous diseases, the characteristics of the disorders, the prognosis for cure, and the general treatment of nervous complaints. After Tissot's return from Paris, a sixth volume containing Chapters XXI to XXIII was published in 1780. Their subjects are different "nervous" diseases such as catalepsy, extasy, migraine, and the disorders provoked by ergotism; the material on the latter is in fact, a French translation of his revised "De morbis ex usu secalis cornutis" published in 1765 in the *Philosophical Transactions* and also known as *Lettre à M. Baker*. Chapters XIII to XIX and XXIV to XXXIV were never published, in spite of the fact that they were announced in the table of contents printed at the beginning of the volume on anatomy; sketches of the projected topics are scattered among Tissot's personal papers, some more elaborated than others.[7] Using the same model as in the published chapters on particular diseases, he had planned to treat others such as apoplexy,

Heimweh, rabies, vertigo, and the convulsions of different organs. Tissot might have used, as for his Chapter XXIII, French translations of his revised Latin letters on medical topics, in particular that to Haller on apoplexy and hydropsy. But, publishing part of them in *Traité des nerfs* became redundant, since in 1780 they all appeared together in a separate volume of translations by M. Vicat with revisions by Tissot.[8]

Traité de l'épilepsie was separately reprinted six times in French, three of which were in Paris. It was translated into Dutch, German, and Italian, for one, two and three editions respectively. The next four volumes of *Traité des nerfs* had five other French editions, as many in German, and one in Italian. The sixth volume, sometimes entitled *Traité de la catalepsie*, had three French editions, but no separate translation.[9]

Tissot worked for about five years on *Traité de l'épilepsie*, or so it would appear from his references to consultations that occurred while he was writing.[10] The organization of the book reveals Tissot's purpose and goals. He moved from symptoms to causes of epilepsy and emphasized curing the roots of the disease, not just alleviating its symptoms when a crisis struck. His aim was first to remove epilepsy as well as any other nervous disorders from the realm of magic, to dispel the old belief that epilepsy was a curse of the gods, embodied in its common appellation of "sacred disease" which is also one of the titles of the Hippocratic Corpus. In some medical circles, but rarely among the lay public epilepsy was treated as a physical problem. In fact, Tissot is recognized being among the first to approach epilepsy from a purely medical standpoint.[11]

Epilepsy, wrote Tissot, was a brain disease which rendered this organ prone to convulsions or spasms carried via the nerves to various part of the body.[12] Tissot noted that what triggered the seizure was so far unknown and that most autopsies revealed no lesions of the brain. He added that many other mechanisms were unknown for now, might be forever, and still were not magic at all.[13] He acknowledged the fact that epilepsy seems to run in families and that some hereditary factors play a role in triggering the brain's spasms.[14] But he rejected the traditional view that the mother's imagination during pregnancy has any influence on the onset of epilepsy in her child, because the placenta contains no nerves and that mother's and child's blood do not mix.[15] He leaned towards explanations that linked errors of regimen or overwhelming emotions to irritation of the nerves leading to a spasmodic brain.[16]

Tissot wrote that an enlightened and persistent doctor should attempt to alleviate if not outright cure epilepsy, especially in the case of young children who are very susceptible to the influence of their physical and emotional environments since their temperaments are not yet settled. What could be a one time occurrence could develop into a life-long complaint if neglected. He insisted that with patience and the regularity of a sane and tested treatment, many epileptics could be cured.[17] He harshly derided the physician who, from lack of interest in such a strange disease, refused to take seriously the suffering of the epileptics and consequently threw the "poor souls" into the arms of charlatans ready to make extravagant promises of cure.[18]

Once Tissot had firmly demonstrated that epilepsy, in spite of frightful symptoms, was an ordinary disease, he turned his attention to giving a description of epilepsy as complete as possible: "...nothing would benefit medicine more than to find in a judicious order all the good observations which are known on this disease."[19] The adjective **good** is of importance. In this book Tissot rejected all marvelous descriptions or cures, reporting first-hand observations only from his colleagues past or present and from himself. He anchored his criteria on the recently accepted definition of a scientifically recognized fact, that is something which is accurately described, with nothing kept hidden or secret, and for which the exact means of the experiment (here the ingredients of the remedy) are spelled out, thus providing the objective possibility of checking the results. His insistence on the veracity of trusted observations is yet another manifestation of the "tournant des mentalités" in the field of medicine. Once Tissot had established that the determinant cause lies in the brain and is conveyed to the organs through the nerves, he looked at what he called occasional causes, such as loud noises, strong odors, pains, tantrums, prolonged arduous intellectual work, or strenuous physical exercise. These irritate the nerves which in turn incite the brain to spasm, creating the disorder of an epileptic crisis.[20]

Tissot employed the most advanced physiology, i.e. the principles of irritability, sensitivity, and irritation. He combined these new notions with the old humoral concepts to come up with a fresh interpretation and treatment of epilepsy. The brain, Tissot explained, acquired this convulsive trait on its own, under the influence of what he called sympathetic causes which he defined as nerves irritated by occasional causes conveying irritation and sensitivity to their roots in the brain. Sympathetic causes can only act when a link exists between the seat of the irritation and another organ in the body. In Chapters I-VI of *Traité des nerfs*, Tissot established that the nervous system provides this link.[21] These sympathetic causes activated by acrid humors due to improper dietetic and hygienic habits continually sting and excite the nerves, in particular those of the stomach, inducing an irritation of the brain, the center of sensations and motion, which pre-dispose it to convulsions. Another source of trouble was an acrid humor which deposits itself on the nerves when its usual path of exit was clogged, so kindling an irritation and a sympathetic cause.[22] By this, Tissot meant that when a normal or abnormal, but regular evacuation was abruptly stopped, the humor flowed back into the body and created a problem. Normal bodily evacuations included menstruation, lactation, urination, defecation, and perspiration; abnormal or pathological ones include catarrhal and hemorrhoidal flux, and discharge from wounds or ulcers.

For Tissot losing consciousness, rather than convulsing or foaming at the mouth, established the decisive factor of the diagnosis of epilepsy. He attached great importance to this definition, since it provided the criterion for distinguishing between true and false epilepsy, real or fake crisis.[23] He warned that the sham epileptic who pretends to have the disease in order to escape work or duty should be dealt with severely, once the stratagem is uncovered by physical or verbal menaces.[24] The true epileptic is indifferent to the threats, while the sham is hard pressed not to react to the testing, and thus is unmasked. Tissot remarked that epilepsy is a very convenient disease to counterfeit since between crises one is perfectly well. In *Traité des nerfs*, Tissot elaborated on the connection between nervous disorders and social expectations pressed on individuals. He was well aware of the escape epilepsy or hysteria offered to those overwhelmed by the demands of society, yet his empathy was not always equally distributed among the neurotics. He showed prejudice toward the lower end of society; all his examples of sham epileptics were from the ranks of servant and the hysteric persons, he described, always belonged to "qualité".

The book is organized around the accepted canons for medical treatises; i.e. observations, description, prognosis, treatment, and recapitulation. Tissot departed from this traditional outline only in content, but not in form; first, by reporting only verified observations, second by inserting psychological and humanitarian considerations into medical diagnosis and prognosis, and third, in the part in which treatments are reviewed, by separating them into three sections: the useful, the useless, and the injurious.

In the section on prognosis, Tissot warned against harsh and quick judgments; epilepsy, he said, like other nervous diseases, gets worse with fear and anxiety. So he advised doctors always to have kind words and to demonstrate caring, especially with hopeless cases.[25] The physician must reassure the patient with solicitude and harmless prescriptions, otherwise the charlatan will take his place with fantastic promises and disastrous results. Tissot could never denounce harshly enough the misdeeds of quacks. Those suffering from epilepsy, as well as the families of sick children, are invariably credulous and hopeful: "a true physician should only prescribe drugs of proven usefulness, since nothing is more deleterious than trusting inefficacious drugs."[26] Aside from wanting to instruct his colleagues on the best way to treat epilepsy, Tissot also hoped to educate them to behave professionally. He described for the physician of the bourgeoisie how to conduct a consultation and why, beyond the immediate cure of the body, the doctor should look into the psychological needs of patient and family. The physician as "directeur de conscience" was already emerging from his writing on nervous disorders, and will appear more clearly in subsequent works.[27]

At the beginning of the section on treatment, Tissot warned physicians to search first for the real causes before prescribing the remedy rather than trying one thing after another, such as bleeding, purging, and vomiting, or using complicated drugs blindly, as these interventions weaken the symptoms without curing the causes. When the sources of the trouble cannot be located, Tissot advised using a mild diet to get rid first of the acrid humors, almost always present in anyone at anytime because of the usual way of life and then to wait for clearer symptoms to surface and provide a better clue on the origin of the disease. Often enough that alone is already sufficient to relieve most of the patient's sufferings: "How many sick would be cured if only put on such a simple diet, and whom violent or ill-chosen drugs have reduced to the most miserable state?"[28] Tissot always emphasized this expectant medicine which can also be a preventive medicine. He also disclaimed the belief that a universal drug against epilepsy existed and stated that such a "remedy" could only be a ploy from the charlatans.[29]

Tissot accepted the practice of prescribing valerian as often helpful to epileptics, but vehemently denied the common wisdom that marriage cured a girl's epilepsy since, quite to the contrary, he had often seen the disease appear a few weeks after the ceremony when the union turned out to be unhappy. Tissot here stood for the new loving family and alluded to women using nervous disorders to escape the pressure of life, a topic he developed further in *Traité des nerfs* and in his manuscript *Des maladies des femmes*. As for useless drugs, he cited explicitly earthworms and peacock droppings. Amongst the dangerous treatments, he viewed the drinking of human blood as offensive and susceptible of provoking more crises out of the loathsome nature of the prescription.[30] He recommended protecting the epileptic against harm during crises.[31] In *Traité de l'épilepsie*, Tissot wanted to help his colleagues dispel superstition, and abandon disgusting cures. Instead, they should adopt a natural, hygienic way of considering and curing the disease. He elaborated on this same approach in his other volumes on nervous diseases.

In the preface to *Traité des nerfs*, Tissot broached the subject of the increase of nervous disorders which he, as well as others of his contemporaries, perceived in their society.[32] Was the supposed increase real, or was it rather a changed perception of normality that led into a broader definition of nervous ailments? Or was society becoming less tolerant of deviants under the pressure of an increased urbanization, with the old support system of the village crumbling away? Or was nervous disorder a product of urban life? Or was it part of the discourse on depopulation, on degeneracy of the human race, and on the idealization of the "noble savage"?

Tissot certainly thought, and he was not alone, that nervous disorders were more frequent in the towns than in the villages. He designated as the culprit the way of life of city-dwellers compared to that of countryfolks. In his view, urban life is more stressful, partly because of the environment (noise, filth, crowding), but mostly because of the demands (expenses, appearance, decorum, patronage). The seventeenth-century advance of politeness and of propriety, exemplified in courtly life regulated like a ballet or in the notion of "honnêteté", was a mixed blessing. The concept of "honnêteté" was issued from the principle of the rationality of Nature, i.e. the Creation of the Judeo-Christian rational God, and from the Greek notion of the Great Chain of Being. "Honnêteté" meant that men and women had to occupy their proper places in the social scale of the Old Regime of Estates and had to behave rationally, according to a rationality imposed by the establishment. The rise of the Absolute State and its attendant bureaucracy provided means for enforcing the new code of conduct. At first, directed to the lowly and their perceived deviants, beggars and vagrants, incarceration in hospitals or in workhouses (Foucault's grand renfermement) was one of the devices of the Absolute State to solve the "unrulyness" problem exacerbated by deteriorating economic conditions. In time, the new norm of rational behavior could be extended to any type of deviation, and led to the incarceration of the undesirable elements of society, be they prodigal sons or ugly daughters of the well-to-do. The question of who was to define the line not to be trespassed became a lively subject of debate, with ramifications reaching into the French Revolution and the scandal of the *lettre de cachet*. The nervous eighteenth century represents a society in transition reacting to feelings of insecurity in much the same fashion as the waning Middle Age was a period in which insanity had been on the rise or the Reformation and Counter-Reformation one of increasing sorcery. It has been argued that the witchcraft craze was the manifestation of a people in the throngs of rebellion, escaping in frenzy to the magical in order to avoid facing the reality of their defeat.[33]

Tissot lived in the Pays de Vaud, a land subject to Bern, with rampant political tensions, not far from a Geneva besieged with social conflicts. He combined the knowledge of his country's past and of its people's soul with his medical philosophy to reach new understanding of inner-thoughts. Thus, aware of the throes of society under the demands of conformism, he tried to apply this insight to the deciphering of the current nervous condition of his patients. Tissot drew the conclusion that their repressed feelings and maladjustment to society's expectations, often compounded with a lack of purpose or calling in life, explained many of their psychic troubles. He developed this theme fully in his chapter IX on moral causes.

In *Traité des nerfs*, Tissot offered his own philosophy of the practice of medicine: "What is it that needs to be changed in this sick person who I am in charge of leading to recovery? What will be the effects of my prescriptions? Here are the two questions that every doctor should ask himself; the two questions on which centers the whole practice of medicine..."[34]   On the next page he added: "...not to harm ought to be the first object of medicine."[35] His preferred line of conduct emphasized observations and reactions which allowed him leeway for controlled experimentations of new treatments devised by analogy.

Anatomy and physiology played a very important role in Tissot's diagnosis: "I am deeply convinced that it is impossible to have an exact idea of a disease if one does not know the parts which are its seat and their functions in the state of health, hence I dare to affirm that the little progress of practice proceeds from the little education of physicians in anatomy and physiology. I have seen that the more one acquires knowledge in these subjects, the more one acquires facilities to seize the causes of diseases, and thus the true indications."[36] Consequently, in the first volume of *Traité des nerfs*, he described the nervous system extensively, including everything that he could possibly know, about the brain, the cerebellum, the spinal cord, and each and every pair of nerves which exit from the spinal cord and their whereabouts inside the body. He used the works of colleagues from classical times to his contemporaries (Galen, Vesalius, Willis, Cheyne, Sydenham, Boerhaave, Whytt, Raulin, Hoffmann, Vieussens, Monro,), and pointed out discoveries as well as errors.[37] In the preface, Tissot noted that since the volume on anatomy had been printed for almost ten years, he was unable to give proper recognition to very recent authors.[38]

Tissot stated specific experiments to buttress what he was advancing about the role of nerves for sensation and motion. Page after page of gruesome descriptions of dogs, cats, pigs, and the like, undergoing the section of nerves in one place or another, getting injections of various poisons and of the effects on their behavior

provide hours of ghastly reading. Since many examples came out
of Haller's research, one can better appreciate his death-bed
torments about the sufferings he had inflicted on animals. Tissot
was not a medical researcher, a fact he regretted, explaining that
his large practice did not leave him enough time to undertake long
and careful experiments. Nonetheless, he attributed a great
importance to the precise knowledge of current medical
discoveries and recommended to his readers to keep up-to-date in
their field; for him this was a *sine-qua-non* condition for the proper
practice of the medical art.

So Tissot described in minute detail the texture and color of the
different layers of the brain; the cerebellum; and all the pairs of
nerves with special attention to their beginning and ending,
because for him a common nerve's root branching to various
organs explained what he called the sympathic causes of nervous
disorders. A nerve irritated in one organ, in turn irritates its co-
axial nerves which transmit this sympathic reaction to the particular
organs to which they are attached. Tissot ascribed to the ganglions
found along the nerves a role of liaison between pairs of nerves,
thus increasing the possibility of sympathic causes.

Tissot noted that an excellent knowledge of the nervous system
served the general practitioner well, even outside of the treatment
of nervous ailments, because the nerves are "very exposed to be
pricked when blood-letting" and a wise physician can watch that
the surgeon bleeds properly.[39] Tissot classified the nerves in three
groups: sense, muscular motion, and vagi. For him, in terms of
nervous diseases, the most critical group consisted of the vagus
nerves leading to the internal organs and it was of the utmost
importance to understand their functioning.[40]

After his chapters on anatomy, Tissot went on to the physiology
of the nervous system, giving first a historical account of the different views on the functioning of the nerves. He was very cautious
about his own choice of explanation for the source and transmission of the motion's and sensation's signals. He clearly did not
want to arouse the censors' wrath nor his colleagues' quarrels, and
wrote in terms of conjectures and putative solutions, using *ab
absurdo* demonstrations to dispose of the systems he did not
endorse. He dismissed mechanical or hydraulic explanations on the
basis of the softness and narrowness of the nerves, the absence of

firm fixed or tied points to allow the nerves to vibrate, their close-ness blurring the mechanical signals, and also the swiftness of the body's reactions. Tissot cited Jaucourt's authority from the *Ency-clopédie*'s article "nerfs" to buttress his argument.[41] The Lausanne Doctor favored the "esprits animaux", yet he warned his readers not to take literally the term spirit which, for him, had no supernat-ural or spiritual connotations. He saw in the expression merely a convenient description for something that was far from being understood. The term allowed him a working hypothesis for the physiology of the nervous system and the linkage of psyche and soma: "the animal spirits are the means not the seat of sensations and motions."[42] In fact, he advanced a model of the functioning of the nervous system in which he likened the propagation and transmission of orders and sensations to shocks transmitted by adjoining balls.[43] Nonetheless, Tissot denounced the abuse of ordinary mechanics for medical purpose and did not exclude the possibility of other theories which would fit better with the obser-vations. He justified his own theorizing on the precept that: "...an ingenious system even if not true is useful in facilitating the path to others."[44] Tissot also strongly recommended the reading of Haller's work on physiology as the best foundation to acquire the correct knowledge necessary for understanding the physiology of the nervous system. He presented his own treatise as an introduc-tion to the subject, and placed his emphasis on the treatment of nervous diseases.

In *Traité des nerfs*, Tissot expounded on the theme of irritability and sensibility he had discussed in *Traité de l'épilepsie*, according to which the muscles have the property of irritability and the nerves that of sensibility. These notions permitted Tissot to propose some definition of death: "the sensibility ends with life, sometimes even before ... the irritability perishes when the organization is destroyed ... it is the persistency of irritability which makes the tenacity of life."[45] In these terms, he transposed the delicate subject of the mind/body connection into a problem of nerves versus muscles. To Tissot, the search for the seat of the Soul was a vain quest. Some-where between the brain and the nerves a difference of organiza-tion was observed and where this difference occurred was the *sensorium commune* that: "established the union between physical man, the machine; and moral man, the feeling and thinking principle; whose immateriality is demonstrated ... [since] ... the soul does not govern the vital functions."[46] And almost tongue in cheek as to discharge the atmosphere, Tissot added that it is not necessary to know the structure of a machine to work well with it.[47] He treated this topic with the upmost caution and struggled to walk the tight rope of free will versus determinism of the flesh keeping in balance his medical integrity and Protestant faith: "it is with the help of this part [*sensorium commune*] that the soul notices all the changes that foreign bodies induce upon that [the body] whose direction it [the soul] received and in turn produces on it [the body] the motions which it [the soul] judges necessary; what is the knot of this union? We will surely always ignore this."[48] But ignorance of the nature of the "knot" does not invalidate observed facts. For example, a person who has lost a limb may still suffer an acute pain in this limb: "the soul suffer in such and such nerve, and it relates this pain to the part of the nerve which is in the limb that suffers, ... it is only the change operated in the brain itself which causes the pain..."[49] or "The nervous fluid is only the means which carries to the sensorium the received impression; it is the impression on the sensorium which is the physical part of the sensation; the notice of this impression by the soul, the change that the soul feels is properly said to be the sensation."[50] Tissot was not going as far as La Mettrie's analogy of man with a machine, although he did admire La Mettrie's medical genius and owned his books; Tissot's position was closer to that of Descartes.

Tissot thought that since simplicity of means is a rule of nature, only one kind of nervous fluid (or material) is required to perform all the functions of the nervous system.[51] For him, the best way to apprehend the actions of the nerves is to perturb them by poisoning. Therefore, Tissot described precisely the effects of poisons inserted in animals by buccal or anal ways, or injected in their blood stream, muscles, or body's cavities. By comparing reactions, he hoped to reach the causes of nervous diseases and to find out which nerves were responsible for what kind of abnormal behavior. Since he used the effects of foreign substances to exhibit the functioning and perturbing of the nerves, Tissot reviewed in terms of the Galenic non-naturals the effects of everyday life on the nerves to propose an explanation for the influences of lifestyle on general health, as well as for some baffling occurrences such as food allergy. He described an allergic reaction to strawberries as a nervous disease induced by irritated stomach nerves or ascribed unexplained internal pains to an inside tactile sense.[52]

Tissot knew that pains can be very real even if their causes remain unknown. The inability to identify causes only betrayed ignorance and did not constitute a license to throw up one's hands and dismiss the complaints. He considered nervous disorders as real illnesses that result from the malfunctioning of the nerves in one or more of their four functions, namely to feel, to determine the actions of the muscles, to help nutrition and to control secretions.[53] The causes disturbing the functions, Tissot wrote, could be physical or moral, or a combination of both. Any pain was a signal of a perturbed function, and no pain should be neglected, especially internal ones. Every normal function was to take place without pain, and Tissot had an even stronger test for functional normality: "everywhere Nature wanted a need to exist, it [Nature] attached pleasure to satisfy it [the need]."[54] He listed some causes of disturbances as the constitution, the passions, the pains, the Galenic non-naturals, the plethora, the over-abundant or suppressed evacuations, the irritating factors, the acute diseases, the chronic illnesses, and the external accidents. The passions (anger, hate, ambition, love, fear...) reflected normal needs turned into fixations which distracted the reason from judging with impartiality. Tissot believed that all human beings have the same number of senses and are able to enjoy all sensations when they are normally constituted. He only objected to the view that all souls have the same needs or are born with the same capacity, hence for him they cannot have the same moral passions which are influenced by circumstances.[55] Upbringing and environment played an important part in the nervous health of men and women.

The duty of the physician was to recognize which causes were at work in the malfunctioning of the nervous system; the doctor, wrote Tissot, ought to observe his patient carefully and to question him or her tactfully to discover the reasons for the illness and act according to his findings to insure his patient's best interest. As in the case of the sham epileptic who feigned the disease to escape duty, Tissot advised looking for the hidden reasons behind the evasion from heavy responsibility into nervous disorders for women who felt inadequate or unable to cope with the demands pressed upon them. Fragility was fashionable, but it could be exploited by a woman refusing to face reality. In such cases Tissot recommended searching patiently for the causes of the rebellion before trying a physical cure for the symptoms: "it is perhaps a true pain for many women to be loved only for a part of their worth," i.e. being loved only for their beauty or their reproductive value with no regard for their intellectual worth.[56] In the way young girls were raised, Tissot discerned the reasons for their subsequent nervous disorders. Their inactivity, be it physical, intellectual or sexual, led to hysteria or vapors, which for Tissot was hardly surprising as inactivity was not the norm of a healthy life. Based on the same assumptions, over-activity of any kind could lead into nervous disorders, a theme he had already explored in *Onanisme* and *De la santé des gens de lettres*. While Tissot showed empathy for fragile females who had not received the proper education to face their duty as human beings, he had little patience with male hypochondriacs whose selfishness and whims were responsible for their troubles. He explicitly noted: "since we owe everything to God, we ought to do what pleases Him most, which is that each human being have a useful vocation and carry it out."[57] To fail in this duty was to betray our human nature willed by God. Nature took revenge through poor health. Tissot did not spare words in denouncing the bad effect the soft life of the parents has on their children's health. He saw in this fact an explanation for the current increase in nervous disorders.

Tissot was not attempting to define from deleterious, yet amendable habits a characterization for a nervous race. He opposed Lavater's static bony or skeletal physiognomy that supposedly revealed national characters and traits.[58] He proposed instead a mobile physiognomy of feelings expressing fear, anger, surprise, joy, etc. which is the same in all humans for each specific sentiment.[59] We have here a hint of the question of nature versus nurture for defining race or personality which later developed into a full-fledged ugly problem when it combined with social Darwinism.

Since Tissot wrote *Traité des nerfs* with a medical audience in mind, he described the influence the Galenic non-naturals have on the nervous system by recounting many cases from his own practice. His concern for the well-being of the whole person was ever present in his investigations of the proper understanding of the role of the non-naturals. Some of the most revealing observations are under the heading of "evacuations". Tissot noted the moodiness of some women before their periods and the fear many experienced at the disappearing of their menses in pregnancy or at menopause. He thought that anxiety about their state was one of the reasons women had nervous troubles during pregnancy or when they reached the age of menopause. The physician's duty was to explain to them the natural changes in their bodies, thus to dispel old tales of curses as well as the so-called poisonous nature of the menstrual blood, a misconception of Arabic medicine.[60] Tissot also reviewed the connection between breast-feeding and nervous disorders. He was well aware of the fashionable pressure exercised on bourgeois women by the new trend of following nature and final causes. He declared: "it would be as stupid to force a woman to breast-feed her baby, because it is in nature's plan, as it would be to deny disease, because our bodies are organized to be healthy."[61] In the first place, the pregnancy could have already been too much for the strength of the mother, so that forcing nursing upon her would only make the matter worse physically and morally. Poor health and guilt might then drive her into nervous troubles.[62] He was especially referring to young brides, married off to satisfy their parents' ambition before they had time to achieve their full growth, who besides had been deprived of an active childhood under the pretext of ladylike behavior.

At every possible turn, Tissot attacked the mores of the well-to-do as the culprit for so many nervous disorders. If only physicians were aware of the causes, they could caution their patients and Tissot hoped that *Traité des nerfs* would enlighten his colleagues on the multifarious facts leading to nervous diseases and on how to cure and prevent them. While Tissot disagreed with some of his colleagues, in particular with Pomme and Raulin,[63] who detected a unique cause (drying and hardening of the nerves) for these ailments which they cured by a unique softening treatment; the Lausanne doctor tended in the overwhelming majority of cases to prescribe the same combination of diet to correct acrid humors and of exercise to fill empty hours. Consequently, he could be viewed as narrow-minded about the causes and cures of nervous diseases as the colleagues he derided. The difference was that Tissot offered hopes of permanent recovery because his treatments were based on a psychological as well as physical knowledge of each of his patients. He had recognized that for hysteric women in particular much of the disorders came from troubled relations with others. He thought that he had the duty as physician to restore normality to women's human encounters. He was ready to be that other, to listen, to care, to probe into the inner feelings of his patients to discover the motivations for their behavior, and then to show empathy, understanding, even affection. Trust in human relations had to be rebuilt before health could be improved. He insisted that the success of treatment laid as much on the trust the patient had in the physician as it did on the proper drugs. He wanted to share his experience of caring and building confidence in sick persons with his medical colleagues to improve their relations with their patients and their ability to cure. Tissot came to define a new role for both doctor and patient: they had to be active partners in the betterment of mental and physical health.

Tissot insisted that in most fatal cases of nervous diseases the autopsy revealed no particular lesions of the brain, cerebellum, spinal cord or nerves. Still, in a few cases, a tumor was found attached to the spinal cord or a nerve; in others, the brain's tissue had degenerated or was bloated with blood, or a clot, even a tumor was present. The sparse evidence was no excuse to deal lightly with nervous diseases which cause real sufferings. More often than not, their causes were moral, such as anger, envy, fear, jealousy, remorse, despair, or sadness, even if their manifestations were physical. Tissot described how anger, by exciting the animal spirits too much, brought redness to the face, a shortened breath, frequent choking and apoplexy. But at the same time, he recognized that anger could sometimes cure by animating the actions of the nerves which did open obstructed vessels.[64] Laughing could be induced by pleasant ideas, but also by ridicule as a way to hide embarrassment; and too much of it could irritate the nerves especially if provoked by tickling and in this case might even cause death.[65]

Nervous ailments were rarely fatal, Tissot remarked, but they greatly affected the quality of life of patients and their family. If only on this account, they should not be neglected. Nobody should laugh at these ailments or call them a chimera. To the contrary, they should be taken seriously and attended to early before becoming incurable.[66]   When Tissot thought that most of the causes of nervous troubles were moral and that nervous disorders occurred when reason lost control, he was the child of his time which admired ancient wisdom, and the friend of Rousseau who distrusted the new mores. Thus, Tissot invoked the authority of Galen to show that the proper usage of the non-naturals was the best way to avoid nervous diseases. According to Galen, regimen acts on the three souls Plato seated in the head or brain (intellect), in the chest or heart (passion), and in the belly or liver (appetite). So, by modifying the regimen one should be able to act on the souls which drive passion and appetite, and to help the intellect, or rational soul, keep the upper-hand. Plato had written that when the rational soul rules the others, a human being is free. Here again Tissot transposed souls into nerves, and wrote that in modifying the physical state of the nerves by the proper diet one can hope to bring about a change in the passions.[67] Recalling the importance Tissot placed on understanding the constraints of social life to apprehend the causes of psychic troubles, his remark about the three-part soul of Plato and about the policing role of the rational soul has a familiar ring to our post-Freudian sensibilities.[68] At the same time, Tissot denounced as causes for the multiplication of nervous disorders, the increase in venereal diseases, in luxury, in sedentary work, in card playing instead of active games for recreation, the ignoramus' rage to write and the women's fury to read: "a girl, who at the age of ten reads, when she should be running, is at twenty a vaporous woman and not a good nursing mother."[69]

In Chapter XII, "On the treatment", Tissot recommended a change in regimen, either to counteract the customary way of life prone to bring nervous disorders, or when no particular cause for the disease could be pinpointed. He also reviewed the most common drugs and treatments used in various nervous cases as he had analyzed those used for epilepsy. He found bloodletting was only useful in the case of apoplexy, which he considered a nervous disorder. Most emetics and enemas were pronounced as being too violent as they over-irritated an already ultra-sensitive system; only very mild drugs should be used. Milk was often recommended to strengthen the body when the digestive powers were weak. When the milk of woman or mare was prescribed, Tissot warned his readers to be sure that her infant or the colt was not deprived of proper food. His preference was for cowmilk, always available and in good supply without risk for the calf. Bathing in lukewarm or cold water could fortify and had no secondary effect, but Tissot discouraged baths in water above a temperature of 35 degrees Celsius, since it excited the functions too much, as could be observed in an accelerated pulse and the redness of the skin.[70] When taking the waters, i.e. drinking mineral water or bathing, was prescribed, the physician had to consider both the quality of the water and of the installations of the spa. Nervous people required comfort, and crude facilities would perturb them. Shocks from static electricity were tried in the eighteenth century to cure paralysis as well as other nervous disorders; Tissot considered this method a heroic remedy of a yet unproven value.[71] From the time of King David, the Bible mentioned that music had been used to appease nervous troubles, so Tissot recommended trying musical cures first, especially since they had no secondary effects. The theme of the secondary effects of a remedy is indeed recurrent in this chapter; it is mentioned already in the article on bathing, and it appeared again about frictions. Tissot always wanted the physician to prescribe only drugs or treatments of proven value and with no side effects. Anything else was useless if not downright harmful.

Tissot concluded the chapter with a recapitulation of preventive means, for him the best cure. A proper knowledge and understanding of the non-naturals' influence on well-being which leads to a healthy regimen is the best way to fend off nervous disorders provoked by urbanization, luxury, and indulgence. So once more, he attacked lifestyle, be it in diet, work, or leisure. These habits were to be changed, at best to achieve a harmonious life within a healthy body and a sane mind, at least to improve the patient's situation. His thoughts on the importance of the link between cultural pressures and the behavior of the disturbed individual as well as the physician's role as guide along the path to mental and physical health turned out to be prophetic. In *Traité des nerfs*, he was developing for the physician what he had already discussed for the individual in his Trilogy: physical or mental health was not a given, it was a process, even better a way of life in which patient and physician have the responsibility to be informed of the consequences of their actions and have to collaborate.

In *Traité des nerfs*, Tissot reveals his mastery of the emerging bourgeois mentality and of the contradictions and rebellions of bourgeois men and women. Tissot provided, as Hoffmann has shown in his thorough study *La femme dans la pensée des Lumières*, the essential link between Bordeu and Pinel in the evolution of the Montpellier School toward new understandings of mental diseases.[72]   The fact (however not mentioned by Hoffmann) that, while a medical student, Tissot had been in close contact with Sauvages throws light on Tissot's emphasis on looking into the patient's "goals of life" as quasi moral causes in order to find the roots of their psychic disorders. Tissot in *Traité des nerfs* as in *Sur les maladies des gens du monde* was pessimistic about the chance of cure from a disease that had been induced largely by the lifestyle of the patients and their entourage. A treatment he could prescribe; a complete recovery he could not procure. He had little hope for the healthiness of the idle adults' set short of a revolution in its mores; yet he entrusted physicians to initiate changes, first in their patients' behavior, later in society, in order to foster better health for all.

Chapter VIII

The Teaching Years

Upon his return from Paris in the summer of 1780, Tissot was preoccupied with the future of his nephew. Marc had studied there with the best teachers and learned the theoretical bases of medicine. While Tissot praised Vicq d'Azyr for his attractive lectures on anatomy and Daubenton for his on natural history, he remarked sternly to Zimmermann that there was no help to be had in Paris for the study of practical medicine.[1] In Lausanne, the uncle could take his nephew along when he went to visit the sick poor in their homes. He surely did that, but this was not adequate training for a physician of the late eighteenth century; certainly not for Tissot who was very conscious of the value of degrees and hospital training for a solid career in medicine. After reviewing different choices (Edinburgh, Goettingen, Leyden, Montpellier, or Vienna), Marc hesitated between Edinburgh or Vienna, and finally chose the former. Tissot resolved to let his nephew go alone because of the distance, but was brooding over the planned separation. In fact, Marc never went to Edinburgh to study medicine. Instead, changes in his uncle's career provided a different site for his medical studies.

In the fall of 1780, an envoy from Joseph II came to see Tissot. Since his visit to the Lausanne Doctor in the summer of 1777, the Emperor had determined to attract Tissot to his service. From his previous contacts with Tissot as well as from what he had witnessed in Vienna of the de Haen/Tissot quarrel, the Emperor understood that Tissot was not to be attracted by an appointment at the Hofburg. Joseph II also knew that Tissot had been on the verge of accepting a position at Padua; so, the Emperor looked into the Habsburg domains in Italy for a suitable post and selected Pavia.

The University of Pavia had been founded in 1361 by Gian Galeazzo Visconti and was well regarded, sometimes even called the Oxford of Italy because of its tradition of excellence in the teaching of Law and Philosophy. A faculty of medicine existed also, and following its reorganization by Maria-Theresa in 1770, it was promising to become a center of enlightened medicine. Among the members of the Faculty were the distinguished naturalist Spallanzani (a correspondent of Bonnet and Haller) and the fine anatomist Rezia.[2] Clinical teaching had been instituted under the leadership of Borsieri, one of the first physicians to write on clinical medicine in *Institutione medicum practica*, published in 1781 in Milan, the same year that Duncan had published *Heads of Lectures on the Theory and Practice of Medicine* in Edinburgh.[3] After ten years at the helm of the clinical school, Borsieri (who became ill soon after his appointment) went into retirement at the court of Archduke Ferdinand in Tuscany where he died in 1785. Tissot was to replace him.

Obviously, Tissot was tempted by the professorship, but, always careful to protect his financial, intellectual and religious freedom, he embarked on a lengthy negotiation over the terms. These included funds for lodging and travel, and the right to consult anywhere in Italy. Tissot wanted to sign a contract with a set limit of years, but he was made to understand that under the very generous circumstances of the call it should be, on paper at least, for life. At 3,000 florins of emolument a year, Tissot was to be the best paid professor. He was granted special permission to be freed of any ceremonies or obligations contrary to his Protestant faith. He asked for and was granted funds for remodeling the clinical teaching facilities. He also requested the right to choose patients from the town-hospital to serve as teaching cases. Tissot was responsible for one course in practical medicine each semester.[4] He also secured for his nephew a privileged position among the students, e.g. to have Marc replace him at the head of the clinics when he himself could not be there.

Tissot gave his nephew the patronage he had so cruelly missed at the beginning of his own career, but this plain nepotism exposed him to accusations of having a double-standard. In *Essai sur les moyens de perfectionner les études de médecine*, Tissot wrote of the bad influence patronage has on the son or nephew of well-known physicians. For this reason, he recommended that the youth study abroad where only their ability and hard work could earn them degrees. In spite of the fact that Tissot denounced any kind of privileges granted by their Excellencies of Bern, he never saw the nepotism involved in his actions on Marc's behalf, especially when back in Lausanne he associated his nephew disproportionately with his own medical endeavors.[5]

Finally late in the spring of 1781, Tissot accepted the professorship of practical medicine in Pavia. The news of his imminent departure for Pavia astounded his Lausanne friends.[6] He had come back from Paris because he suffered from *Heimweh*; no one had suspected he would go away so soon. The negotiations had been carried out discreetly by Baron von Cronthal who, for the occasion, had taken up residence in Switzerland. Count Firmian in Milan had countersigned everything for the Emperor and the Archduke.[7]

The reasons for Tissot's acceptance of this post are complex. As disclosed in his correspondence, the medical studies of his nephew weighed heavily in his decision, but Tissot also considered his own professional situation. When he returned from Paris, he was warmly received in Lausanne by his friends; his return, however, was taken for granted by their Excellencies. Tissot's medical father, Haller was no longer there to prompt the tight-fisted Bernese to a more generous disposition, nor was he there to remind their Health-Council of the services Tissot was performing in the Pays de Vaud. Furthermore, the death of Haller had turned the Lausanne Doctor into a wholly mature physician, ready to make decisions and accept his role as teacher. Tissot was now eager to meet students in the classroom and the hospital, and to train them for a new kind of medicine: enlightened expectant medicine and *post mortem* dissection.

Another factor in the decision was financial. By the 1780s, Tissot's pecuniary situation had changed, although it is difficult to pinpoint to exact circumstances for the change. *Traité des nerfs* sold well, but still poorly in comparison with *Onanisme* or *Avis au peuple*; and from his correspondence one gathers that Grasset, his publisher, was not generous. Allusions to lawsuits occasionally crept into Tissot's letters before his departure for Pavia. His brother had met with financial difficulties after returning from military service in the East Indies and settling in Geneva; Tissot might have helped him too generously. When he wrote to his wife

from Pavia, especially during his second year, Tissot wrote
frequently of money, of *lettres de change* she was to request, since
his professorial emoluments were tied up elsewhere. Unfortunately, the letters have been censored and most details about his
financial situation are crossed out with a heavy pen.[8]

Speculating that Tissot's financial difficulties might have come
from faulty investments, I searched for a clue in Lüthy's well-
documented study of Huguenot banking activities and network.[9]
Lüthy wrote that several wealthy Vaudois participated in the
enterprise of the Genevan bankers. The Vaudois chose to enter
merchant-trade and their operations were quite successful; if Tissot
had invested in these deals, he would not have been in financial
straits.[10]   Lüthy also discussed a financier, Rudolf Emmanuel
Haller, who was neither from Geneva nor a Vaudois, although his
name and his family's relations suggest a possible connection
between his not always successful banking practice in the 1780s and
Tissot's money problems.[11] My conjecture is that after his father's
death, Emmanuel, who was already in the merchant-trade business
in Amsterdam, found his own financial inheritance to be meager
(the physiologist Haller had never been rich except in fame and
children) while the intellectual and sentimental heritage had more
lucrative potentials. Tissot might have committed some money to
Emmanuel's hands, since young Haller was moving to Paris and
entering into association with Necker. But in 1781 Emmanuel was
implicated in a bankruptcy in Amsterdam and Tissot might very
well have suffered some losses in the process.[12]

Whatever the reasons, Tissot's decision to accept the professorship at Pavia marks a definite change in his attitude toward what he
saw as his role in the field of medicine. As a private doctor, he had
been concerned with groups of individuals sharing similar health
problems. As the occupant of a chair and holder of an official
position, he now turned his attention decisively to safeguarding
public health, first in the training of competent physicians, then in
the licensing of able medical personnel, and finally in proposing
rules for public hygiene. In his fifties, enjoying reasonably good
health, Tissot felt that his youth's ambitions to become a reformer
of medicine could be realized in Pavia where he was expected with
great anticipation.

Tissot immediately began to refresh the Italian he had learned while a student at the Academy in Geneva. His reasons were not academic, since he was to teach in Latin. Latin fluency was indispensable for a student of medicine, as he wrote in *Essai sur les moyens de perfectionner les études de médecine*. French was the language of the elite and of diplomacy; all the correspondence between Baron Cronthal, Count Firmian and Tissot had been in French, except for the act of nomination which was in Italian. Tissot wanted to know Italian well enough in order to have contacts as directly as possible with the patients and the staff of the San Mateo Hospital. Most hospital surgeons knew little or no Latin and the poor certainly knew neither Latin nor French. Tissot had to learn their language to converse with them and to built the bridge of trust he thought necessary to accomplish his medical task. Earlier in his career Tissot had found out how useful it was to know the *patois* of the Pays de Vaud when he had to care for the poor of Lausanne. It was very important for him to be able to communicate with the common people in their native tongue. Tissot certainly mastered enough Italian to use it in scholarly pursuits, such as reading Frank's treatise on medical police in an Italian translation. Neither this nor his success in teaching Italian medical students offers any clue for his fluency at the bedside of peasants who spoke only a Lombardian dialect.

Tissot and his nephew left Lausanne for Pavia on 9 October 1781.[13] They stopped in Turin, where they were received at the Court of Savoy, then went on to Milan, where Count Firmian assured Tissot of the continuing support of Archduke Ferdinand. Uncle and nephew finally arrived at their destination one day before the semester began.

From Pavia, Tissot wrote regularly to his wife.[14] Fortunately, the "censor" left intact the details about the lectures and the rounds of the hospital; these accounts are all the more precious since the letters Tissot wrote to Zimmermann while in Pavia never reached their addressee.[15] On 27 November 1781, Tissot wrote to his wife: "This morning, I gave my first lecture wearing a Spanish gown, I anticipated fifty to sixty students, there were four hundred fifty to five hundred persons who were well taken in."[16] At first, Tissot's lecturing style was as stern as a Calvinist sermon, with no stylistic flourishes. Moreover his voice was dulled by emotion, since Tissot had not anticipated such a large audience. A few weeks later, however, he wrote to his wife: "...neither the lectures, nor the hospital rounds are giving me any difficulty..."   He then commented on the great number of students who had come from all over Italy, and how he had to change the rounds at the clinical wards to accommodate so many students within the allotted space. He also described the setting of the university.

The classical buildings erected by Maria-Theresa where Tissot taught are still standing, despite many wars, and today house the Humanities at the University of Pavia. He noted: "There is a large room with a huge fire, where the professors meet before going to and after coming out of their auditorium I always find some charming men there. The lay professors dress in their Spanish gown there, and take back their sword when they leave, and this gown goes over any coat's color. I have not yet parted with my grey coat..."[17] Tissot did not mention whether he himself wore a sword; meanwhile, he let his wife know that he was not indulging in frivolous expenses, one detail about his pecuniary straits that the "censor" overlooked. Tissot had only good words for the academic situation in Pavia, praising the authorities of the San Mateo Hospital for their cooperation in his efforts to upgrade clinical teaching.

As weeks passed, Tissot relaxed in the classroom, and the students began to appreciate the clarity of his style. They recognized the validity of Tissot's mode of teaching which called on personal experiences and active readings rather than passive compilations of famous books or commentaries on ancient medicine. They discovered the erudition and vast practice under the modesty and amiability of the foreign professor who managed not to stir up jealousy about being the best paid faculty.[18] Spallanzani wrote to Bonnet in Geneva about his newest colleague: "Everybody in Pavia is very satisfied with him. His lectures are very instructive and very advantageous to the youth who have rushed from all parts of Italy to benefit from the Swiss Hippocrates. Besides his learning which certainly is very extended, Mr. Tissot is the most polite and likeable man in the world."[19] Tissot had been loved by his patients, wealthy and poor alike; he had now the appreciation of his colleagues and students. Even when one takes into account the superlative tone of the eighteenth-century epistolary style, the testimony of this Italian student conveys true admiration: "Mr. Tissot is really delicious ... his practical views are beautiful, wholly reasonable, sanctioned by the works of the masters of the art and confirmed by his own experience ... What more could one wish in a lecture?"[20] The phrase "confirmed by his own experience" is the key to Tissot's teaching and writing, he only spoke of what he had himself verified. This student went on to describe that Tissot taught every morning for "five quarters of an hour", reading from manuscript notes and that afterwards he led the rounds in the clinics. The description he gave of Tissot's attitude at the bedside in the clinical wards is exactly the method Tissot expounded in his inaugural lecture and personal notes and which he later published in a more elaborated form in *Essai sur les moyens de perfectionner les études de médecine.*[21]

In his inaugural lecture of 27 November 1781, delivered of course in Latin, he began with a brief history of clinical teaching, attributing its debut to François de la Boë, a French Huguenot physician, who taught at Leyden in the seventeenth century. In learning the history of one's specialty, Tissot saw a means for emulation and humility at the same time: emulation in the progress made over the centuries in understanding the physiology of the body or the treatment of diseases; humility in view of how much still remained incomprehensible. He also stated his priorities for the rounds in the clinical wards: "It should not be forgotten that the healing of the sick is always the first objective, and that teaching is only the second."[22]

Tissot continued with the first contact between patient and aspiring physician; he stressed the urgent need for compassion, decency, and kindness in this verbal and physical encounter. Testifying to his determination to move away from the artificiality of scholastic medicine and to embrace the "natural" way, Tissot spelled out a number of questions to be asked in a logical or natural order as the first part of the contact.[23] The questions concerned the country of origin or residence of the patient, its quality of air, its type of climate, its prevalent diseases. This was the typical Neo-Hippocratic approach to medicine and was exploited on a large scale by the Société royale de médecine in its questionnaires to French country-physicians in an attempt to elucidate the mystery of morbidity and pestilence.[24] Before the nineteenth-century germ theory of disease was articulated,

miasmas and atmospheric conditions, in accord with the Hippocratic tradition, were considered to have decisive roles in morbidity
and pestilence.

The second step was observation and physical examination of
the patient, specifically the eyes and mouth, the face and its
complexion, the abdomen, the respiration, and a careful pulse
taking to determine its qualities. The pulse, Tissot said, exhibits
the vital forces, telling the physician whether, and how much,
nature needs to be helped to assure recovery; in this he placed
himself squarely within the vitalist movement of the Montpellier
physicians Bordeu and Barthez.[25]

Under the professor's guidance, the medical student performed
the questioning and the physical examination. In a spirit of learning and not of humiliation, said Tissot, the professor should elicit
by his pertinent questioning of the student the right questions to
ask from and observations to make of the patient.[26] Then, the
student gave his prognosis, diagnosis, and treatment of the disease.
The student was to state the reasons for his conclusions, to give a
short review of what was known about the disease, and occasionally
to quote authoritative treatises. Tissot advocated simplicity of cure
and remedy "because nature is simple in its ways."[27] The medical
student was responsible, once his treatment was approved by the
professor, for instructing the hospital personnel of its implementation. No other student should meddle in the process. Tissot
declared that one visit per day was sufficient in most cases and
should be kept that way so as not to tire the patient. Only in the
eventuality of special symptoms occurring at a time other than that
of the clinical rounds should the student return to the wards.
When the patient was cured, Tissot said, the student was to attend
to his discharge from the clinics to the convalescent room. And he
added sternly: "When the patient died, the student who took care
of him will perform the dissection."[28] Tissot insisted that an
autopsy be performed after each death, to verify the diagnosis and
to look at all the parts affected by the disease. Tissot's systematic
program of *post-mortem* as an integral part of the clinical teaching
at Pavia was among the first to be established. In fact, from the
beginning of his career, Tissot had performed autopsies of his
deceased patients, and it was jokingly said that his patients were

lucky to be perfectly dissected when not perfectly cured by their doctor.

Another point that Tissot described in his inaugural lecture was the diary the student had to keep of the history of the case. The diary had to contain the diagnosis and prognosis along with justifications, the prescribed treatment and its effects as well as the bodily occurrences. After reading what had been written on the subject of his patient's disease, the student had to write for his own use a "précis" of the specific disease and its variations so as to increase his general knowledge through specific cases. This mode of compiling information was not unique to Tissot; it was inspired partly by a Baconian view of cumulative knowledge that would shed light on the solution of problems, and partly by a spirit of systematization of medicine that would allow comparison of success and failure for specific treatment and illness and might uncover patterns of recovery.[29] This can be seen as a prologue to the nineteenth-century statistical approach in medicine. What was novel with Tissot and others, such as Duncan in Edinburgh, was their insistence on objectivity. Physicians had to report only rigorously observed medical facts, not just those observations which fit their own particular scheme, while excluding those facts which did not buttress their own understanding of diseases. In his personal notes on how he was to conduct his teaching at Pavia, Tissot spelled out specific conditions for choosing patients for the clinical wards: "I will admit only one well-defined case of each common disease in a way to insure that the students will be exposed to a variety of illnesses during their two years of clinical training."[30]

When Tissot arrived in Pavia, one of his first steps was to inspect the hospital and the clinical facilities, and consequently to request either new locations for the teaching wards or extensive repairs and remodeling of the old wards.[31] Prior to his coming, he had been given what amounted to a "carte blanche" for the reorganization of the clinics. Once Tissot was in Pavia, would the authorities live up to their agreement? Among Tissot's personal papers are the drafts of the reports he made to the authorities of the city of Pavia after the first few weeks of clinical teaching and, perhaps, again after a few more months.[32] In them, he alluded to an earlier report which is missing and was probably written at the time of the negotiations to bring him to Pavia. Tissot had to scale down his project of clinical teaching. He had hoped for separate wards for men and women, of at least twelve beds each, large enough to accommodate all the students (at minimum twenty-four) during their rounds of visits without disturbing the patients with noise, over-heated and over-vitiated air. Instead, he had to satisfy himself with rooms in which only eight patients could be admitted, and with so narrow a "ruelle" between the beds that the less advanced students were to take turns to follow the visits once a week. With this reduced number of patients and a larger than expected group of students attending the clinical training, not every terminal (fourth-year) student could have, as Tissot had wished, his own patient to follow to recovery or death. Instead, Tissot devised a system of team learning, in which he paired students to take turns at the bedside of one sick person and to assume responsibility for the diagnosis, cure, and eventual autopsy.

Tissot described a few peculiarities of the existing building. He requested the demolition of a wall obstructing the windows of the apothecary room and asked to have special provisions made to the effect that the wall could not be rebuilt at a later date; he also required that the adjacent house, identified as the Belcredi House, henceforth not be used to lodge a locksmith, coppersmith, candle-maker, or any other trade which generated noise and dust.[33] He wrote about the orientation of the building and how the dissecting room was too cramped and exposed to the southwest. He would not tolerate the overcrowding around the dissecting table, because it was unhealthy and worthless for teaching purposes.[34] The southwest orientation, which exacerbated the summer heat, was less important to him, since the university and the dissecting room were closed from mid-June to late October.

Tissot never complained of a situation that was not quite as promised. On the contrary, he wrote to his wife: "the Marquis de Botha, chief director of the hospital, is quick to have everything I asked carried through and, in general, the more we move forward, the more we have reason to be satisfied."[35] He hoped that the improvements he suggested for the clinical wards would be met and implemented during the summer recess of 1782 and the clinics readied for the October reopening of the University. If we can believe Joseph Frank, only the women's ward was built according to Tissot's specifications.[36] Still, the number of students attending the clinics grew from forty at the time of its founding by Borsieri in 1770 to seventy when Tissot taught and to a peak of one-hundred and fifty students under Frank.[37] These figures are corroborated by Tissot's notes, in which he wrote of sixty students following the rounds the first year he taught.[38] The pioneer work of Borsieri on the importance of practical medical training was bearing fruit. In two years, through creative means in circumventing inadequacies, Tissot built a model of clinical teaching that Pinel praised.[39]

Through his teaching, Tissot discovered a new dimension to his medical dedication. His contacts with students of the clinical wards made him conscious of the importance of dialogue, of direct exchange without the mediation of written words.[40] Medicine was coming alive through observations and physical examinations of suffering bodies. Tissot was to be most remembered by his students for the teaching he did at the bedside, for his original attitude toward the interaction between patient and physician, for his use of observation and examination, for his correlation of diagnosis and prognosis, and for his careful autopsies.

During the Christmas recess of 1781-82, Tissot and his nephew travelled through northern Italy. Eynard mentioned a travel diary of Tissot covering his stay in Italy, but the diary appears to have been lost.[41] Tissot was invited by the Senate of Venice to visit the city; the reception he received surpassed all he could have imagined. He wrote that the town physicians attended on him from morning to night as if he were a king. Tissot, who had thought that republics were less subject to the spell of hierarchy and subservience, shortened his stay in Venice to the limits of politeness. He went to visit Padua where, among his colleagues of the Medical Faculty, he felt at ease and enjoyed the intellectual atmosphere, but was much annoyed by the admiration of the non-academic populace. To avoid all this fuss about his person, Tissot registered at the gates of Vicenze as Marc d'Apples and his governor; this stratagem let him travel in peace and return to Pavia in time for meeting his classes.

The news of his triumphant reception in Venice and of successes in treating an epidemic of bilious fever in the region of Pavia increased Tissot's popularity among the students. Nonetheless, Tissot remained objective, almost harsh in his assessment of them.

He wrote to a friend back in Lausanne: "I have already told you and I repeat it, mediocrity is common everywhere, everywhere there are beings of true merit: there may be some difference in the sharing out, but, without having seen it all, I believe I have seen enough to be convinced that our country is not the worst, and one thing is certain, it is this one which up-to-now I prefer to all others I know."[42] Here Tissot was writing as much of intellectual conditions as of the climate of Pavia, which his friend supposed to be always sunny. Certainly Tissot would rather have endured the biting north wind of Lausanne than the fog from the river Ticino which dampened everything in Pavia; he would have eaten potatoes rather than rice.[43]

At the end of the first academic year Tissot and Marc left for Lausanne to spend the summer months there. On their way home, they stopped in Milan so that Tissot saw Count Firmian and discussed with him the situation in the clinical wards. Whatever the Count promised Tissot, implementation was prevented by the turmoil in the Lombardian administration which followed the Count's death. In Lausanne, Tissot felt the warmth of friendship, and his old acquaintances found him still the same modest, devoted friend whom neither honors or flattery had changed.[44] By September, uncle and nephew were on the road again. Tissot had promised to visit the Countess of Albany in Rome and the Queen of the Two Sicilies in Naples.[45] Queen Maria-Carolina tried to keep him at least six months and said that she would arrange everything with her brothers.[46] He responded that his duty was to be on time in Pavia to teach the fall semester. Even so, they parted on good terms; Tissot praised the Queen's intelligence and gracious behavior toward them and the Queen gave snuff-boxes to him and Marc. Later from Pavia, he wrote to his wife that all the news about his stay in Naples printed in *Gazette de Berne* were false. He had never seen any patients outside the royal family, and the only gifts he had received were those he had already described, he added: "We would have had to come back in pilgrim's style, if I had not had letters of credit on Naples, Rome, Florence, and Leghorn..."[47]

On his way back to Pavia, Tissot stopped again in Rome. It was during this second stay that his portrait was painted by Angelica Kaufmann, a well-respected portraitist.[48] Tissot also had an audience with Pope Pius VI who had initiated the meeting and let it be known in advance that Tissot was dispensed, as a Protestant, from all ceremonials towards his Holiness.[49] He wrote to his wife that he had been presented to the Pope who kept him for more than a half-hour, but did not report the subject of the conversation nor that the Pope gave him a complete set of the gold medals minted so far during his Holiness' reign.[50] Tissot never kept her informed of intellectual matters, only describing everyday routine, such as playing badminton with Marc inside their apartment where the ceiling was so high that it was difficult to push the bird all the way up. Gossip was endemic: "One does not expect the Emperor anymore, and we ignore what is transported from the Chartreuse to Milan, it can only be Church ornaments of which one might perhaps mint golden and silver coins."[51] He was more generous with details about landscape and countryside which he admired, but the Italian cities did not attract him as he found them dirty and overcrowded.[52]

In March of 1783, Tissot was called to the Court of Savoy in Turin; he did not want to go lest he lose time from teaching. He felt that his foremost obligation was to the students, as he had already privately decided to relinquish his professorship. On the order of Archduke Ferdinand, he went reluctantly, acquiring one more reason to long to be back in Lausanne where their Excellencies were not in the habit of blatantly ordering him around. He returned very tired: "I had to see more patients that I wished to ... yet I am pleased by the money I have earned during this short trip."[53] Soon, he fell sick, and Marc replaced him at the hospital. The sickness dragged on, and Tissot became worried about dying away from Lausanne. On 15 April 1783, he wrote to his wife a letter which is in fact a testament, but the "censor" applied his hand so heavily on it that it is impossible to make sense of the instructions. Tissot wrote that he would be much more reassured and calm once he knew that everything was in order. He did for himself what he said a good physician should always do: tell his patients of the prognosis of their illness, for if the physician thought the issue was fatal, the patients ought to know and should have time to put their affairs in order.[54] *Heimweh*, combined with overwork and latent tuberculosis, was worsening an ear infection.

After his illness, Tissot announced his resignation. Neither the pleading of students nor the offer of additional monetary rewards from the authorities could induce him to stay. Even appeals to his duty toward the students left him unmoved. In his eyes, he had fulfilled his obligations. He had taught clinical medicine for two years as he had always intended. He had tried hard to get the promised new clinics, although only the one for women was actually built. Under the circumstances new assurances were not very credible. As for private reasons besides his own health, now that Marc had completed his medical studies, Tissot was ready to return home and use his influence for setting his nephew up there. In the company of Marc, he left Pavia on 21 June 1783. Two years later he published *Sur les moyens de perfectionner les études de médecine*, the fruit of his experience at Pavia. A marble plaque placed in one of the auditoria commemorates Tissot's teaching at the University.

Chapter IX

The Pavia Watershed

The decade of the 1780s bustled with calls for reforms and attempts to implement them. An urge to improve society was felt by liberal citizens and enlightened monarchs alike. This feverish reforming activity was a sign of a "fin de siècle" atmosphere ripe with potential for both the best and the worst of innovations. In the lands of Louis XVI and Joseph II, for example, toleration edicts and economic reforms raised hopes and ushered dissent. The last years of Tissot's life aptly reflect this Janus age in which people rushed to champion changes in the name of progress as well as of tradition. His own reform of medical studies and his call for public health measures best exemplify the thrust of his last medical activities.[1] These same topics were also the center of preoccupations of other medical and political authorities. Therefore, Tissot's published and unpublished views on these matters shed light on the rationale for both the general consideration and his own concern for the public good.

The Pavia sojourn marked a turning point in Tissot's life and medical endeavors. The responsibility of teaching had forced him to look concretely at his art, to reflect on the purpose of medicine and the training of physicians who would deliver health and happiness. He became even more aware of the failings of traditional medical and political thoughts when he was confronted with the reorganization of the Pavia Hospital. Tissot redirected his preoccupations to emphasize practicability and feasibility. He devoted his time to the social and political aspects of the use and abuse of medicine and he entered the realm of public health.[2] He still wrote because he enjoyed it, but he published very little. *Essai sur les moyens de perfectionner les études de médecine* was the last original work on medicine he gave to the public, although during the final years of his life he wrote and published the biography of his

deceased friend Zimmermann.[3] Revisions of his previous books
appeared mainly as several editions of collected works.[4] This failure to publish any new work is especially puzzling since his
personal papers include several nearly-complete treatises.[5] A
partial explanation for Tissot's meager publication record after his
teaching stint may be his commitment to promote his nephew's
career. Marc published two pamphlets before his uncle's death:
the first on instructions to persons caring for the sick and the other
on the respective benefit of home-care and hospitalization for the
poor. Both works are in manuscript form among Tissot's papers in
his copyist's hand, with numerous revisions in his own hand. He
certainly spent much time on these publications, but gave the credit
to his nephew.[6]

The experience abroad changed Tissot in another aspect. During
his extensive travels throughout Italy, he discovered barren countryside and overcrowded cities sharing a common poverty. He
observed almost everywhere the enfeebling effect of swampy atmosphere, even in the Kingdom of Naples.[7] He saw distress around
Pavia and at the hospital much more vividly than what he had seen
in Lausanne where habitude and custom had blunted the truth. To
be sure, the Pays de Vaud was not short of poor or of unhealthy
places, but the familiarity of the sites had dulled his perception of
the needs while their Excellencies of Bern had seemed inclined
toward enlightened paternalism. From Venice to Naples, the
different states of eighteenth-century Italy were grappling with
problems arising from increasing poverty, due to archaic modes of
production in agriculture and manufacture compounded by latent
demographic pressure ready to explode in spite of apparent
depopulation. Authorities in the various states seemed well-
disposed towards reforms; new agricultural ventures were tried in
Tuscany, Piedmont, or the Two Sicilies, and some changes in the
penal code were introduced in Lombardy. In spite of these
thoughtful and perhaps wishful reforms, "the people misery:
mother of diseases" (Frank's catch-phrase), was haunting Tissot.
Back in Lausanne he dedicated his last years' efforts to denouncing
the vicious circle of poverty breeding disease. He also wrote on the
development of agriculture and transportation, two subjects dear
to the Bernese.[8] He revised his letters to Baker and to Hirzel to
emphasize the dietary importance of wholesome food and proper

cooking or baking. For Tissot, medicine became more than the healing of individual bodies, it became a social call to heal society: only a concerted action of citizens and authorities could accomplish the task. In Lausanne as elsewhere, the political climate of the 1780s was darkening, while the privileged hardened their defense of or tried to preserve the status quo. Tissot was diffident as he had to face the decision of whether to work for reform within the system or to break from it.

In the 1760s, Tissot had been a sort of physiocrat wanting to improve the lot of the peasantry, "the most useful portion of society". He had seen in the Pays de Vaud, and again even more vividly in Italy, the attraction of the urban centers for young male and female peasants who, deprived of land to cultivate, sought employment away from their village. In the Lausanne of the last decades of the eighteenth century, as in many other towns, opportunities for them were few except as domestic servants. Tissot saw in domestic as well as mercenary military service a degradation of the individual. At first, he insisted on the consequences of urban living for the physical health of immigrants, the stale air, the humidity of streets and dwellings without sun, the polluted water and food, but he soon broadened his attack to include the artificiality in the urban life of the wealthy who hired the servants. Tissot blamed them for the moral depravity of their domestics who aped their masters' fancy tastes. He denounced high society's own perversion in bartering their liberties and responsibility for vain trinkets. For him, service of any kind spelled dependence, and dependence was unhealthy physically and intellectually.

This interpretation of Tissot's writings of the 1760s might not square well with his later timorous position toward the stiffening Bernese rule during the revolutionary years. Even so, in the 1780s, Tissot was still inspired by physiocratic and democratic thoughts. As their Excellencies' policies for the Pays de Vaud were directed at increasing agricultural production in a combined effort to expand the tax-base and to better their subjects' condition, Tissot clung, in the 1790s, to his view of a benevolent and enlightened Bernese government. His vision of independence and dignity was blurred by the excesses of the revolutionary urban populace; he lost his hopes for bourgeois rule, as he watched anarchy ravaging France. He became convinced that reforms from above rather than from below were the road to the just and healthy world he had advocated in his Trilogy. Tissot never doubted of being able to persuade the Bernese authorities to implement public health regulations and to reform the dispensation of health-care.

While Gibbon was denouncing the tax exploitation of the Pays de Vaud, Tissot remained confident in the future, to the point of blindness toward the shortcomings of the present.[9] He thought that their Excellencies's past achievements which had often been motivated by the social humanism of Calvin[10] would be extended to include liberal policies towards partnership in medical, political, and economic endeavors. His own religious faith motivated his thinking and he deluded himself in believing that others did likewise.

Tissot transposed to the body-politic the gaze of the Neo-Hippocratic physician. He observed the symptoms of a deeply seated malaise due to the cleavage of society, each order tugging for its own profit, neglecting the health of the whole. Applying his definition of individual health (as the happy harmony of all physiological functions) to society's health, Tissot arrived at a cautious position favoring gradual reforms and a program of cooperation between all parts (or organs) of the body-politic for the common good. One part could not be allowed to suffer or to dominate without affecting the whole. As seen earlier, Tissot was a partisan of expectant medicine rather than heroic medicine, of diet and exercise rather than purge and bloodletting for physical ills. Consequently he recoiled at the excesses of the revolutionaries, as bloodshed and expulsions could not cure political imbalance. He advocated a new regimen adapted to the needs and desires of a changed population that was no longer satisfied with passivity. Partnership was the key to Tissot's solution for reform, a partnership including authorities, experts, and concerned citizens that would construct a better world for everyone.

Tissot applauded the calling of the Estates General, after the failure of the Assembly of Notables. He saw the possibility of a renewal of policies brought about by the intervention of the provincial delegates, independently of the Court and the ministers whom he judged impervious to innovative solutions. Summing up his views of the Revolution he wrote to Zimmermann: "I had seen from too close the abuses in the French Government and the misery of the people not to sense the need for reform; I saw with pleasure the convocation of the Estates General. The huge preponderance given to the Third Estate diminished that pleasure giving me some fears; yet I had liked to keep some hopes, which I kept until 11 July 1789."[11] Tissot's hopes were dashed by the behavior of the Parisian populace and the ineptitude of the Court: "One of the parties inspired only horror and the other showed neither genius, nor even the most common intelligence, nor unity, nor steadiness; and it just inspired pity without interest."[12]

Tissot and Zimmermann seemed to agree that the domestic events in France were the problems of the French. They limited their own concern to the safety of Switzerland and the integrity of the Empire threatened by the revolutionary propaganda of words and deeds. They wished for a recovery of nerve by all political authorities so that they could calm tempers and lead their peoples into better times; but their hopes were illusions. By 1794, the two doctors came to realize that abuses had lasted too long, the pressure of frustrations was too high to be contained by ordinary means, that only exhaustion of one of the warring parties would bring some peace to the Continent.

Tissot could never really decide for open rebellion; he only manifested occasional impatience, and mostly tried to reconcile his medical dreams with the Bernese reality, in particular in his work within the Collège de Médecine. He had envisioned the Collège, on the model of the Société royale de médecine, as an independent institution for the regulation and enforcement of public health measures as well as for the licensing of properly trained medical personnel. Officially, the College had no teaching mission, it was to have in the Pays de Vaud the power, formerly held by the Health-Council of Bern, to regulate the practice of medicine. Tissot was its first vice-president and Marc d'Apples one of its members; and since the Bernese Bailiff, residing in Lausanne, was always automatically its President, their Excellencies kept control over its decisions.[13] Although this arrangement provoked many incidents and caused much tension, it nonetheless represented some progress towards autonomy and speedier action.

Tissot had dreamed of being the Hippocrates of modern medicine, but he could hardly fail to realize that the Neo-Hippocratic medicine of which he was a partisan had embarked on an

irreversible course of change. He was too tired, too old, too preoccupied with the day-to-day task of the Collège to make a complete
break from what he sensed was an obsolete style of medicine. His
were the burned-out ambitions of a young man eagerly coming out
of his village to conquer the city and change medical care. Now he
was a mature man; he had tried his best at Pavia, but sickness and
Heimweh had shortened the endeavor. Back in Lausanne, Tissot
tried to apply the weight of his prestige to reform the medical institutions of his country. He also took time to answer the many
letters of consultation sent to him from all over Europe, most of
them about nervous disorders as *Traité des nerfs* had made him a
much sought-after authority on the subject. But he had no more
ambition for international fame. Only when sitting alone at his
writing table would he commit to paper his thoughts of a new kind
of medicine which would engage everyone in the betterment of
health.

   Initially the disturbances of the French Revolution were hardly
felt in Lausanne, as only a few émigrés arrived, among them some
physicians who requested the right to practice. Bern liberally
granted the patents for the Pays de Vaud, on the pretext of the
similarity of language; the Collège de Médecine resented this
infringement on its rights. Tissot had to walk a tightrope in order
to displease no one. Some of the notes Tissot left about the deliberations of the Collège de Médecine betray some impatience
toward obstruction of his wishes. Tissot had earlier let it be known
that the attitude of acquiescence shown by students and colleagues
in Pavia had made him uneasy. He longed to be among Lausanne
friends who would dare to contradict him. Although he did not
expect to win approval merely because he was a celebrated physician; I am of two minds, however, on just how well he could, in fact,
accept personal affronts to his authority. The following incident is
an amusing illustration.

   In 1785, Antoine de Servan, an early French liberal, had taken
up residence at Lausanne, and shifting his interest from politics to
science, had become a devotee of Mesmerism.[14]   Servan was
demonstrating Mesmer's animal magnetism tub for his friends and
the curious. Charles Bonnet, having heard of wondrous cures by
this method, wrote to Tissot about Mesmerism.[15] However, being
almost blind, Bonnet did not want to travel to Lausanne to observe

Servan's demonstration; he asked Tissot to do so. Mesmerism was used to cure nervous disorders, a subject close to Tissot's medical expertise, so he obliged and went with Marc to watch the experiment. After one session, Tissot wanted to see another. When he and his nephew presented themselves at the door of the meeting place, they were barred from entering, Tissot for taking notes and Marc because he had smiled.[16] Tissot was angered at the incident as much in the name of scientific objectivity as on account of the rebuff he had suffered. So Tissot and Bonnet were unable to decide on the validity of the claim of Mesmer; they refused to participate in the debate over animal magnetism without solid and fair observations of the phenomenon.

One joy for Tissot was his namesake, the first son of his nephew, born in 1785. In spite of the fact that Tissot had inoculated him twice unsuccessfully, little Auguste contracted smallpox in March 1790, and died. Tissot who had thought the child immune to the disease was broken. He wrote to Zimmermann: "Nothing will ever lighten the burden of my affliction ... your friend is nothing, not good at anything anymore ... I am not asking for consoling, there is none ... if you still love me, pray that my time of distress be abridged, since nothing can soften it, and the necessity to hide my pain is worsening it, if that can be."[17] Tissot had kept a record of Auguste's progress and wrote in a weak hand below an entry of the child's height: "How could I know it was the last time I was to measure you my little Auguste."

The German physician Frank and Tissot had from time to time exchanged letters. In his autobiography Frank mentioned a correspondence going back to at least 1771.[18] Frank had written to Tissot upon his appointment as his successor at Pavia, requesting some advice.[19] They were interested in the same problems of public health policies and of teaching medicine at the bedside. Frank came to visit Tissot in Lausanne in August 1791. He was travelling with his son Joseph who was also a physician. Frank briefly recorded the visit in his autobiography: "I wish simply to recall that this journey provided for me the pleasure of making the personal acquaintance of my great predecessor at Pavia, the famous Tissot of Lausanne, and of enjoying his instructive company for three whole days."[20] Joseph also left an autobiographical account of that trip and of the meeting with Tissot. His description is more personal than his father's. Although he noted how much Tissot had been affected by the death of little Auguste d'Apples, he added that Tissot was always ready to discuss medicine, seemingly the only way to draw him out of his melancholy. Joseph reported that he listened with rapt interest to their conversations and also that Tissot asked his father to read aloud from his manuscript on the spine and its disease, commenting: "Ah! how beautiful!"[21] According to Joseph, Tissot had hoped to find in his father a physician friend of the stature of Haller... but Joseph might have overstated the case. Frank was too busy chasing success to take the time to correspond at a level above that required by a politeness which served his own best interests, namely to secure Tissot's favorable opinion.[22]

During the last years of his life Tissot buried himself in work to hide his grief. He kept revising *De la médecine civile* with the hope of implementing its reforms through the Collège de Médecine. He frequently became ill with fainting spells; as months passed his handwriting weakened and his notes of the Collège's meetings are an indirect record of his decline. When Tissot became convinced that tuberculosis was undermining him, he embarked on the writing of a treatise on etisis, which he described to Zimmermann: "I have looked again at my teaching notes from Pavia and I have made them into a huge work of 600 pages, the case-history of the author, naturally, occupies eight or ten pages of it which I will add to my next letter."[23] Tissot gave his Montpellier measles case as the beginning of the problem, and his grieving over his grand-nephew's death as an aggravating cause.[24] In an earlier letter, Tissot had already described his illness, how he had lost weight, had frequent bouts of fever, was coughing and spitting blood; he diagnosed it in English as "galloping consumption". At first he had refused to take care of himself; after several months, he had finally followed his nephew's advice to take "Kermès minéral" [an expectorant] and his health had improved so much that he was better than he had been for the last four years.[25]

The Revolution was spreading, but much as Tissot was annoyed by pretension and injustice, he could not subscribe to violence as a mean to right the wrongs of the world. At least for his own country, he still entertained hopes for reform within existing institutions that would adapt the old order of corporate responsibility and benevolent paternalism to a new situation of personal duty and active participation. He had the utopian hope that reason and justice would prevail to bring an orderly transformation. These were the dreams of an old man, informed by his younger enthusiasms as physician of the poor denouncing the injustice of poverty and now chastened by the weight of fear of lost control over his own exploded reforms turned revolution. He perceived what it would take to implement his program, how revolutionary it was in fact, and became afraid. He was afraid first for himself, of the retaliation of a government he had loved enough to want it to improve; second, he was afraid of the excesses he saw perpetrated in the name of the justice he advocated. To the end of his life, Tissot appears to have opted for the status quo, while confiding to paper his social conception of health and medicine.

Public health came into the limelight in the second half of the eighteenth century primarily because of the fear of depopulation and the perceived necessity to halt this threat to the wealth of nations.[26] Only a better medicine might decrease mortality and a better medicine implied hygiene. Public health was recognized as the best hope for increasing population, since natality was thought to be at its highest level, mortality had to be blamed for the decline.[27] The Philosophes had already argued for health as a right, health as a part of the pursuit of happiness. Health, attained and maintained through curative and preventive medicine, became the focus of attention.[28]

Tissot reinterpreted the individualistic message of the Philosophes into the happiness and well-being of society through public health. He concentrated the intellectual efforts of his last fifteen years on transforming the established medical institutions; as he wanted them to serve his new demands for public health. Medical faculties and hospitals first attracted Tissot's attention because of his duties at the University of Pavia; then, upon his return to Lausanne, he focussed on the entire environment which could not be dissociated from its effects on human life. Tissot recognized that curative medicine alone was not enough. Restoring health had to take second place to preserving health. So, he turned to hygiene and to medical police which he defined as "public hygiene". Tissot also included in his vision of medical police articles on the government's duty for provisioning the population with enough wholesome food at affordable prices for the prevalent wages. He was well-aware of the fact that destitution bred disease. After his return from Pavia, because of the poverty and wealth he had seen side by side there, Tissot became steadily more involved in the politics of medical matters. The fact that medicine became politicized characterized an age deep in factional struggles epitomized by the French Revolution.

Tissot left voluminous notes about transformations to the Lausanne Hospital and the training and licensing of medical practitioners.[29] This material reveals an image of Tissot of greater breadth than the portrait of the fashionable doctor that emerges from his books of the 1770s, although the liberal dimension and revolutionary tone could already be discerned between the lines of his writings on the health of classes of individuals.[30] Tissot objected to the mismanagement of resources, be it due to carelessness or inertia of custom. Whatever the resources (financial, intellectual, physical, or political), he intended them to be used to their best potential, without waste, but also without exploitation.

Initially in Pavia Tissot had struggled with the Faculty over the reform of medical education when he had advocated changes in curriculum, examination procedures and the ensuing favoritism. His clinical experience led him to his second objective: the transformation of the hospital from a *mouroir* to a *machine à guérir*.[31] During the last decade of his life he waged a subdued fight against the inertia of both the Republic of Bern and the Lausanne Council of the Sixty, of which he was a member, in the hope of improving health-care.

Lastly, Tissot undertook to review and to challenge the entire conception of good health, from living conditions to medical care, from birth to death. In this attempt, he extended the role of the Galenic non-naturals from a private guide to bettering individual health to a general standard for promoting public hygiene. Tissot added to his innovative use of the non-naturals his constant emphasis on the dignity and worth of each individual human life; the result was *De la médecine civile*.[32] He, therefore, reached out to a social conception of health and medical care, which I will analyze in the next three chapters. The Pavia watershed is here: on one side the Enlightenment's concern for the individual, on the other the revolutionary advocacy for public hygiene and societal reforms.

Tissot died early in June 1797, after a month of lethargic living during which his wife had died without his showing any sign of grief.[33] That December French troops entered Switzerland (called in by the "Patriotes Vaudois") and swept away the Bernese domination of the Pays de Vaud as well as the Old Regime of Switzerland.

The Old Order and the Old Medicine were gone. Tissot did not live to participate in the new order, nor was he, for a long time, recognized as one of the heralds of the new medicine.[34] Still, Tissot's published contributions to the new concept of health were seminal to the work of his successors.[35] As for his ideas confined to manuscripts or found in the minutes of the Collège de Médecine, in spite of the fact that they had little or no immediate influence, they are a precious witness to the times.

Chapter X

Institution of the New Physician

The word institution is used here in its eighteenth-century meaning of foundations. The "new physician" that Tissot wanted to see trained was of two kinds: a country-surgeon for the peasantry, a physician for the bourgeoisie. In his writings, the definition of each kind evolved with changing circumstances in his career as well as in society.

In the 1760s Tissot had recognized the importance of qualified physicians, surgeons, midwives, and apothecaries for the general well-being of the population.[1] This concern for the people is one manifestation of the "tournant des mentalités".[2] Whereas reasonably qualified or indeed well-trained medical personnel were practicing in the towns, villages too often remained in the clutches of outright charlatans or well-intentioned incompetents. Tissot fought for strict regulation and enforcement of the decrees of the Bernese Conseil de Santé. But in view of the scarcity of physicians, the enforcement of the regulations presented the villagers all too often only with the alternative between their own familiar healer or nothing at all.

In the 1780s Tissot, as vice-president of the Lausanne Collège de Médecine, became involved in the proper licensing of medical staff.[3] The Minutes of the Collège de Médecine contain many reports of quarrels over who could practice medicine and many instances of villagers petitioning to keep their "medicinemen", even though these practitioners did not meet the regulatory requirements.[4] The Conseil, as it had in the past,[5] issued regulations on the practice of medicine in the countryside in an effort to check the activities of the quacks rather than to try to displace them with qualified physicians and surgeons as Tissot had advocated in 1765 *Plan d'instruction pour des médecins de village*.[6] The Bernese authorities were following the same course of actions that the French royal ministers had adopted in their fight against quackery, namely repeated decrees as if these periodic reappearances would engrave their enduring validity in the population's mind.[7] A determined medicalization of society had to wait until the 1780s. It took the persistent efforts of physicians such as Tissot for the ship of the state to change its course from enacting decrees to implementing reforms.[8]

Tissot had included in *Plan* provisions for medical instruction of midwives. He was aware of the long-term effects on health that proper or bad care at the time of delivery had on mother and/or child. He did not doubt the dedication of the matrons; but he questioned their ability to act properly, specifically their capacity to reach medical and anatomical decisions and courses of action based on sound grounds. He feared that they remained bound by their traditional training, the transmission of lore and folk medicine from mother-to-daughter. Tissot aimed to instruct these women in the enlightened techniques of child delivery; for he knew the attitude of the peasantry toward childbirth: it was a female province. In *Plan*, written in the 1760s, he recommended training midwives to serve in the villages in accord with popular mores; in the 1780s, when he wrote treatises on the health of children and women for the specific use of physicians treating a bourgeois clientele, he directed his advice on childbirth to the physician rather than the midwife, in step with the changing medical mentality of the bourgeoisie. Tissot was not alone in denouncing the loss of life or health due to poor care at birth; Venel, his colleague in Yverdon, joined him to advocate to their Excellencies the founding of a school of midwifery, a goal that Venel realized in 1778 in his hometown.[9]

The last decades of the Ancien Régime witnessed a vast medicalization of childbirth due to the efforts by surgeons to displace the matrons rather than to educate them as competent midwifes.[10] In nearby Savoy, the surgeon Dussaix appealed in 1776 to Victor-Amadeus III, for support in his crusade against the superstitious practices of the matrons.[11] Dussaix' request was met with laughter by the King, who was too busy with his Italian domains to remember his poorest subjects in Savoy. The King was quite willing to invoke the help of religion for the welfare of infants and decreed special instructions to the matrons about their responsibility to baptize those who were in danger of dying before the priest could christen them in the parish church and thus ensure their eternal happiness in Heaven.

In 1785, Tissot published *De l'instruction des chirurgiens pour les campagnes* as an appendix to *Essai sur les moyens de perfectionner les études de médecine*. He mentioned in a footnote that he had extracted the present essay from a larger piece entitled *Mémoire sur les moyens de procurer au peuple les secours les plus utiles dans les maladies* which he had composed in 1776 at the demand of the Conseil de Santé.[12] In fact, the *Mémoire* Tissot submitted was essentially the same document as the 1765 *Plan* mentioned earlier. He had only changed the title and added a few lines to update it. A close look at both documents reveals that one (*Mémoire*) is a clean copy with only minor revisions of the other (*Plan*) in Tissot's hand.

While the published *De l'instruction* closely follows the *Plan*, there are a few significant changes. The word surgeon replaces physician, indicating a scaling-down of the original project. Midwifery is no longer mentioned: childbirth is not a disease.[13] Tissot included instruction in basic rules of hygiene as an essential part of the village surgeon's training. In the twenty years since Tissot had written *Plan*, hygiene had been recognized as an important factor in the well-being of individuals. Since Antiquity, rules of hygiene had been emphasized in guides to the conduct of life for the wealthy who could afford to watch over the quality of their food, drink, and surroundings. Tissot portentously extended the availability of preventive measures in the form of hygiene to a larger segment, if not explicitly to the entire population, by insisting on teaching hygiene to practitioners who served the villagers. He was thus among the first to envision generalizing the special health care reserved for the few to all levels of society. When Tissot updated his work to include instruction in hygiene for his country-surgeons, he was moving toward a social conception of health which, building on Revolutionary Institutions, would blossom in early nineteenth-century France.[14]

To the list of prerequisites for admission to study, such as being a fluent reader and writer of one's language, but not Latin, superfluous for a surgeon, Tissot added that the candidates should know "their religion", so as to be protected against succumbing to popular superstitions and to the temptation of using spells and magic formulae in their medicine.[15] He may have wished to affirm the religious spirit that informed his medical vocation, in a period (the 1780s) that was becoming increasingly secularized. In the 1760s, when he wrote *Plan*, he might have been less aware of the importance of belief in medical care, be it credence in superstition, materialism, or Christianity. In the 1780s, after his stay in Catholic Pavia, he became quite explicit on the subject.

Tissot's idea was not to train a medic of inferior quality, but rather one specifically formed for a particular task. In terms typical of the Enlightenment, he argued that, as a result of the peasants' uncomplicated life, diseases in the countryside were plainer and simpler than those affecting city-dwellers; besides farmers had a stronger constitution which better responded to medication because they lived closer to nature in a less polluted environment. Therefore, the country-surgeon faced with less complicated diseases did not need training as elaborate as that of the town-physician.[16] Previously Tissot had denounced malnutrition and exhaustion as causes of many diseases in the countryside. Because of his distaste for the effete aristocrats Tissot now came to idealize country-folk as portrayed in the Rousseauist pre-romantic image of the unspoiled peasantry.

Tissot's country-surgeon was not to be left to care for the population of the villages completely without senior medical help. In *Avis au peuple* (1761), Tissot had tackled the problem of consulting at a distance and had given instruction on how to deliver an intelligent and valid oral or written report to a physician. He repeated that such instructions were part of the course of study of his innovative practitioner.   He thought that a well-trained country-surgeon would be better equipped than a well-intentioned layperson to give the necessary information on the symptoms, duration, former and current treatments of the present disease as well as a reliable history of the patient's constitution. Incidentally, this method of reporting illness is still used today in Alaska and in Nambia where villagers elect one of their number to be instructed in the right way to question and observe a sick inhabitant, then report to the distant physician who will be able to decide whether a visit is necessary or not, thus saving lives, time, and money.

Tissot advised training persons who were willing to return to their villages; known previously by their future patients they would already enjoy a degree of confidence that would facilitate their serving. He wanted his surgeons to receive some training in agriculture which they could pass along to the peasants, introducing them to new ways of cultivation that would increase their food supply. He emphasized here again that good health started with ample provision of wholesome food. To be cost effective, Tissot proposed that this type of medical school be organized within community hospitals autonomous from academic faculties of medicine. He thought that two years of study would suffice to provide the rudiments of physics and chemistry; botany and pharmacy; anatomy and surgery, specifically the skeleton and reduction of fractures; physiology and pathology; and hygiene. All of these should be directed to one principal object: the simple description of the most frequent acute and chronic diseases and their course of development, completed by clinical training in the observation of the pulse, bodily evacuations, and all propitious and deleterious symptoms, so that nature could be intelligently aided in the recovery of health.[17] In *Plan* and *Mémoire*, the course of study included the teaching of the surgical technique for treating harelip since, Tissot noted, this was a condition often encountered in the Pays de Vaud. Even today, harelip occurs among Vaudois in greater proportion than for the general population of Switzerland.[18] Tissot proposed that two physicians, one surgeon and one apothecary, were the only personnel required for his country-surgeon school. A small library would be an asset and he advised buying: "Stork's treatise which should be translated ... *Avis au peuple* ... Buchan's work ... for surgery, Dionis' excellent treatise and the observations of the wise La Motte ... Verdier should suffice for anatomy ..."; yet he deplored the limited choice.[19] Such a school would both further health-care for the rural people and open up career opportunities for smart villagers. Tissot's *Plan* was two-pronged: it improved medical practice and it gave ambitious young peasants some alternative to domestic or military service.

Tissot thought that the people were clever enough to recognize their best interests and choose the qualified country-surgeon rather than the quack, once the former was available in the village. The choice was to be made on the success of cures and the cost of drugs. Tissot based his optimism on the reception of *Avis au peuple*, in which he had advocated simple, sure, and inexpensive remedies. *Avis* which was directed to the elite citizenry was successful; *Plan* which called on the state went largely ignored. Apparently *Avis au peuple* owed its success to being addressed to persons who understood individual endeavors for their own good or for that of their immediate neighbors. *Plan* was directed at the Bernese authorities who had not yet comprehended the severe consequences of only enacting decrees rather than training qualified personnel to replace the quacks. By repressing quackery, the decrees in fact created a vacuum of medical care unrecognized by their Excellencies; therefore *Plan* as well as the repression could only meet with failure. Very seldom does Tissot betray signs of impatience at the inertia of Bern. When his recommendations were neglected in one form, he presented them again in another. This explains his drafting several essays on the same subject in a span of twenty years (1765-85). For his last try, he went public by appending a revised version of *Plan* to *Essai sur les moyens de perfectionner les études de médecine*; in this way he hoped to reach beyond the border of the Republic of Bern and to move to action some more innovative government. The Corps Legislatif of the Consulate may have been inspired by *De l'instruction des chirurgiens pour les campagnes* when it created in its decree of 19 Ventôse An XI (10 March 1803) the *officier de santé* who was to receive mostly practical training.[20]

When in 1781 Tissot was appointed professor of clinical medicine at the University of Pavia, it was agreed that one of his duties was to write out his ideas on medical studies to serve the modernization of the Faculty; during his stay there, Tissot wrote some drafts for the proposed reform of the medical curriculum. In the introduction to *Essai sur les moyens de perfectionner les études de médecine*, he stated that he had been prompted to write it by a request from Count Firmian, but only upon his return to Lausanne had he found time to complete the task. Tissot's contribution to the renovation of the medical curriculum is not exclusively to be sought in the material he prescribed to be taught; in great part it is to be found in his search for the correct didactic method to motivate the students' medical curiosity. Tissot had acquired practical knowledge in pedagogical methods, first in acting as tutor to his nephew, then in Paris when he listened to medical lectures with Marc, and finally in Pavia where he himself taught with success.

From the Paris lectures Tissot learned that too strict a regulation of the topics fostered stagnation, crippling exploratory minds and their dynamic attempts at enlarging their purview. From the Pavia experience, he remembered that medicine progresses through the inquisitiveness of students who had to be encouraged to search further than what they had learned from lectures or books. Finally, he contrasted these experiences with his own student days at Montpellier and with what he had learned about medical training at various faculties when he had explored possibilities for his nephew's studies. Yet, the French system was the most familiar to him.

While Tissot's ideas for the clinical training of a new kind of physician are expounded in this chapter, the setting of the clinical wards where the actual teaching took place will be treated in the next one, together with Tissot's plan for the construction of clinical facilities as part of his reflections on the uses and abuses of hospitals. The best way to measure innovation in Tissot's view of medical studies is to compare his opinion with the accepted notions of what constituted medical education in France in the second half of the eighteenth century. Although separated by nearly two centuries, two important perceptions of medical studies, i.e. Lavirotte's article "Docteur en médecine" for the *Encyclopédie* and Gillispie's *Science and Polity in France at the End of the Old Regime*, offer the pervasive image of Parisian supremacy.[21] Albeit both mention the growing role the Montpellier Medical Faculty assumed in the training of physicians and in changing perceptions of medical practice and expectations, they both wrote mainly of the Paris Faculty as the embodiment of French medicine. The same holds true for Coury's essay on French medical studies in O'Malley's *The History of Medical Education* with perhaps some more emphasis on the role of the Montpellier graduates in the establishment of the Société royale de médecine. Ramsey's *Professional and Popular Medicine in France (1770-1830)* provides a more balanced view of all French medical institutions.

To embark on medical studies, wrote Lavirotte, the aspiring physician had first to have acquired a master of arts degree, which meant principally that he knew Latin. At the Paris Faculty, the course of study was four years, at some other institutions it was only three. The professors were chosen from the members of the

Faculty, which implied that all of them were not teaching simultaneously. Teaching positions changed every year and were not held
in great esteem; private lessons enjoyed more favor as they were
more lucrative for the professor and more rewarding for the
student. Ordinary classes were held in anatomy, physiology,
pathology, chemistry, botany, materia medica, surgery, and obstetrics. After two and a half years of study, the student was ready to
take the four required examinations (physiology, pathology,
commentary on Hippocrates, and hygiene) to obtain the license
degree. Once *licencié*, the student was allowed to attend the
consultation for the poor. Another examination, taken six months
later on the subject of materia medica, conferred the degree of
bachelor. At the beginning of the third year of medical school, the
student defended his first thesis in the form of a disputation on a
general topic or an aphorism of Hippocrates. In January or February of that same academic year, the anatomy test was taken,
followed during Lent by the defense of a second thesis on anatomy.
Meanwhile the student was still enrolled in class-work. At the
opening of the fourth year, the bachelor defended a third thesis on
a point of pathology, followed in January by a six-day examination
in surgery on a cadaver. A fourth thesis on a topic of medical
surgery was defended during Lent. Then in July or August at the
end of the fourth year of study, the aspiring doctor took his final
examination. Focussed on medical practice, it spanned four days,
during which the candidate was questioned by all the *docteur-
régents* of the Faculty who cared to do so. Then, added Lavirotte:
"The act of the doctorate is nothing more than the ceremony in
which the president gives the hat to the *licencié*."[22] Tissot had
reported identical information. The title of *docteur-régent* was
given after a new doctor had presided over a thesis defense; it gave
him the right to deliberate during the Faculty Assembly.[23]

In the program of study described by Lavirotte, medical students
took their first examination after five semesters of study. In
emphatic terms Tissot rejected this practice.[24] In its stead, he
recommended strict examinations at the end of each year of study.
He grounded his argument for changing the testing schedule on
the preposterous ignorance of the physicians churned out by the
existing system. Tissot was also concerned with favoritism. He
wrote that professors showed complacency for their colleagues'

sons and nephews and gave them unmerited degrees.[25] He added that too many students were given their licentiate degree despite poor showings at the examinations. He attributed this lack of knowledge to the laziness and poor motivation of the students as well as to the leniency of the professors. Tissot wrote that a degree was to be earned by merit, not by pity, since often the professors passed a student for the simple reason that the "poor devil" at great cost had spent (and lost) almost three years of his life at the university and could not switch careers so late. Tissot also denounced the indifference of the professors who assumed that many of these students would practice in small towns from which no one would hear of their poor performance. Furthermore, the study of medicine is a comprehensive enterprise; each step has to be completely assimilated before the next one is undertaken. For him, only the satisfactory completion of yearly examinations on the material just covered guaranteed cumulative learning and if this result was not obtained, only one year was lost in repeating the course work, a small price to pay compared to a lifetime or to the dire consequences on future patients. A second failure terminated the student's enrollment.[26]

Tissot placed the responsibility for success on both student and teacher. The student had to do his part: attend classes and study the materials, both regularly. He opposed dictation of what he called a *compendium*, i.e. an abstract of the material.[27] His reasons were the waste of time and the insult to the intelligence of the good student who was smart enough to compile his own compendium from attentive listening and good note taking. Compendia were only crutches for the lazy students who studied them the night before the examination, then regurgitated their content in front of the professor without having digested it, only to forget everything by the next day! The professor had the duty to prepare a well-informed and up-to-date lecture on the material and to deliver it in a lively manner. Tissot had learned at Pavia how contagious the enthusiasm of the professor was and how a cheerful voice rather than a cold and morose one kept students attentive. He thought that professors should present their own lectures and not merely comment on or read from an established text.[28] Tissot certainly practiced what he preached; as several sets of original lecture notes are among his personal papers.[29]

In the 1780s medicine was a rapidly changing field; Tissot's purchases for his personal library show that he was familiar with the new texts which, more often than in the past, were original contributions and not merely commentaries on the so-called classics of medicine. A large portion of his letters with either Haller or Zimmermann are devoted to the review of recent publications. Tissot perceived how quickly a textbook could be outdated and yet could give a false security to a professor who did not feel compelled to search through his own medical experience and that of his contemporaries for his teaching material. Tissot was in fact advocating the researcher as the best teacher. Chosen by a professor at the beginning of his teaching career, the best and most advanced book on any subject in medicine would, with each passing year, fall behind the state of the art into obsolescence.

Tissot wanted students to acquire both a solid knowledge of and a critical attitude toward published data. For him, the printed word was frozen information, the milestone only of a stage in the progression of medicine and the art of healing. Still, Tissot was no book-burner of the Paracelsus' type: books were a necessary part of the intellectual baggage of the physician, yet not sufficient in themselves.[30] Curiosity and observation, backed by sustained studies of the human body and pharmacopoeia, provide dynamism to the profession. Tissot proposed to train a new breed of doctors, who would expand bookish and scholastic study into direct observation, examination, and experimentation at the bedside of the clinics' patients. Tissot might be partly in debt to Baglivi, whose *Opera Omnia* in its 1745 edition he owned, and to Zimmermann's *Von der Erfahrung in der Artzneykunst* for his views on the pre-eminence of observation over theory.[31] After four semesters of proven learning of the usual curriculum plus medical police, the student was to embark on the study of clinical medicine for which Tissot advocated a two-year program before the would-be physician could obtain his final medical degree.

Crowded enrollments at the Pavia clinics had forced Tissot to devise a system of teams of medical students for the care of a single patient at a time. Reflecting on the experience, he concluded that in their first year of clinical rounds students benefitted more by watching the process than by getting involved in the verbal or tactile dialoguing between patient and aspiring doctor. After a year, the students felt more at ease with their duties in the clinical wards and learned more from the exercise. Furthermore, two years of training offered a chance to see at least one case of almost all the most common acute diseases a physician might expect to encounter in his medical career. Tissot knew that the teaching clinics, compared to a town-hospital, allowed for more precision in diagnosis and treatment because of their small size and protected environment. He was also aware of the draw-backs which restrained the experience the student got by walking the wards of a large hospital, as he had done at Montpellier. The professor of clinical medicine had the responsibility to choose among the patients of the town-hospital the cases best suited to provide illustrations for his lectures and examples for the training of competent doctors.

Tissot suggested that an advanced student check the happenings of the day each evening with the surgeon in charge, in particular the admission to the hospital of an interesting case that should be immediately transferred to the clinics to provide better experience in the regular morning rounds of visits. To this he added in a footnote: "Many sick from the town or the country came to the hospital, for they knew they were cared for with the greatest attention."[32] At least in Pavia, the hospital was no longer the place to avoid, it now offered hope for recovery. Yet, Tissot knew that not every patient would be cured; but, at least from the point of view of teaching, the death of a patient should not be seen only as a loss of life, as it could also become a learning experience when an autopsy was performed. At the *post mortem*, a correlation between symptoms and pathological findings, such as the identification of the affected organs, could be discovered and be of great help in future diagnosis and treatment. For him, such a systematic program of careful autopsies should be promoted by every clinical medicine professor dedicated to the advance of his art.

In *Etudes de médecine*, Tissot still defended fluency in Latin as a prerequisite for medical studies.[33] In the 1780s, confronted with a rising tide of vernacular writings, Tissot was advocating a scientific idiom that transcended political partisanship reflected in the supremacy of any modern language. He was aware of the weight the French tongue was developing in cultural and diplomatic affairs. Because of his many contacts abroad, he was informed about medical publications in different languages. He felt that he was missing a great deal by not knowing all these languages. So, he took a rearguard position of defending Latin as the privileged vehicle to convey medical knowledge in the classroom as well as in the library. He also based his argument for Latin proficiency on economy and efficiency. He knew that only a clear and precise knowledge of a language permits one to apprehend all the subtleties it conveys. The average person, in Tissot's view, could only attain this level in a few languages, especially when that person also wanted to excel in something else, medicine for example. With all the books being published in different vernaculars, the physician who wanted to keep up-to-date had to master Dutch, English, French, German, Italian, Spanish, and Swedish or had to rely on translations which were often of inferior quality, and/or "passport" for the translator's own views, often at variance with those of the original author.[34] On the contrary, if Latin was still cultivated as it should be, a single language would suffice. A few years as a young boy spent at learning Latin would render accessible all the new as well as the old knowledge. Time was precious to Tissot who believed none should be wasted. It is in this spirit that he insisted also that the history of medicine ought to be taught to stimulate students to surpass their masters; yet, in his "whiggish" perspective, emphasis should be placed on the facts that led to new discoveries; dead-ends were to be avoided.[35]

In the year of its publication, *Etudes de médecine* was re-edited three times in French and translated into German and Italian.[36] This book did not enjoy the success of Tissot's other works, and yet it was published at a time when the importance of clinical teaching was recognized in places such as Edinburgh, Paris, and Vienna; and when the directors of some hospitals felt the need to provide this experience to medical students.[37] Perhaps the fact that Tissot had withdrawn from his professorship before the publication of his book and that others had published treatises on the same subject while holding chairs of clinical medicine can explain its lackluster success.[38]

Tissot had advised the aspiring physician to go to a foreign university to get his training; nevertheless he wanted the local physicians, accredited by governmental authorities, to have the last word on who was licensed to practice in their jurisdiction. In *Etudes de médecine* Tissot had praised the success of the licensing examinations administered in Geneva; later, he tried to institute similar ones in Lausanne under the aegis of the Collège de Médecine.[39] Consequently, Tissot transferred his interest in the teaching of medicine to the licensing of properly trained medical practitioners who should be the new physician he had described in *Etudes de médecine*; a physician who listens to nature, who interacts orally and physically with his patients, who cures and cares for the whole person.

The first task of the Lausanne Collège de Médecine was to establish a census of all the persons who were, in one way or another, practicing medicine. Then the Collège had to call each of them to present for verification the degrees, certificates, or letters-patent that qualified him or her to practice. It was to set up committees for oral examinations for checking the claim of each practitioner. The tests were to be at different levels depending on the candidate's type of practice, i.e. surgery, medicine, midwifery, apothecary; and they were to be offered every six months in April and October. Over the years, such testing would insure the quality of health-care. Emulating the practice of the Société royale de médecine, a report by Tissot mentions the Collège's desire to appoint correspondents in the Pays de Vaud in order to be kept informed on all medical matters, such as the name of all practitioners, occurrences of epidemic or epizootic disease, or abuses of practice.[40] But Tissot complained of the difficulty of finding reliable correspondents, due to the lack of good training for country-surgeons: he never missed an occasion to drive home his point concerning improvement through education!

In 1785, the Conseil de Santé of Bern had decreed new regulations for the practice of medicine and in 1788 it required from the Lausanne Collège de Médecine that these serve as guidelines for licensing. The Collège met the Bernese demands with strong resistance. Under the pressure of the events in France, the whole fabric of relations between the Republic of Bern and the Pays de Vaud was becoming increasingly frayed. Tissot, as Vice-President of the Collège, was caught in the tangle of enforcing the regulations his medical standards demanded, without relying on the heavy-handedness for which the Bernese were, by now, openly hated. He often felt powerless to satisfy colleagues and rulers. The Minutes of the Collège de Médecine, although graced with very polite sentences, disclose signs of protest: "Following up on the letter with which their Excellencies of the Conseil de Santé have honored the Collège de Médecine about the two ordinances ... the physicians of the afore-mentioned Collège, after having read on their own with the greatest attention the said ordinances, have met for deliberations under the Presidency of the Magnificent Lord Bailiff; and the Collège so assembled take the liberty of presenting to the illustrious Conseil de Santé very respectfully, yet with the frankness that the good of the matter appeared to them to require..."[41]

For some particular occasions and under special circumstances, Tissot requested for the Collège the right to meet without the Bailiff's presence.[42] He argued that the Bailiff should not be bored and disturbed with petty medical matters, but in fact he was requesting more autonomy and power. This was brought home more firmly and explicitly, when Tissot requested that the "Premier Médecin" alone have the authority, without the Bailiff's endorsement, to bar from the licensing examination "...persons of whom the ignorance and imbecility are so stunning that it is useless to have it recorded by several witnesses...", or to validate the medical degrees earned by young men of the Pays de Vaud in Strasburg, Montpellier, Leyden, or Goettingen "which are very good universities." Control of examinations and licensing should belong to the physicians "...as it is practiced in the towns of aggregation."[43]

Practitioners turned down by the Collège tried to get their license to practice in the Pays de Vaud approved by the Bernese Conseil de Santé. Tissot wrote in the Minutes of the meeting of 21 November 1796 of such a challenge by a "maître de violon" who had presented himself to the Collège to be licensed as a physician with doubtful certificates "scratched over letters", he specified.[44] The question of jurisdiction had always been a very thorny matter; time did not smooth relations; quite to the contrary. Tissot defended what he felt to be the integrity of the Collège de Médecine, but he never questioned the validity of the Bernese rule over the Pays de Vaud in political affairs; at least he did not commit any such thought to paper.

Tissot's notes concerning the Collège convey more than the politics of medical matters in a time of revolutionary changes; they elaborate on the proper training of physicians i.e. a university education checked by a recognized medical board; and they render more vivid his fight against quackery and the hopes he placed in his country-surgeons to stamp it out. Yet they also testify to the failing health of Tissot. The notes dated after 1794 are in a more and more blurred handwriting, although the sharp intellect persists to defend the competence of the Collège and to uphold its standards.

In *Etudes de médecine* as well as in his leading role in the Lausanne Collège de Médecine Tissot consistently followed a path of reform, trying to better existing structures from within. This accommodating spirit may be the mark of an aging man in an atmosphere of *fin de régime*, but it could also reflect a mature mind's wisdom which can differentiate the possible from the impossible. In this attitude Tissot was a forerunner of the meliorists of the early nineteenth-century movement of French hygienists. The 1790s were a time for revolution, and the old reformer, although he had struck revolutionary notes, was ignored by revolutionaries as well as by the old guard government. To the one he appeared too timid; to the other he was an embarrassment. Tissot's last proposals went largely ignored by his contemporaries; they were too close to home to be comfortable and when their value was recognized in the new medicine of the new century, they had been melted into the common intellectual heritage.

Chapter XI

The Liberated Hospital

In the late eighteen century, the role and purpose of hospitals were radically transformed. In the past, hospitals had been of two kinds best described by their French names: *Hôtel-Dieu* and *Maladrerie*.[1] The first were charitable institutions meant to receive those poor who, for whatever reasons, were unable to care for themselves or common folk travelers for whom inns were too expensive. *Hôtels-Dieu* functioned as temporary relief agencies for those who were not recognized residents of the town, or as permanent abodes for the paupers who were. *Maladreries* received victims of certain types of diseases, deemed most contagious. The Lazar-house was one example which fell into disuse when leprosy faded away in Europe late in the Middle Ages. Another was the pest-house which was open only in times of epidemics. Usually situated outside the walls of the city, the plague hospital was staffed by salaried surgeons and care-takers whose wages were drawn from both public and charitable purses. These establishments had a poor reputation, largely because they were not kept up during plague remissions, but also because their staff was attracted not as much by compassion as by greed. The reward was quick since they often inherited the personal belongings of the hospitalized dead. But theirs was an awful task: entering the pest-house was as good as entering death's antechamber, when the "cures" were bloodletting to the point of fainting and the opening or burning of the buboes. As the plague endemic caused less frequent surges of the dreaded disease and syphilis spread, the plague-hospitals were often turned into institutions for those sick with the great pox. The mercury-based remedy for syphilis was no easy ride into recovery either. Thus, it is no surprise that under such circumstances the hospital, whatever its type, was regarded by the poor and the wealthy alike as a place to avoid. Such hospitals offered nothing that could not be provided at home, as long as someone was willing to carry out the task at the patient's house.

At first sight, the multiple rebuildings or foundings of hospitals meant to cope with the mounting problem of poverty seem to indicate a stiffening of traditional views on the nature and function of hospitals, that is the repression and control of the swarms of poor.[2] The monarchs who had built palaces for themselves in the late seventeenth and early eighteenth centuries as a symbol of the absolute state's ascending power, decades later shifted some of their attention away from their own grandeur to the needs of their people and created magnificent hospitals to replace the outgrown, outworn medieval hospices, as an embodiment and reflector of their prestige and wealth;[3] and in the 1760s Lausanne did the same for its poor.[4] The perennial problems of sanitation, ventilation, or ease of service did not receive any innovative treatment in the conception of these hospitals.[5] The main objective behind their construction was to house the poor, the disabled, the aged, or the very young, that is to deal with poverty in the usual, old-fashioned way. The "tournant des mentalités" had not yet reached the hospital and the concerned authorities. In the Germanies where monarchs, secular or ecclesiastic, and city councils vied for power, one can to this day observe their competing efforts in the Juliusspital and the Burgerspital in Würzburg.

In Paris it took the terrible disaster of the fire of the *Hôtel-Dieu* (1772) to prompt officialdom into consulting the experts: rationality, economy, and scientific attitudes entered the studies of the design and aim of the hospital through the channel of a specially appointed Commission of the Académie royale des sciences. In the fourth quarter of the eighteenth century, the hospital became the focus of investigations on how to improve its functioning and to transform it from a *mouroir* to a *machine à guérir*.[6] The surgeons, who often had a more direct experience of hospital, were among the first to call for reforms.[7] The investigations and proposals of Tenon for Paris are a good example.[8] It is therefore possible that the persistent animosity between the two groups prompted the physicians to undertake innovations, out of the fear of being bypassed and excluded from an amelioration that certainly would enhance the prestige and expertise of the group who fostered it. Ackerknecht's and Temkin's studies corroborate this view for a somewhat later period, the Revolution, with its forceful change in the conception of hospital for which the surgeons provided a potent motivating force.[9] A concerted effort on the part of physicians, surgeons, architects, and scientists led to studies and projects for a new type of hospital building from which the pavilion-hospital emerged in the nineteenth century.[10] Eventually, in the twentieth century, the pavilion-hospital, thought cost inefficient, was abandoned. The effectiveness of its design for cutting down the spread of infection went without recognition.[11] This lack of foresight is now deplored, as witnessed by the participants in the program "Dossier-Santé" broadcast by the television chain Europe 5 in July 1989.

Physical structures and their functions were not the only points under investigation; the debate also addressed the hospital's geographic location (inside or outside the city), its purpose within the medical police, and the central question of its admission policies.[12] These pioneers wedded the old conception of the hospital to new ideas about medicine and social justice, notably on the proper treatment of curable diseases; on the relations between patients and doctors; and on the role of the hospital as the proper locus for cure and for medical training. They were bringing forth the hospital as we know it, the liberated hospital.[13] The traditional view did not immediately give way to the modernized concept; often both co-existed under the same roof. This dual character of the eighteenth-century hospital creates difficulties today in the interpretation and evaluation of its evolution. It begets two almost opposite line of thought: one views the hospital in its repressive role, the other emphasizes the liberating effects of the modernized hospital which procured, or hoped to procure, better health for its patients.[14]

The question of admission was twofold, at once medical and socio-economic. It was generally recognized that the high mortality rate of the hospitalized sick had disastrous effects on the profession of medicine. The aspiring as well as the seasoned physician in accord with the Hippocratic tradition avoided cases which offered no hope of recovery. This view also applied to hospital admissions for the Neo-Hippocratic school of medicine developing in the eighteenth century. As a consequence, only the sick with a chance of recovery within a short period of time were admitted (for Tissot this meant on the order of three weeks including convalescence, a much shorter period than the two to three months commonly accepted) while those recognized as incurable were denied entrance except in special institutions such as Guy's Hospital in London. The same rules applied to contagious patients. The contagion of some forms of venereal diseases and of smallpox, for example, was discerned, but not that of tuberculosis or of any of the bilious or putrid fevers. The contagious sick were to be cared for at home or in specialized hospitals, such as the *Maladrerie* of the past. The important point here is not which diseases were admitted or what cures were administered, but what changed in the role of the hospital. It was now perceived, and for Tissot this was the main point, as the locus for cure and recovery, a place of temporary abode to regain strength to meet the demands of the market-economy. The healing emphasis in the conception of the hospital displaced its socio-economic role as a place set apart for the confinement and/or control of the poor.

As long as the hospital was an uncontrollable breeding ground for infection (and this control is again of pressing concern today), anyone sick and able to receive adequate care at home was restored to health in familiar surroundings, and if needed, with help from a *Miséricorde* (the purpose of its personnel and money was to offer better health care at home). It was argued that the loving care of relatives was more beneficial than the mercenary care of the hospital attendant.[15] The question of the nurses or hospital helpers was a crucial one also in the reform of the function and service expected from the new hospital.   Traditionally in Catholic countries, the nurses had been recruited among the religious orders, for example the sisters of Charity. Their training and supervision, when engaged in hospital service, were left to the discretion of the superiors in the Order. The sisters of Charity had mixed feelings about the medical reforms the physicians and surgeons wanted to introduce. The issues of the importance and professionalization of nursing, because of political circumstances, erupted acutely during the French Revolution. These issues re-surfaced time and again during the nineteenth century, amidst continuing discussion of the improvement of hospital care.[16] Since the Reformation, religious orders and their hospital services had been abolished in Protestant countries and the problem of recruiting nurses had been confronted earlier, but was not really resolved before the mid-nineteenth century. Still today (without conflicts between the secular and the religious), the team relationship of physicians and nurses, and their respective roles in patient care, brings up discussions of purview, competence, and training.

The inevitable proximity of other sick crowded in large wards, often several to one bed, was justly perceived as complicating any disease to the point of hampering diagnosis and proper treatment. The trauma and shock of separation from family, the worry about the financial well-being of dependants provoked by hospitalization were seen as adverse conditions hurting the patient's prospects for recovery that were serious enough to weigh heavily against admission. But the facts of life then as now were such that some people could not be cared for at home (even with the help of a *Miséricorde*) because they were too poor to have a home or were so isolated in the anonymity of the large city that no one could be found to carry out reliably the physician's orders.[17]

Cost-effectiveness was also considered in the discourse over hospital admission. Because home care was more economical than hospital care, it should be encouraged as much as possible. "The fire that warms the broth of the sick, warms their family; the meat that is used for their broth nourishes the family ..." wrote Dupont de Nemours.[18] Nevertheless, cost efficiency and rationality of treatment were also used in favor of hospitalization as the best means for cure and recovery. The advocates of the renewed hospital wanted to make it a place for the poor first, then also for the not-so-poor such as the servants of the wealthy, and even for the wealthy themselves. The arguments for the admission of servants were that they could not be cared for at their master's house when their sickness deprived the household of their help and obliged the master to hire extra hands for nursing tasks that could be had at a lower cost within the hospital. Wealthy patients, remarked several hospital reformers, could receive better care in special quarters of the hospital than in their homes. Consequently, some of the blueprints for hospitals incorporated private rooms for the wealthy admitted as paying patients, in addition to the usual large dormitories or public rooms. Sharp criticisms were levied against the old hospital and its indiscriminate policy of admission and boarding of the sick. Privacy and separation of diseases were recognized as important factors to be considered in the new building. Strong complaints were also heard about the custom of accommodating several patients in one bed.[19]

Separate maternity wards were planned to train medical personnel and to guard the prospective mother from contagion and indiscreet looks. The indiscreet looks were probably prevented, but contagion certainly not! Until Semmelweiss' discovery of the etiology of puerperal fever was widely accepted late in the nineteenth century, women delivered in hospital or at home by physicians were more likely to die from puerperal fever than women who gave birth on their own or with the help of trained midwives, always less inquisitive and interventionist than physicians.[20] In the past, the violent insane had been routinely institutionalized, but curing was not the main purpose of their hospitalization. Like the beggars and vagrants, they were locked up because they were perceived as a nuisance; now their specific needs were beginning to be understood through new studies of medical care.[21] Surgical cases were perhaps the worst off in the old system and surgery rooms would not change for some more time. No differentiation was made between pre-and post-operative stages. Surgery was performed in the midst of the ward itself, sparing none of its boarders the horror of surgical interventions without anesthesia, antisepsis, and asepsis. The death toll was as atrocious as the sufferings.

Most of the inquiries concerning hospital's betterment were directed at the situation in urban centers, where poverty and sickness were more apparent and considered more prevalent than in rural areas. Country hospitals or better dispensaries were sought to solve the problem of the sick and the maimed of the countryside, too far away from towns to be transported to their hospitals over rough roads and in primitive vehicles. In *Avis au peuple*, Tissot argued that help should be found locally to be effective.[22] This argument of proximity served also to promote decentralized hospitalization in the cities and the conception of smaller hospitals situated in various neighborhoods.[23]

These reforming studies followed two paths which led to different and complementary goals: the curing and the teaching hospitals; both stressed observation of pathological phenomena and application of newly formulated scientific theory and experimentation to the problem of hygiene.[24] Advocates of these institutions saw in a renewed hospital the best place for the implementation of their programs of reforms. The motivations behind these inquiries were a remarkable mixture of compassion for the destitute; of fear of contagion (only too real in towns); of enlightenment on the part of academic, royal, or medical authorities; of rationality in the face of waste in life and resources; and, not to be over-looked, an always present sense of mercantilism and emerging capitalism that saw wealth in a healthy population. As the century neared its end, these studies increasingly reflected the thinking of physiocrats and liberals such as Dupont de Nemours; they also pertained to the hopes of hereditary improvement of mankind through better health provided by physical and mental hygiene of a new kind, most cogently articulated in the Idéologues' theory of medicine and the work of Cabanis.[25] That hope was shared and shaped by Tissot in his efforts to obtain better health care for all levels of the population.

The importance of these studies has often been masked by the scant success they seemed to have enjoyed in their own time. The French Revolution swept them away together with the Old Regime and the revolutionaries were not often ready to recognize debts to predecessors. The liberated hospital which was emerging from these proposals came too late or too early, like many other enterprises of the reign of Louis XVI.[26] Nevertheless, these studies were not done in vain; they served as the unacknowledged basis for many real or virtual reforms of the nineteenth century.

Tissot's thought and career cannot be dissociated from the general current of medical reform; his contributions should be evaluated in their eighteenth-century context, and should not be easily discounted by a twentieth-century perception of the provincialism of the Lausanne doctor. This neglect of Tissot's influence is reinforced by a certain disdain for Old Regime medicine fostered by the sweeping changes brought to the art by the revolutionary and imperial physicians of Paris. It is also common for those newly introduced to Tissot's work to point to its similarity to the better known work of Frank. But the reverse is closer to the truth: Tissot taught clinical medicine at Pavia in 1781, Frank succeeded him in 1785; Tissot published *Essai sur les moyens de perfectionner les études de médecine* in 1785, whereas Frank's *Plan d'école clinique* appeared in 1790. Ackerknecht noted: "Tissot was an inspiration for the great Johann Peter Frank..."[27]   One cannot understand Frank independently from his less assertive predecessor.

When Tissot turned his attention to the issue of public welfare transcending individual health (the well-being of the few cannot be met without that of the whole), he focussed first on the hospital. Tissot hoped and worked for a hospital which would serve the purpose of restoring health, to the poor first and then to all classes of society. He envisioned a "liberated" hospital which was freed from its oppressive image as a pauper work-house and its perennial problem of insalubrity. Such a hospital effectively liberated its clients from diseases and returned them to productive lives. Tissot saw hospitals foremost as curing places and, when a medical Faculty was organized in the town, as a teaching institution. In fact, he wanted to extend the hospital's teaching role also to patients. He hoped that sensible care dispensed in the reformed hospital would by imitation foster changes in the ways health-care and hygiene were provided at home. The patients who improved in a cool atmosphere, drinking refreshing herb tea alone in a clean bed, cared for by a trained nurse would soon learn to reject the sweltering heat of their customary dirty featherbeds and hot strong drink. Tissot despaired that the *Miséricorde* alone could ever achieve such results. Rather, he saw the *Miséricorde* and the hospital as partners in promoting health: the former by preventive measures (giving out food, fuel, or clothing), the latter by curative interventions.[28] Once properly managed, hospitals would be the best places in which to receive the correct treatment prescribed by a physician for a particular illness. In a renewed hospital one would find trained personnel ready to follow the physician's instructions precisely; that would rarely happen in the home where the relatives usually gave in to the sick's wishes or tried the suggestions of well-wishers. Nevertheless, Tissot was well-aware of the argument (e.g. by Dupont de Nemours) that the *Miséricorde*'s help was more effective than that of the hospital, since it spared the trauma of separation from family, of exposure to the many infections of the hospital, and that the help offered to the sick poor through the *Miséricorde* extended to their families and benefited many in the home rather than just one in the hospital.[29] Not a physician, Dupont de Nemours was skeptical of the hospital's effectiveness in curing diseases; he could not share the physicians' hopes for a reform of the hospital, nor did he anticipate Tissot's dream of educating the people to take better care of themselves. Yet, Tissot, who did not deny some validity to the argument, remarked that often the homes of the poor were cramped, humid, stale, and lacked the consistently competent care and tranquility that only a reformed hospital could provide. As the physician of the poor he knew only too well what their habits and prejudices were in the case of sickness and that the money given for drugs and nutritious food was often spent on drinks and sweets that "only feed a fever". Tissot also pointed to the exhausted state to which hard work and malnutrition reduced the poor and he insisted on the responsibility of the hospital staff to see that they discharged only those people who were totally cured and once again fit for the harshness of the work-place. Tissot wished to transform the hospital from a place of confinement for the outcasts, misfits, or undesirables of society or one of death supervision into a liberating institution where the sick (poor and rich alike) went first, not last, to regain health and strength before going back to their homes and their trades.

When time came for Tissot to look into the best setting for clinical teaching, he remembered from his Montpellier's days, how much he had learned by walking the wards of the hospitals and realized how much more could be taught by properly organizing the wards with an eye for the best clinical learning experience. This led him to reflect upon the hospital of his time, and on how it could be transformed to offer better service to individuals and the community at-large. He based his reflection on the different professional situations in which he had lived. The first was the experience he had acquired in Montpellier on the rounds in the wards and in the home visits to the poor he cared for as the assistant of a qualified physician. The second came from serving as physician to the Lausanne poor; he had seen how health-care was provided through charity organizations. The poor were cared for at home or in the Lausanne Hospital, and, when necessary, in Bern at the Inselspital.[30] At mid-century, the Inselspital was praised for its organization and its well-qualified staff.[31] The third source of Tissot's practical experience was in Paris, where he had the leisure to evaluate the quality of medical education as well as the state of the hospitals of the French capital, including the establishment founded by Madame Necker in 1778 which had an undisputed reputation for its excellent management and low death rate.[32] Tronchin was still living in Paris at the time of Tissot's visit and might have introduced him to the problem of private health-care for the poor; the Genevan Doctor freely gave advice, drugs and, even money to the Parisian indigent.[33] Fourthly, Tissot's experience at Pavia proved by far to be the most decisive in the formation of his thought on hospital reform; it was also the most successful. The combined political and financial situation gave Tissot enough clout to be able to implement his view while he was professor there. In 1785, when Frank succeeded Tissot in the chair of clinical medicine at Pavia, he was able to build on this success, even though things had deteriorated somewhat between Tissot's departure in 1783 and his own arrival, as one can gather from the derogatory, and probably exaggerated comments made by his son Joseph on the state of the clinical hospital when he arrived with his father in Pavia.[34] The same success was not to be met by Tissot in 1789 Lausanne, where the political climate, as things turned out, foiled the project.

In *Etudes de médecine*, Tissot presented a formal exposition of his thought on clinical teaching in its locus: the clinic. In this book he often referred to the situation at Pavia, always adding however that in the present work he was writing of an idealized situation. He had no particular medical faculty in mind; he was ostensibly striving only to describe the best auspices and to draw the best blueprints for the inside of the clinical hospital.[35] He did not worry there about facades, windows, or staircases, but about the construction and size of beds, the ease of service, the amount of air per patient, and the heating system. Most importantly, he planned enough space around the beds to accommodate the students and the professor without impairing the view of the student or discomforting the patient. For Tissot, it was the architect's role to attend to the structural design and the physician's duty to concentrate on the medical organization. Throughout the work Tissot emphasized that the medical student had to learn the essential interaction between physician and patient at the bedside of the sick in the clinical wards. This new emphasis on the active relationship between physician and patient represented a crucial step in the development of the medical profession. It indicated a shift from an art of discourse to a science of dialogue and stressed the need for listening, examining, and observing. It propounded an active rather than passive role for the sick. This attitude contravened those of traditional medicine, still prevalent in the late eighteenth century; to wit the custom of consulting at a distance and by third party, or the practice of diagnosis and prescription after a mere glance at a urine bottle. Tissot's advocacy of an active role for the patient assumed a dynamic interplay that could only be realized through mutual esteem. His call for the physician's prerequisite regard towards all the hospital patients took many forms. It was embodied in structural reforms such as individual beds, privacy of curtains and wide "ruelle", clean and appropriate clothing and bedding, cleanliness and convenient location of latrines, individual rooms for the contagious or the agitated. It was also manifest in the attitude of the physician toward the patient which ought never to be affected by the adequacy or inadequacy of the surroundings. He insisted here again on the kindness the doctor had to show when he was questioning or examining a patient. This courtesy fostered reciprocal good feelings and created trust between doctor and patient and a more congenial atmosphere for the cure.[36] Patients, feeling secure and understood, were more apt to relax and regain their strength through the help of the art and of nature. With the same kindness and quiet atmosphere in mind, Tissot also wrote of the role of the helpers of the hospital. If they did not carry out the orders of the physician in the same considerate manner, success in healing and recovery would be hampered, even annihilated. The sick had their role in this mutual enterprise; they had to answer as precisely as possible their physician's queries concerning their complaints so as to facilitate his diagnosis and treatment.

In the second part of *Etudes de médecine*, entitled *Mémoire sur la construction d'un hôpital clinique*, Tissot elaborated on the physical setting of the clinical wards and on how to foster an atmosphere of caring by the proper environment.[37] Before engaging in the details of space and interior layout, he stated that the purpose of the clinic was not only to teach medical students, but also to cure patients, though he conveyed it in an indirect way, a clinic without a convalescent room was not complete. He stressed convalescence as a stage in illness prior to full recovery. He observed that many patients, deprived of the opportunity to convalesce, relapsed into weakness or languor because they were sent home too soon and exhausted themselves with work, while others kept in the sick ward fell prey to hospital fever and died. If a compromise had to be made because of space exiguity, only one room for men was to be built, since the clinics would admit only acute diseases which more often afflicted men than women.[38] Tissot did not elaborate here on the differential frequency of acute diseases between the sexes, but he later gave a clue to his thinking on this matter in *Des maladies des femmes* in which he described men more prone to accident (an acute condition), while women's constitutions predisposed them more to chronic ills which did not belong to the purview of his new hospital.[39]

Next Tissot wrote of the size of the rooms, paying special attention to their height: "...a high ceiling is healthier than a low one because it allows the vitiated air to rise well above head's level... ", he used the work of Lavoisier on breathing to estimate the cubic footage "no less than five toises" necessary per patient, insisting that the sick needed more fresh air to recover than the healthy did to sustain life.[40] The problem of ventilation was treated very carefully, but revealed no ground-breaking innovations. He described cross-ventilation through windows and small openings near the ceiling, fitted with mechanisms allowing for easy opening and closing. He recommended the use of a machine of Sutton, but not that of a fireplace, to activate ventilation, as the open fire presented more inconveniences than the benefit of the draft created.[41] He gave special attention to the orientation of the wards; they should face the "winter-south", procuring the maximum of sunlight in winter and the minimum of heat in summer. The wards must have a stove, placed against a wall away from the beds.[42] It was to be rekindled twice a day to give as even a heat as possible. Tissot warned of excessive heat in the ward, for he viewed it as increasing putrefaction and infection. The temperature of the room should not exceed 10 or 11 Reaumur grades, i.e. 55-57 Fahrenheit or 13-14 Celsius.

The wards were to be fitted with single-size iron beds, dark colored linen curtains, a closet with robes of washable fabric for the patient to wear when they used the "chaise percée", and a supply of fresh water. He wanted portable bathtubs instead of bathrooms which were often too far away for the strength of the sick. The wide "ruelle" would easily accommodate the bathtub, while a curtain hung between the beds would assure privacy. Cleanliness was imperative and the wards were to be ventilated, swept, and sprinkled every morning before the round of visits and again every evening. Windows were to be kept open during good warm weather.

The number of beds per ward was to be adapted to the size of the room and the number of students. Tissot wanted the students to see enough cases during their two years of clinical observations, but he did not want them to become bored and tired by very long rounds. He always tried to combine the patients' comfort with the students' learning; therefore he suggested leaving at least three and a half feet between beds. In addition, Tissot wanted the clinic to have a few individual rooms, three at most for each ward, where contagious patient would be received. These private rooms could also be used to lodge newly inoculated patients, giving the student-physician opportunities to learn the technique of inoculation.[43]

As for the supporting structures, Tissot thought that the apothe-cary of the main hospital could serve the clinics very well, saving space for two rooms of great importance (in his eyes): the assem-bly and the dissecting rooms. The assembly room, furnished with benches "because everywhere the students are not seated there is noise" and with a table, a bookcase and a fireplace, would serve as a gathering-place after the round of visits.[44] In this room, the professor would be free to elaborate on some cases or to rectify some prognosis without upsetting the patients. The students would also have leisure to question him and to exchange opinions among themselves. This assembly room would also serve as an out-patient clinic at set hours, offering more training, in particular, with the treatment of chronic diseases. The dissection room was to be in the shape of an amphitheater to allow the best possible view of the process. It could be smaller than the auditorium usually reserved for the regular anatomical demonstrations, as it would seat only the students of the clinic, but he insisted that the clinic had to have its own room for performing the necessary *post mortem*. Tissot had nothing special to say about the helpers, nurses or surgeons, of the clinical wards, "since this was regulated for each particular hospital".[45] He did treat this subject in *Médecine civile*.[46] In his conclusions and as an illustration of the possible, Tissot wrote that so far the best clinical school was in Edinburgh.[47] He was indeed very well acquainted with Scottish medicine as he owned, for example, the books of Cullen and Duncan on clinical training.

As mentioned before, Lausanne had its own hospital, an ancient institution, with all that this implied in the eighteenth century. The Hospital stood between the Castle and the Townhall, linked to each by steep staircases and tortuous narrow streets. At the time of the Reformation and of the Bernese conquest, the jurisdiction of the Hospital (finances and services) had gone to the Town-Council. Civil benevolence had replaced religious charity, and help to the poor had been organized along the lines of neighborhoods or *bannières*, political entities with elected representatives on the Town-Council. Each neighborhood had its own pauper fund, physician, surgeon, and apothecary, and their services were coordinated by a *Miséricorde* and supervised by the official physician of the poor. This officer was appointed by their Excellencies of Bern, and the incumbent was entitled to a stipend in money and in kind. The Hospital was to serve the poor of all the *bannières*.

In the early 1760s, the old building was declared a disgrace to the city, and projects for a new one to be built on the same site were sought.[48] The old Hospital was now perceived as an eyesore at the foot of the elegant silhouette of Castle and Cathedral. The Town-Council's many tractations of the past over the crumbling state of the Hospital changed tone and became serious deliberations on how to finance the construction of a hospital worthy of the generosity and status of the city elite. Taking a lead from what had been accomplished elsewhere by monarchs in Berlin, Copenhagen, or Vienna, and by bishops and burgers in Bamberg, Lübeck, or Würzburg, the influential citizens of Lausanne wanted also to build a palace for the poor, as a show of commendable concern for their fate. The discussions about the construction and the financing of the new Hospital illuminate the mentalities at mid-century; their essence, captured in the minutes of the Town-Council, reveal how much the Councilmen were concerned with the improvement of appearance; they insisted on the erection of an elegant dwelling to   enhance   the   city-scape.   However,   they   demonstrated no empathy, nor even the slightest curiosity, for what was to take place behind its walls. At this time, it was only the building itself that was perceived as inadequate for the status of Lausanne; the services provided by the hospital were no matters for discussion.

Tissot, who lived just across from the Townhall on the square of "La Palud", certainly knew of the Town-Council's deliberations.[49] Tissot was then still considered a young physician, albeit one of promise and possibly even renown, but not one to be consulted, even as physician of the poor.

In 1761, the Town-Council adopted a project of total reconstruction. There would be no more *ad hoc* solutions nor botching up of the old structure; instead a brand new hospital would be built. A contest open to all resident architects was announced. The Council then faced the task of raising money for the new construction. Several schemes were discussed. It appeared soon that the favorite means (and a customary one at the time) was a lottery.[50] In fact, three lotteries were organized successively in 1761, 1764, and 1768. Each winning ticket was assessed a 10% tax on its value for the Hospital building fund. About half the cost of the reconstruction was covered in this manner. The Council decided not to solicit private donations, nor to appeal to Bern for a subvention, lest their Excellencies might seize the occasion to extend their writ to matters concerning the Hospital. It decided against the renting of pews in churches, and arranged that a legacy to the workhouse be attributed to the reconstruction fund. The first lottery tickets proved hard to sell; the second one sold better; however the last lottery was near to impossible to place. The Public Purse and the different Poor Funds were even forced to absorb the purchase of a third of the tickets. Lastly, in 1767, the Town-Council adopted a measure by which the amount of money required to buy the Lausanne letters of bourgeoisie would exceptionally be lowered from 4,000 to 2,500 florins for the year 1768.[51] The monies thus raised would go to the building fund.

By 1764 some money for the reconstruction being available, the Council pushed ahead with concrete decisions about the new Hospital. The resolution to erect it on the same site as the old Hospital was confirmed and I found no record of any discussion about the desirability of building it on the outskirts of town to prevent contagion or to improve its hygienic conditions. Its current occupants (the director of the Hospital, the boys and girls schools, the workhouse, and the confined poor) were to be temporarily accommodated in rented quarters. In 1765, two projects for the new Hospital were submitted by two local architects: Crousaz and Fraisse. The spring of 1766 saw the demolition of the old Hospital and the decision of the Council to adopt Fraisse's plan, because the projected cost he submitted was less than Crousaz estimated for his own. By September 1769, the beams of the roof were in place and the workers received a special bonus. The construction had been slowed down by changes in the accepted blueprint. The architect Fraisse came back with a fifth floor to be added for esthetic reasons. The Town-Council argued hotly on the issue, since the initial project already had eleven unused rooms on the third floor, to be left unfinished for the time being. The construction costs were inflated by the esthetic demand and the Town-Council was reluctant to spend more money than had originally been allotted, knowing full-well that raising more funds was nearly impossible. Nevertheless such was the power of urban esthetic arguments that the plan for a fifth floor was accepted. Finally, on 21 June 1770, the Director moved back to the Hospital. The construction had been achieved without major accident. The total cost came to 255, 315 Florins of which 101,250 had been raised through the admissions to the Lausanne Bourgeoisie and 145,000 by the three lotteries. The balance came from a bequest of 6,000 Florins, interest, and petty transfers within the municipal finances.

The Town-Council's minutes are replete with discussions about architectural matters, but hardly any about the services the Hospital was to render. It was simply taken for granted that it was the building called hospital which was defective, while its services were not at all questioned. Hence, the kept poor, the workhouse, the boy's and girl's schools, the Director, and the teachers all moved back more or less to the same kind of rooms which they had occupied in the old dwelling; the additional space offered by the reconstruction was left vacant and unfinished. No innovative use of space was attempted. Architects and fund-raisers were the main protagonists in the reconstruction of the Hospital. Medical experts were hardly consulted or heard during the discussions and, as already mentioned, not even Tissot, the physician of the poor, was asked his opinions about what a hospital should be. This is somewhat puzzling. Perhaps some reasons other than sheer traditionalism are to be considered.

The Lausanne Council did not see why their Hospital should duplicate the services offered at the Inselspital. If they were to consider admitting to their institution the sick, currently treated at home with the funds of the *Miséricorde* or in Bern at their Masters' expenses, then the purse of the Hospital would have to foot the bill. The Town-Council felt that they were already paying enough taxes to Bern; they had learned from the proverbial stinginess of their Excellencies to be parsimonious with their own funds.

Perhaps it was also that Tissot was not too keen about getting involved in the process of the reconstruction. His wife's first husband was the principal organizer of the lotteries and a prominent member of the Town-Council. Also, in the 1760s, Tissot was mainly concerned with the plight of the peasantry, as reflected in *Avis au peuple* (1761); it was to take the Pavia experience and maturity for him to argue effectively for reform of the hospital.

The Town-Council was proud of its new Hospital, of the harmony of its front facade, of the imposing simplicity of its entrance gate flanked by two wings. On the outside, all of the elegance of the eighteenth century was there to be admired, but none of its inquisitive and reforming spirit was applied to the services performed inside the Hospital. Years went by, rooms stayed empty; nothing was done to complete the interior, not even the planned fireplaces that would have kept dampness and cold away. The traditional services of a hospital were not sustained in any better fashion in the new dwelling than they had been in the old.

So far, Bern had not meddled with the Hospital of their subjects in Lausanne. Their Excellencies held physiocratic thoughts in high esteem, and thus were mainly interested in promoting agricultural ventures. They were more pre-occupied with the health of the peasants than they were with what was happening to the urban sick poor. Only when the traditional use of hospital became a hotly debated topic by the members of various Academies, by physicians and by architects, did their Excellencies begin to be concerned with the use of the Hospital of their subject-city. In 1788, the report from the Commission of the Académie Royale des Sciences and Tenon's *Mémoires sur les Hôpitaux de Paris* were published. That same year, on September 18, their Excellencies of Bern addressed a rather stern note to the Lausanne Town-Council to the effect that within a year they should see to the "proper" use of their hospital building.[52] After decades of complacency the Bernese elite had been shaken into action by the specific memoirs; the "tournant des mentalités" had reached them insofar as the purpose of a hospital was concerned. Bern was also looking into the possibility of using some space in the Lausanne Hospital to spare resources at their Inselspital.

The relations between masters and subjects had become much more tense over the years of domination. The Town-Council took five months to recognize the legitimacy of the admonition, stifled as they were by the perspective of losing the complete supervision of their Hospital. A commission which included three physicians, among them Tissot as the Collège de Médecine's representative, an architect, and some councilmen was formed to study the situation. They held their first meeting on 18 February 1789, and met every week thereafter until an oral report was presented to the Bailiff two days before the deadline.

Tissot moved quickly into his new responsibility and on 7 March 1789 he presented to the Commission *Notes sur l'Hôpital de Lausanne*.[53] Before writing *Notes*, he thoroughly inspected the facilities; he drew an inventory of all the occupied rooms, their utilization, their state of repair, of cleanliness, and their habitability; he also counted the empty rooms, finding sixteen of them, among the best of the edifice, if one excepts the apartment for the Director. The hygienic conditions were deplorable in the quarters for the transient poor. Men and women were lodged together in a dirty room; the latrine cabinets opened directly into the room, without even a door. The schools were situated on the fourth floor of the East wing for the boys, and on the fifth floor of the West wing for the girls with adjacent lodging respectively for the Master and for the Mistress. The Master complained that his classroom was very damp and lacked sunshine because of the neighboring buildings height. The *Discipline* [pauper-workhouse] was situated above the boy's school; its quarters were also without much light. Its boarders manufactured clogs and vine-sticks. The ground floor rooms, which Tissot found to be more like cellars than real rooms, were too humid to be healthy but were nonetheless used to lodge the fourteen kept paupers. The service stairs were dark and steep, and often covered by running water, as they were in fact on the day of Tissot's visit. He lamented that more than half of the building was empty, and it was the sounder half! The only redeeming observation in the report was that the food served to the charges was in sufficient quantity, of good quality, and should be kept that way; this proves that the monetary resources of the Hospital were not the problem. The problem was the old-fashioned conception of the purpose of a hospital.

In *Notes sur l'Hôpital de Lausanne*, Tissot spelled out a plan to take advantage of the empty space and convert it to a curing hospital. He reminded the Council of his experience in Pavia, and summarized for them his further studies on the functions of a hospital. He proposed to take in his own hands the responsibility, first for the supervision of the remodeling, then for the direction of the hospital of the sick. Tissot proposed a new allotment of space. Within the same structure, he housed the Director, the workhouse, the confined poor, the two schools and their teachers. He added dormitories and private rooms to accept fifty patients at a time, specifying that each should be in a single bed. Taking Tenon's figures for Paris as a basis for his estimation and assuming further that the cure of the average patient would require a hospital stay of three weeks, Tissot concluded that fifty hospital beds devoted to the sick would amply serve the needs of Lausanne in normal years exempt of epidemics. Private patients, such as foreigners and servants, for whom treatment at home was impractical or costly, could be admitted to the Hospital for a fee. So, Tissot acknowledged the wish of their Excellencies of Bern to see some space allotted in the Lausanne Hospital for sick outsiders. Tissot reported that a fifty-bed hospital should prove to be a very manageable task for the physician-director, and should not strain the existing resources by its special demands for surgeons and nurses. The apothecary needs of the curing hospital could be met by the existing *bannières'* pharmacists.

Tissot submitted in an eleven-point proposal, a detailed program of repair, remodeling, and improvements from which the following highlights delineate the contemporary tensions between salvaging the past and ushering the future.[54] The hospital building was to be rid of dampness by proper sewage and cross-ventilation. The first floor rooms, which were vaulted, were to be used as warehouses and cellars, never again for the purpose of lodging, except for an occasional raving mad person whose isolation was necessary to ensure the peace of the other patients. All the second floor rooms should be panelled with wood, fitted with heating stoves or fire-places. This floor could then easily house the fourteen paupers. The capacity could be raised to twenty-four if they were to be boarded two-to-a-room, yet never two-to-a-bed. The *Miséricorde* should look into the number of poor kept on the dole at home, and have them moved to the Hospital for a more efficient use of the poor fund and of the building. The Hospital's servants should perform their duties with more exactitude to improve the cleanliness of the Hospital. A decent dormitory for the transient poor had to be set up. Two windows should be opened in the blind room of the workhouse to improve its hygienic conditions. All the empty and unused apartments of the Hospital should be converted into rooms for patients with acute diseases. At the end of his report, Tissot repeated his offer of service to help with the setting up of these rooms, with the choice of proper furnishing, and with the formulation of all the regulations pertinent to a curing hospital; he also reiterated his willingness to serve as director of the sick patients floor of the Lausanne Hospital. Thus, without disturbing the current users, the building could be turned into a hospital of the newest conception. Tissot hoped to transform an elegant, half-empty building into a show piece of enlightened medicine. However, the day of philanthropic pursuits and enlightened medicine had passed; it was now a time for quarrelling over prerogatives and sovereignty between the Lausanne Councilmen and their Excellencies of Bern, a quarrel inflamed as time went on by the tremors of the French Revolution.

The Town-Council argued back and forth at length on the issue, on how to finance renovations and innovations, and how to keep Bern away from the affairs of the Lausanne Hospital. In spite of Tissot's efforts and willingness to oversee the realization of the project of upgrading the Hospital, the tergiversations of the Town-Council led the Bailiff to reject the oral report. On 17 May 1790, their Excellencies served the Town-Council with a renewed demand for a written report, this time within two weeks.[55] Their Excellencies, known in all other matters for their slow pace, were not about to tolerate any foot-dragging from their subjects. Fearing the approaching wrath of their Masters, the Lausanne Council now acted swiftly and presented a full written report within a week. Only palliative measures were considered and no action was taken concerning the general revision of the allocation of space and resources of the Hospital advanced by Tissot. The final report proposed only to sanitize the room for the transient poor by building a partition to separate the sexes and painting the wooden beds to destroy the vermin. The report contained no mention of creating rooms for the care of the sick. The Hospital's traditional services were only marginally improved. The Bernese acknowledged the report on 1 July 1790 and declared themselves satisfied.[56]

The Town-Councilmen had won and kept intact their prerogatives over the Hospital. Sadly however, both Lausanne and enlightened medicine had lost. All this seems rather strange and puzzling: why were Tissot's counsels not heeded? In the 1790s, he was a well-respected and honored physician throughout Europe; his advice had been sought by foreign governments. The clue is perhaps to be looked for in his personal life. On 15 March 1790, little Auguste d'Apples, Tissot's dearest grand-nephew, had died leaving his great-uncle broken. That loss was a terrible blow to his morale and hampered all his activities for months, if not until his own death. He lost the drive to push his project for the Hospital, and the Town-Council's narrow-mindedness prevailed. Lausanne had to wait until after the turmoils of revolution in the Pays de Vaud were settled to see a liberated hospital in its midst; by then, Tissot was in his grave.

Tissot failed in the concrete world; nonetheless as a witness of the Enlightenment preoccupations, he left plans for a liberated hospital and an admonition to realize it: "Let us no longer refuse to those of our fellow humans who suffer under the double burden of pain and poverty one of the greatest privileges that wealth can bestow, that of being in their illnesses treated with exactitude, served with intelligence, and assisted by all possible means!"[57]

After that defeat Tissot, in the privacy of his rooms, worked until his death on *Médecine civile*.[58] He wrote it for the attention of the civil authorities who ought to watch over the well-being of the population. Tissot never completely gave up on convincing the authorities of his country of the value of his suggestions. He waited for his hour, but the revolutionary events of France also disturbed the political climate of the Republic of Bern and rendered obsolete the advice of an aging doctor.

Médecine civile goes beyond the scope of our immediate concerns with the reform of the hospital and it will be the topic of the next chapter. Nevertheless, some remarks about its points on hospitals are in order here. In it Tissot took up anew many of the themes treated in *De la construction d'un hôpital-clinique* and adapted them to the situation of a town hospital. The admission of patients was no longer to be determined by their worth as teaching cases, but by their recovering chances after a short stay in the hospital.[59] Tissot described the process of admission in as much detail as he had that of questioning at the bedside. Here too kindness and respect, from the sick's initial admission through their whole stay, were stressed as a matter of human concern and for the pragmatic reason that a trusting patient more easily volunteered information that could be used to prescribe the best possible treatment.

A new concern emerged in *Médecine civile* that was only alluded to in *Construction d'un hôpital-clinique*, namely the importance of professional nurses, trained specifically for the position. Tissot foresaw the need for qualified personnel that a strictly medical hospital would generate. His extensive experience in the clinical wards of the Medical Faculty of (Catholic) Pavia directed his attention to the supportive role of nurses. He wanted them to become, through proper training, true partners in the purpose of a modernized hospital and its healing process. Tissot's nurses were secular professionals much like the surgeons and physicians who, having escaped the rigid constraints of the Church in the Middle Ages, had developed professions of their own.[60] Consequently, he proposed to have the nurses paid a regular salary rather than having them levy a fee directly on their patients. At first, Tissot wrote of the nurse or watcher as a male, but soon afterwards, giving the qualities required of an excellent nurse, he noted: "In general women accomplish this task much better then men".[61] He based his judgement on his experience in training nurses for his private patients. He recommended to physicians that they took seriously their apprenticeship: "Good nurses are infinitely precious to the physician"; and he enumerated the eight qualities good nurses should possess: "precision, honesty, cleanliness, modesty, tranquility, kindness, fidelity, and paramount, reliability in making their account of all events in the ward and of the state of the patients".[62] In his eyes, the nurses, who had the responsibility to see that the prescribed treatment was dispensed correctly at home or in the hospital, were indispensable for the recovery and well-being of the patients. He saw qualified nursing as an integral part of the service of the liberated hospital.

The movement behind hospital reforms is one more manifestation of the "tournant des mentalités". The study of Tissot's writings provides a textbook case for understanding the new conception of the hospital, as an institution for curing and teaching rather than one for death or confinement. Studying his reform's proposals sheds light also on the importance of religious background for the eighteenth-century attitude toward medical modernization. Tissot's original contribution could be debated endlessly, with chronologies of books published and reforms implemented. However, this would obscure the main thrust of research which should be to understand how and why almost simultaneously at Edinburgh, Paris, Pavia, Vienna, or elsewhere, things began to change. And the modernization of the hospital and of medical studies took hold.[63] Tissot's proposals alone would not have moved the medical establishment of Ancien Régime toward reform. Yet, nourished as they were by a new hope for health care and public hygiene, his contributions, like those of others (Cullen, Duncan, de Haen, Frank, or Tenon), pointed in a new direction away from obscurantism, fatalism, and inertia, toward a brighter and healthier future of reason, education, and progress.

Chapter XII

Physician of the Society

For Tissot, the city was a living organism, a close symbiosis of buildings and people, in need of specific health-care as would any other living creature. Applying to society what he had advocated for the individual in his early books, namely to watch lifestyle and regimen with a view to fostering better health, Tissot devised a comprehensive approach for the betterment of society. Based on his own extended conception of the time-honored Galenic non-naturals, he articulated for the city a remarkably innovative program of civic improvements and far-reaching public health measures meant to tame urban excesses and to promote a pleasant environment for the enjoyment of every inhabitant. Tissot acutely perceived the {r}evolution of the late eighteenth-century civilization, from agrarian to urban, from particular privileges to general rights, from absolute rule to concerted action. He therefore wrote *De la médecine civile ou De la police de la médecine* as a blueprint for a rational (natural and sensible) way to achieve healthy surroundings for the happiness of all.[1] In his scheme, Tissot assigned to his new physician, in concert with the most enlightened citizens, a major role for advising political authorities on how to recognize health hazards and eliminate these through proper public health measures. In this manuscript written mainly in the 1790s under what appears as a very Old Regime title, in the style of the German cameralists, Tissot combined echoes of enlightened paternalism with tones of liberal democracy to strike new cords of social medicine and civic improvements.

The concept of Medical Police can be traced back to the seventeenth century and is mainly of German ancestry.[2] George Rosen saw its early manifestation in the work of Seckendorff and its culmination in that of Frank and Mai.[3] Medical police flourished best, and in various forms, within the context of enlightened despotism.[4] It would seem natural that Tissot be attracted to the idea, as he lived under the Bernese oligarchic Republic, a political regime with a strong bent toward enlightened despotism.

From Tissot's organization of the material to the role he assigned to Magistrates and physicians, his interest in public health emerged as something more than the cameralist preoccupation with the increase of population and wealth, which founded work-houses, invalid hospitals, and economic or medical societies.[5] The traditional medical police had aimed at regulating the life of the people from womb to tomb, at managing symptoms of ill health. Tissot brought a distinctively new attitude to the project. As previously noted, Tissot's Swiss Protestant background prompted his thoughts and actions to follow somewhat different paths than those of other physicians of the "coterie". His position can be compared to Rousseau's within the Philosophes' circle. Both men were very much part of and embodied many of the idiosyncracies of Philosophie, yet they had an originality of thought and method rooted in their Calvinistic and republican upbringings.[6]

The Lausanne Doctor is often perceived as a vulgarizer of medical doctrine and practice rather than a reformer; yet a case for his having a deeper motivation than mere popularization can be made on the basis of his calls for individual responsibility in health matters. Tissot had no intention of placing a veneer of medical knowledge over crass ignorance; he wanted to educate every stratum of the population in the advantages of good health. He is thus part of the "tournant des mentalités" which moved the frame of Western thought from a fatalistic attitude toward the misery and ignorance of the masses, to active innovations in the care of the person, then to a transformative organization of society in which all levels would participate and everyone would be concerned and enlisted. His success, even modest, at improving hospital and clinical medicine encouraged him to propose a revision of the concept of medicine in the social sphere. In Tissot's scheme, preventive medicine should investigate the social causes of disease to remedy the symptomatic ills of society: poverty and pollution which breed poor health. *Médecine civile* is an attempt in this direction, with its choice of subject (the environment) and of approach (the Galenic non-naturals).[7] Soon Tissot discovered even deeper causes: social injustice born out of misunderstanding the worth of each human life. This attitude appears clearly in his entry on jails.

In *Médecine civile* Tissot is occasionally carried away by his long term goal of a safe, peaceful, orderly, and enjoyable environment for everyone.   Clashes between private versus public hygiene appeared, for example, in the way he treated the wet-nurses here and in *Des maladies des femmes*. He is coming to grips with a view of society very close to nineteenth-century meliorist attitudes exemplified in the attempts at clearing out slums and at bringing forth a polite and genteel society.[8] This is not too surprising since he wrote most of *Médecine civile* in the 1790s, in the immediate post-revolutionary mood of "no more uproar from the masses", an atmosphere the bourgeoisie of talents, which he favored, wished to see established, now that they had broken the Old Order. Tissot disliked rowdiness as much as idleness.

Médecine civile was to provide Tissot's new physician the social motivation and medical knowledge to identify the causes of poor health, then to prescribe corrective and educative public measures. This was a credo in the power of knowledge, a credo made plausible by the agricultural, technical, and medical advances of the preceding decades, a credo which the *Encyclopédie* had meant to foster. Dearth and famine could be averted with newly discovered techniques of crop rotation and improved tools; the Franklin stove and the Argand lamp could cut down on the risk of fire and the pollution of air in confined space such as hospital rooms; smallpox could be checked by inoculation, and dropsy helped by digitalis; examples could be multiplied; yet it is better to let Tissot speak through *Médecine civile*, first situating this work in his career and evolving medical philosophy.

A lifetime's harvest of medical experiences had taught Tissot that the best cure was often a preventive cure. As physician of the poor in Lausanne he had observed and cared for several outbreaks of what was then called bilious fever. He did not know the exact cause, but his medical instincts led him to suspect more than environmental and climatic factors in epidemics. Miasma was a convenient and easy way of pointing to a cause so general that nothing particular could be done to counteract it.[9] Tissot refused passivity as a response to questions of health, so he dealt in *Médecine civile* with direct measures to prevent the spread of diseases through foul water, spoiled food, or bad living conditions. While Tissot chose not to address in *Médecine civile* the subjects of sexuality, reproduction, and marriage, i.e. regulation of private life, in spite of his unequivocal denunciation of masturbation, Frank did so at length.[10] According to Foucault, Frank's attitude was in character with his time: "Sexuality is not only to be judged, it is also to be administered."[11] Tissot wrote only on the regulation of brothels and the prevention of the spread of venereal diseases. By the 1790s, Tissot's view on the medical consequences of onanism had evolved. He considered them as much less dangerous than the threats on the environment that increased urbanization and nascent industrialization were creating. Besides, onanism was a mostly private pollution and abuse of one's own body, while industrial and urban pollution were general abuses of the public domain. Tissot did not advocate improving morality through public intervention; nor did he promote a repressive control of behavior under the cover of public hygiene. He wanted to safeguard the environment and to foster respect for the commonwealth of land and people. In many instances, Tissot was torn between the path of enlightened despotism and that of liberal political economy, between improvements imposed by the state and betterments that resulted from the free pursuit of knowledge as it replaced ignorance and prejudice. In fact, *Médecine civile* suggests that Tissot held views that in the nineteenth century would be called liberal.

In the late 1780s, when Tissot began writing on medical police, he might have drawn some inspiration (would it be only his alternate title) from the early volumes of Frank's *System einer vollstandigen medizinische Polizei* since he owned its Italian translation.[12] In these volumes, Frank showed strong sympathy for enlightened absolutism as means to enforce measures of public health. In character, temperament and education, Tissot differed sharply from Frank; Tissot's work on the same subject favored a different and more liberal way of dispensing regulations. Nonetheless, Tissot's and Frank's respective *Medical Police* display fascinating parallels in their treatment of many common points. Both doctors were addressing urgent contemporary problems and were dealing with medical concerns shared widely by European physicians and politicians. Only a very close chronological comparison of their actual drafting could perhaps settle who influenced whom. Recalling that they exchanged many letters, that Frank succeeded Tissot at Pavia and visited him in Lausanne in 1791, a certain coincidence of views on medical teaching or on public health measures could be expected.[13] My purpose is not to sort "small change" and to render to Caesar what belongs to Caesar, but to analyze Tissot's thought on public health as the culmination of his own efforts as physician to better the health of the general population. That his views are echoed in or from others' demonstrates how representative Tissot was of the general re-thinking of medical endeavors in the closing decades of the Ancien Régime.

With his age, Tissot believed in the capacity of human beings to behave in their best interest if only this interest was known to them. Passing decades and more experience of the world showed him that individual and personal enterprises are not always the most efficient. Tissot came to recognize that established authorities had a role and possibilities for action, on a large scale, that the individual lacked. He first disclosed this position in his reply to the King of Poland's invitation to become Court Physician in Warsaw, then later in his advice to his friend Zimmermann upon his acceptance of the post of Court Physician at Hanover.[14] Moreover, his reputation as a successful physician brought him consultations and advisory requests from foreign and local governments about matters of public health such as inoculation to check smallpox epidemics.[15] When he became the Vice-President of the Lausanne Collège de Médecine, he recognized even more the importance of public health, social medicine, and regulation of the medical profession.[16]

Tissot's opening statement faithfully reflected one facet of the spirit of his age with its concern for man in society, a man "corrupted" by society, forced to promulgate laws to protect himself from the detrimental influence of societal life: "As soon as a gathering of men forms in any given place, one has also a number of circumstances which influence their health and to which no individual can escape without the help of the whole of society."[17] Next and without ambiguity, he ascribed the task of identifying propitious and pernicious environmental conditions to the physician, whose duty it is also to propose appropriate regulations to assure the health and well-being of the whole population. He defined what is medical police and how it rightfully belongs to the competence of the physician by the expression: "the medicine of the citizenry as a whole".[18] Whereas previously Tissot had written about particular groups of people, here in *Médecine civile* he addressed the problem of social life under different circumstances: urban life; military life; industrial settings; hospitals; and jails; each requiring its own proper medical police. To Tissot, urban life was the most important since cities, towns, and villages "contained the majority of human beings and of which the other groupings are only emanations."[19] For him, the government was to implement the public health program planned by the physicians: "since the official authorities have the power to enact regulations and to disburse money from the public treasury while too often private persons would be frustrated in their attempts if the magistrates did not help them."[20] Tissot's writings often reflected intellectual and political currents. *Médecine civile* bore the mark of the French Revolution, specifically of the *Déclaration des droits de l'homme et du citoyen*, when Tissot mentioned the selfish tendency of individual interest and worried that personal liberty may contravene the general good guaranteed by the social contract and prevent the enactment of medical police.[21] Speaking of "true liberty", he wrote: "if that contract [of true liberty] is the reciprocal engagement of each citizen doing nothing that can harm the others: so to hamper the harmful will of the individual is to insure the liberty that this will violated."[22] All things considered, Tissot noted, the objection to limits imposed on individual freedom can be raised against any law; it is only the short-sighted person (who can be found in any group, including the Magistracy) who will take a stand for no curbs on individual freedom. Citing in French from the Italian version of Frank's *Medical Police*: "It is incomprehensible to me how anyone can hope to retain natural freedom in social life without curbs", Tissot concluded: "what seems to be mere severity is, in fact, dictated for justice and humanity."[23] Always an admirer of Rousseau and perhaps the only doctor whom the writer trusted, Tissot argued the validity of medical police on premises very similar to those of *Contrat Social*: a small personal inconvenience for the greater good of all.[24]

Tissot wrote that "in the interest of order" he would divide *Médecine civile* in two parts. In the first, he would treat the general causes which destroy the health of the population and the means to preserve health by combating the causes of its destruction. In the second, he would address the ways of restoring a health that is in jeopardy. The first part corresponded to ordinary hygiene and dealt with the Galenic non-naturals: air, food, and drink were more apt to be improved by a comprehensive medical police enforced by official authorities; exercise, sleep, and the passions are more dependent on the choice of the individual's lifestyle, although Tissot noted that some regulations can be useful in these areas by providing quiet nights, inviting walkways and pleasant surroundings. The second part, which I will discuss later on in this chapter, dealt with medical institutions and professions.

Many times in previous works Tissot had emphasized the importance of an historical survey of the subject under study before treating it in its current context. Accordingly, he devoted his first chapter to **La médecine civile des anciens**.[25] He reviewed the laws of nutrition for the sacerdotal class that prevailed in Ancient Egypt and the pertinence of the Mosaic Laws to the Hebrews' choice of settlement. Tissot considered these laws the oldest and wisest sets of health rules that had come down to us: "and one sees by the wisdom with which these laws are suited to the land and climate that in each country one has to bend to the local circumstances".[26] He also reported that the necessity of pure water was recognized in Greece, where burials were prohibited within towns. Tissot described the Romans' concern for water and air and how they constructed sophisticated systems to bring pure water and to drain through closed sewage pipes swampy grounds that contaminated the air. The Roman magistrates supervised the food supply (in particular grain), seeing to its quality and quantity. Tissot praised their foresight for insisting on the importance of proper storage as that problem remained crucial in the eighteenth century, bad wheat caused much suffering and disease. The topic attracted considerable commentary, Tissot himself had contributed a medical point of view to the debate.[27] According to Tissot, after the Fall of the Roman Empire, not much attention was given to the proper storage of good grain, and only recently had interest arisen again. He praised their Excellencies of Bern for their prudence, in this matter as in many others, throwing in a bit of flattery to entice them to listen.

After this review of public hygiene in Antiquity, Tissot turned his attention to the ubiquitous problem of providing clean air, pure water, and wholesome food. His historical introduction set the stage for his treatment of perennial problems: burial grounds and open sewage infesting the air and water; spoiled and meager food enfeebling the population. Examples from Antiquity were cherished and respected in enlightened circles. Tissot thus cast his advice in a mode congenial to the frame of mind of those able to implement it.

In chapter 2 **De l'air**, Tissot listed humidity, heat, and putrid vapors as the three circumstances that render air the most noxious and he noted that they appear every time human beings congregate. Man himself, Tissot explained, produces these putrid vapors through breathing. As illustration he recalled the famous "Black Hole" incident that took place in Calcutta in 1756, where, within a few hours of incarceration in a confined place, 120 out of 146 Englishmen died.[28] Only the renewal of the air, he held, keeps it able and fit to sustain life, and only its circulation could insure its regeneration. In order to help ventilate urban centers, he proposed to pull down all remaining fortified walls that turned cities into jails and had, anyway, become obsolete as defenses; in their stead esplanades should be created where the population could conveniently get fresh air and exercise.[29] He urged that, when feasible, new streets be built or existing ones widened to let the north wind sweep through.[30] For Tissot, humidity was the culprit for many unhealthy situations; to remedy the problem, he proposed: "paving streets, with proper slopes to permit drainage of used water, as unpaved streets can never be kept dry, and the fetid mud sickens the children who breathe its vapors."[31]

On consecutive pages Tissot made seemingly contradictory remarks reflecting his awkward position when confronted by the pull and push of the process of modernization. While he could not completely forget tradition, he still incorporated in his work the best innovations or discoveries of his contemporaries: "Large trees create an obstruction to air circulation and in consequence to its renewal, they should therefore be cut down in cities where they also generate humidity..." and "Inghen-Houze demonstrated that the vapors produced by plants standing in the sun constituted the most healthy and purifying kind of air."[32] Tissot used the discovery to advocate sunlight's contribution to healthier quarters while his objection to trees was based on their effect of screening wind and hindering aeration. He was so eager to convince his audience of his prescriptions' correctness that he lost sight of such contradictions. He held that breeze and sunlight were the best ways to keep a location fit for a healthy life; they were also the surest means to render a new building habitable. Tissot described, examples in hand as was his wont, the kind of diseases that can strike people living in humid or freshly painted rooms.[33] He also cautioned against the danger of leaded paint which he had already pointed out in *Observation sur la colique de plomb*, and added examples from Lavoisier's work to buttress his warnings.[34] It is obvious from his remarks on "air vital" that Tissot was familiar with Lavoisier's research on respiration and its importance for hygienic conditions.

In the late eighteenth century, it was still necessary for Tissot to mention a third cause of air corruption, namely "pestilent emanations" which not only made the air unfit to sustain healthy life but also brought disease and infection (plague). He warned of the danger of improper disposal of human and animal excrements: the content of chamberpot should never be thrown out in the streets; complaints against such a practice were made often by pedestrians in Paris.[35] He wrote that each house should be equipped with latrines hooked up to covered drain pipes and that the excrements should be removed at night, adding that the noise of the operation was less hazardous to health than the vapors infesting passers-by and merchandises during the day. Tissot also addressed the problem of stables and manure; the police should banish dung and garbage dumping to outside the city-limits, and should not show any complacency in this matter in any neighborhood. He noted: "a pestilence does not appear every time a garbage heap is left to rot in the streets; yet, it is precisely this apparent safety that breeds false security and lets one believe that what does not kill at once is inoffensive."[36] As an aside he remarked that he was opposed to the custom of having patients suffering from phthisis live in stables as a way of cure: the stench could only enfeeble them further.

Continuing his rounds of offensive smells, Tissot turned his attention to corpses: human and animal. "Burial grounds are of such an importance for the sanitation of towns that I will treat the topic in a separate chapter."[37] He was not alone in denouncing the danger of city-cemeteries and of graves inside churches.[38] In this chapter on air, he drew attention to the health threat inherent to the trades that used animal or vegetal matter, as this material presented a risk of putrefaction and in consequence of infesting the air by its fetidness. In an added note, he also warned against the danger they represented in regard to fire and explosion, and reported an accident involving tallow smelting.[39]   He recommended that all these dangerous trades be practiced at the outskirts of town. Market squares and all food shops were to be placed under an inspection system to insure that they were maintained free of decaying foodstuff and disinfected with vinegar.

Rag shops were also denounced as nests of infection, because of the filth of the old garments they stored. Their stench was sickening, wrote Tissot, as he recalled an episode from his Italian days: "I don't believe that I could have stayed twenty-four hours in the Rome Ghetto, and especially in the Synagogue, without catching a malignant fever."[40] While the remark may seem antisemitic and antisemitic sentiments were rampant in the eighteenth century, it should be noted that Jews had been massacred or expelled in 1348 from Savoy (which then included the Pays de Vaud) on the pretext that they were "bouteurs de peste"; this had been so fierce that Jews were still largely absent from eighteenth-century Lausanne and Geneva. Tissot was thus not attuned to the restrictions imposed on Jews by Gentile society and to the difficult living conditions in ghettoes. Resuming his general remarks on offensive smells, Tissot saw human, animal, or vegetable waste and corpses as the principal sources of pestilence, although he recognized that still others existed such as hospitals and jails which he would discuss in separate chapters.

Then, Tissot turned his attention to several types of buildings intended for congregations of people, specifically churches, theaters, factories, and schools. The medical police should be mindful of the proper ventilation of churches and theaters; and even more importantly, it should watch over the sanitary conditions of factories and schools: "because too often the workers' health was sacrificed to the interest of the owner."[41] Since in the late eighteenth century, Lausanne had few workshops devoted to large-scale production, Tissot's caring for the factory worker was probably a direct consequence of his British contacts. In discussing the safety of manufactures, he was sensitive to recent trends and their possible abuses and had a keen grasp of the problems into which unchecked industrialization could lead. Tissot was especially concerned with the schools where the worker children spend their days. Schooling would be beneficial to them only if they received basic education and trade-apprenticeship in well-ventilated, clean, and properly heated rooms. He contrasted this ideal with the current situation: "If the persons in charge of the medical police would only visit these schools, they would see the pupils' wan faces, smell the stench of stale air, and would then attend more scrupulously to this part of their charge."[42] The corporal and mental well-being of the children was paramount to Tissot; for him children were their country's future and should be of concern to the political authorities as well as to the private family doctor, for whom he had written *Des petits enfants*.[43] After attending to the protection of city dwellers, Tissot turned to salubrity in the countryside, noting that the corrupted air of the country would flow into town and vice versa. Everywhere putrid emanations were to be arrested or prevented: "Swampy grounds which breeds fever should be drained and turned into fertile meadows."[44]

In the last section of **De l'air**, Tissot spelled out measures to prevent the spread of epidemics. His major concern was not childhood epidemic diseases, such as chicken-pox or whooping cough; rather his preoccupation was with fevers, dysentery in particular. He first noted: "Facts have proven that food shortage and filth caused many epidemics, even when there is no general famine, a real dearth could exist in some households, and fever in a single family could infect the whole town which is a fitting punishment for letting a few people starve in the midst of plenty ... many observers have noted that corrupted air from a poorly ventilated, over-crowded factory spread disease"; to buttress his point he cited observations made by Dr. Ferriar in Manchester and published in 1790.[45] Tissot argued that even if poverty and over-crowding in a neighborhood or factory would perhaps not breed fever to the whole town, these facts should not be neglected. The magistrates should enact the proper measures: the resources of the poor fund should serve to correct the origin of the problem, that is to improve the lodging and diet of the poor, instead of offering palliative actions by treating poverty-induced sickness in the hospital. He was adding a social dimension to preventive medicine.

Tissot was as critical of slow action in the face of epidemics as of rash declaration of a contagious disease's outbreak after a few deaths had occurred in a neighborhood. He thought that panic had a disastrous effect; however once an epidemic condition was acknowledged, the measures to check it should be available to everyone. The magistrates should post the names of the physician and apothecary responsible for each neighborhood; they should insure that help was available to those needed it. When a community was too poor to support a physician on a yearly basis, the government was responsible for sending one promptly in case of epidemics. He remarked also that the role of the medical police did not end with enacting the right measures in times of epidemic fever; it also included seeing to their enforcement.[46] For Tissot, the terrible mortality of some epidemics resulted as much from poor food, bad air, filth, and lack of rest as it did from the deficiency of medical help or the inferior quality of the drugs dispensed.

In his third chapter *Des aliments,* Tissot dealt with the provision, storage, preservation, and sale of food. "It is more important to see to the salubrity of food and drink than to the accuracy of weights, scales, and measures that serve to their sale, since adulterated or spoiled food are truly poisonous ... a rascal falsifies the measures, while it takes a criminal to sell rotten and altered merchandise which threatens the life of others."[47] Tissot wanted grain-control to be very strictly enforced, because the quality of its components and its preparation affects its nutritional value. In the past bread was (and in the twentieth century we tend to forget this) the main source of nourishment for a large portion of the population. He added that if poor bread did not kill immediately, it nevertheless weakened the people who ate it; these persons unable to support themselves became public charges. He reviewed the many circumstances that render grain inedible.[48] Tissot warned of ergoted rye, the most dangerous cause of disease because of the nervous and gangrenous ills it provoked.[49] It was not enough to watch the quality of grain and flour; the medical police should also supervise the bakers to be sure that they incorporated no dangerous additives such as chalk or white lead into the bread. Tissot wrote down a method to detect these adulterations that ought to be prosecuted severely.[50] The magistrates should anticipate needs: "Public provisions would prevent, not only hoarding and speculation in times of scarcity, but also malignant and putrid fevers always present in famine and enhanced by the consumption of bad food."[51]

Under most circumstances, Tissot condemned monopolies, favoring a free-market economy. But he was ready to make a concession in the case of grain. He believed that the State justifiably could grant a monopoly of grain importation, for in this case, private enterprise replaced State enterprise. Tissot viewed governments as being above suspicion of not dispensing the best possible services.[52] He noted that in countries that also cultivate potatoes, the proper provision of grain was not as crucial, but should not be neglected "for bread will always be the healthiest food for the person who works at heavy tasks."[53] Tissot was (for the eighteenth century) uncommonly fond of potatoes and when he was in Pavia missed this food.[54] The Bernese had introduced potato cultivation early in the eighteenth century at the same time that they had pushed for increased dairy production.[55]

From bread, Tissot moved to other foods and their proper handling. He first turned his attention to meat. He was mainly concerned with the "hidden" corruption of meat, i.e. meat from sick animals, which the unsuspected buyer would take in good faith. Tissot advised to inspect regularly herds and flocks for detecting any epizootic or endemic diseases, thus preventing the sale of contaminated meat.

Next, Tissot investigated the quality of vegetables. He was mainly concerned with the accidental consumption of poisonous varieties. He saw ignorance rather than malice in the sale of toxic plants. He argued that mushrooms which, in some provinces, were the main causes of these poisonings, should be banned because there existed no safe method to distinguish between good and poisonous ones and "anyway they are difficult to digest and have little nutritive value".[56] Tissot reported that in the Pays de Vaud mushrooms were not a favorite of the people and that he saw only five accidents related to them in his forty years of practice; but, in some countries, Piedmont for example, where they were in favor, they occasioned every year many and frequently fatal poisonings.[57]

Even today, the problem is severe enough to warrant weekend opening hours of the Geneva Health Institute for the voluntary inspection of the mushrooms gathered mainly by the Italian guest-workers.

Noting that the selling of fresh fruits had often been prohibited, when diarrhea occurred at the end of the summer, Tissot branded this practice mistaken. He recalled the position he had argued in *De febricus biliosis* and in *Avis au peuple* where he had prescribed with success fresh fruits in times of dysentery. Accordingly, the authorities must assure the abundance and cheapness of ripe fresh fruits on the market, not their prohibition.

Tissot also advocated the drinking of milk, which he held to be the healthiest of food, provided it be pure.[58] From petty deeds of diluting it with water to the dangerous practice of making some from water, starch and sugar, or of adding a lead component to butter to stretch its weight, he described a continuous spectrum of abuses of dairy products. He wanted the medical police to supervise all dairy products, including the "lait vénal" [wet-nurse's milk], reporting that this was done in Sweden and some part of France. The medical inspection of hired wet-nurses would save the life of many infants whose mothers had no milk or refused to nurse them. Here, he described the wet-nurse as a commodity on the market to which "the magistrates should pay special attention as to any others that are in short supply, because shortage favors cheating."[59] In *Médecine civile*, Tissot distinguished between private and public health; since he was attending to public health, he refrained from dictating private conduct, such as the right to hire wet-nurses; but because he wanted to have only safe and healthy goods offered to the public, he sometime went so far as to equate human resources with merchandise. This same attitude of private versus public health crept in again in *Médecine civile* when he addressed the problem of brothels and pubs; more on these will be said later in this chapter. These were cases in which the long-term benefit blinded him to the short-term harshness of his prescriptions.

Continuing his systematic review of the non-naturals, Tissot considered beverages in his fourth chapter *Des boissons*.[60] He suspected that some correlation existed between good health and plenty of unpolluted beverages, including water. The most terrible late-summer epidemics of putrid fever seemed to occur in years of drought or when, the preceding fall, the grape harvest and wine production had fallen short.[61] Wine, in many instances, proved to be a more hygienic beverage than water and easier to preserve. The Pays de Vaud, then as now, is a wine-producing country, so it was to be expected that Tissot discussed wine first. He began by cautioning against dangerous ways to "improve" wine, deploring the use of lead-based ingredients supposed to sweeten the bad vintages. He described the ills produced, when and how fraud occurred, and the means to detect it. He added that recent progress in viticulture had permitted the production of better wines that were less often in need of "improvement". He warned of the hazards that arise from the material used in the storage or production of fermented beverages. Again he meant lead. Several eighteenth-century authors studied lead poisoning and recognized it as the source of colics which had previously been attributed to climatic conditions. The British physician Baker was a pioneer in this field, and the only book published by Tronchin, Voltaire's famous physician, was on that topic; both physicians happened to be Tissot's correspondents.[62] Writing also on the subject of beer, Tissot commented that given the abundance of wine in the Pays de Vaud and the frequent shortfalls in the grain harvest, it would be unwise to increase beer production and to push its consumption.

In the next article on hard liquor, Tissot worried more about its quantitative than its qualitative abuses; as it was "good for nothing" he saw no inconvenience in prohibiting its sale. Still, he realized that an absolute prohibition was impossible to enforce, so he suggested restricting both the number of shops allowed to sell liquor and the quantity to be served to an individual: no more than one to one and one-half ounces to the same customer at one sitting. He insisted that strict regulations be placed on the sale of poisonous burning alcohol (now recognized to provoke blindness).[63]

Tissot opened his article on water with the following remark: "If the Police ought to pay so much attention to beverages which are not really necessary, one will judge how much care it should give to water which is of top necessity."[64] In Lausanne, the supply of pure water had always been a problem; the rivers Flon and Louve were of very unpredictable flow and quite polluted; the lake stood too low to provision the city; an aqueduct brought water from a distance, but it was time-worn and contaminated. Tissot insisted that a sufficient supply of water should be provided for drinking (for humans and animals); cooking; washing; fire-fighting; and, often neglected, for a stream to run through the streets to clear away the filth of garbage as well as for sprinkling the streets in hot weather to reduce the level of dust, to cool the atmosphere, and to clear up some of the miasma of stale air.

The quality of water had a direct influence on the health of the people, especially that of the children who should not drink anything else. Tissot reiterated a warning he had sounded in *Des petits enfants*, in which he recommended no wine or fermented beverages before the age of five. Bad water would throw children into languor for their entire life. Then he described how to determine the suitability of a water source. Once more he warned of the danger of leaded pipes and vessels. This time he quoted Tronchin, who had observed terrible colics in Holland where rainwater was collected from leaded roofs, and he refuted, with the help of the English physician Percival, the opinion of Heberden, another English physician, that lead and copper containers were harmless.[65] Always systematic in his investigations, Tissot then took a close look at utensils for cooking and storing food. He wrote that the magistrates should be concerned mainly with crockery belonging to inns; regulation of utensils would provide useful guidelines for private homes. He mentioned a recently introduced method of tinning which used a no-lead alloy, charging the Police to promote this new process.[66]

In the next article **De la sûreté du mouvement et du repos**, Tissot addressed safety problems of commercial and recreational traffic which he approached from the non-naturals, motion and rest; sleep and wakefulness. He looked into urban infrastructures and developed ideas on city-planning and civic improvements with a view to creating healthier and more pleasantly livable towns. He declared: "Exercise is necessary to health and it is essential for health to be spared all strenuous excesses, so one of the duties of the Magistracy is to arrange for public works meant to facilitate exercise and to prevent work burden."[67] He described in some detail what he meant by public works. He extolled the advantage of esplanades at the outskirts of town where merchants, artisans, and their families, drawn by the pleasantness of the surroundings, could get away from the stale air of workshops and narrow streets. Good roads running from towns to villages across the countryside would not only invite sedentary people to take longer, healthier walks, but also facilitate the task of the farmer bringing his produce to town or of the carter conveying goods from one place to another. Tissot held the medical police responsible for easing the labor of the population by every possible means. To that end he wanted benches, with raised shelves, to be built at crossroads so that peasant women coming to the town-market could, when they stopped for a rest, readily unload and reload the baskets they carried on their head.[68] He also advised draining swamps close to roads to cut down on foul emanations, the risk of falling into them... and to prevent their use as a convenient place for dumping a cadaver after an assassination.[69] Fright provoked troublesome accidents; the magistrates should minimize their occurrence by implementing proper regulations Tissot had in mind fire prevention, street lighting, ice breaking on streets and stairs as well as mad persons and rabid dogs that create fright by the disorder they propagate.[70]

In the *Médecine civile* article on hospital, Tissot wrote of the special needs of the insane. He thought that only the wildly insane who threatened public tranquility should be interned in special rooms where they would be treated with decency and gentleness. Here again Tissot was addressing public, not private health and did not elaborate on the subject of cure which he had attempted in *Traité des nerfs*.[71] Tissot, wishing to preserve public peace and promote public health, adopted a repressive attitude bound to bruise our twentieth-century civil sensibilities. Any offensive conduct or object was to disappear from the public eye; the medical police was to allow only a polite and polished atmosphere in public places for the enjoyment of everyone.

Tissot wrote that rabid dogs were not as common as popular opinion claimed. Very often people cried rabies without proof, and the tumult they created, running after a supposed rabid dog gave rise to more harm than rabies itself. So Tissot advised that a special force be maintained to take care of "rabid" dogs and to disperse any mob that congregate around or chase after these dogs. If the dogs had to be killed to check rabies, it ought to be done with decency; and all other dogs were to be kept indoors for six weeks after the incident and watched for signs of rabies. His concern about the way dogs were treated, and killed if necessary, reflects the emerging mentality which saw the world of animals and plants as partners with human beings, rather than inferiors without feelings or souls. The new mentality was specially strong in Great Britain, it had resonances too in the works of French-speaking authors such as Rousseau.[72] Though at first the motivation behind this change of attitude toward animals was religious, when a different understanding of Nature was later accepted, that attitude became one more aspect of the secularization of thought and mores.[73]

After these different suggestions on how to deal with rabies and its scare, Tissot added: "One may allow a person to have as many superfluous jewels, clothes, and furnitures as {s}he wishes, this is only harmful to that individual, but ought one not to prevent {her}him from keeping superfluous animals that clutter streets and squares? ... wealthy {wo}man with fancy taste, put all of your money in trinkets if you so wish, but do not increase the price of the bread of the poor because you feed by luxury or vagaries animals that are useless."[74] The gentry had been keeping pets for centuries, but the habit was now spreading to the bourgeoisie in the cities. This raised the question of the legitimacy of possessing useless animals, which were often better fed than the servants.[75] Tissot had never been favorably inclined toward the useless, and he saw pets as such. He did not seem sensitive to their potential value as centers of affection; he only viewed them as eaters of somebody else's food. Or perhaps he was aware of the growing fondness for pets which threatened to displace the renewed interest in children and tried to counteract the trend. Evidently, Tissot was reacting to a new habit, since he had no past example of regulation of pet-owning to offer. Still preoccupied with sumptuary laws, he declared that the medical police should be concerned only with the quantity of food and drink, and not with clothing, jewelry, and furnishings. Food and drink affect health; the other items do not. The question of the beneficial or detrimental influence of luxury was hotly debated in the eighteenth century. Some (heirs to Colbert) vindicated the manufacture and sale of luxury items as a way to boost the economy; others (including the physiocrats) rejected them to advocate the production of goods for general consumption.[76] Tissot took a median position; only the over-consumption of food was harmful to the over-eater's health and to that of the public in general, which was deprived of necessities by the luxury of the few. He wanted regulations to improve public health, not manufacture and trade as commercial ventures. Tissot recalled the Roman laws about the number of people attending a dinner party, and the amount of money allowed to be spent on one banquet adding: "But who today would think of proposing any such thing? It is already venturing much to recall the fact."[77] He only suggested strict laws against drunkenness, since intemperance accounted for the most frequent injury to the people's health. Drunkards were an object of scandal and fright in the streets, causing harm to innocent lives; so Tissot wanted to see the tippler jailed until sober and heavy fines levied against the merchants who sell liquor late at night.[78] The punitive attitude toward drunkards constituted one of his lapses from even-handedness in his treatment of different social groups. The rich could get drunk in the privacy of their rooms, but the poor drank at public places and needed to walk back to their homes, possibly causing scandal along the way. The intemperance of the poor was more visible and seemed of more consequence to their health and to the well-being of their families, than the abuses of the wealthy were to their relatives. Besides, in the late eighteenth century, as for that matter still in the early twentieth, poor people had not much choice in entertainment and relaxation, other than drinking. Tissot did not always master the ambiguity of intertwining liberal thinking with paternalistic views.

Besides drinking places, Tissot denounced brothels that exercised a long-lasting corruptive influence. He held that the mistake of an instant turned into a lifetime misery for the individual and his family by infecting his spouse and procreating languishing children; he quoted Buffon to buttress his argument.[79] Tissot, who in *Onanisme* had depicted the ravages of excessive sexual activity, mustered here even stronger arguments to ban brothels. As a private vice masturbation harmed only the individual, but the depravity of brothels concerned the public as much as any source of pestilence.

Arguing for censoring licentious prints and tracts that incite lust, Tissot wrote that the freedom of the press did not include the freedom to print the rambling fantasies of a sick mind: imagination and thought should always remain free, but, their fruit ought to be checked before they are printed. He then candidly admitted that others had thought of banning another kind of books as dangerous, namely his *Avis au peuple sur sa santé*. "As painful as I find this sentence of Dr. Schraud, famous Hungarian professor of medicine, it is my duty to report it here", he added in 1795.[80]

One of the most interesting and innovative articles of *Médecine civile* is entitled **Des prisons**.[81] In his earlier writings Tissot had called health the most precious property of man, woman, and child; without health no other possessions could be acquired or enjoyed. Poor health even undermined the possibility of earning one's own living and of pursuing happiness on this earth. To Tissot, it was the duty of the medical police to see that all persons, even prisoners had access to good health, first by environmental measures promoting salubrious surroundings, and second by providing the means to keep or regain good health.

In **Des prisons**, Tissot addressed the purpose of jailing, the grounds on which imprisonment could be justified, and how society could protect both its fabric and each of its particular threads, free citizen and prisoner alike. This duty of the magistrate to protect, noted Tissot, was even more "solemn" in the case of the prisoners (who could not take care of themselves) than in the case of the free persons (who can better control the circumstances of their life and health). The punishment meted out by society in jailing someone was the privation of free action. This could be justified on the grounds of the safety of society when a person was suspected of a crime, or as a punishment for very serious offenses against society. Unfortunately, Tissot did not elaborate on what he meant by **serious**, a factor limiting the understanding of his conception of society and social behavior. He wrote that incarceration did not entitle the prisoner to gratis subsistence, nor did it authorize the jailer to mistreat the captive; rather in the only just and reasonable imprisonment, the convict was to earn his/her own living for which no one else had to pay.[82] Tissot noted that such a prison existed in Bern at the Chalvair and that more should be organized; he mentioned the existence of such a prison in Philadelphia. Tissot was probably referring to the Walnut Street

Jail reorganized in 1794 which emphasized hard labor as a means of correction.[83]

Tissot did not address the question of torture or corporal punishment which he doubtless abhorred (both harmed mind and body) since he explicitly argued that the only acceptable punishment for a crime was separation from society by imprisonment. For him, society would be liable to the prisoner for any loss of health while in jail: "One cannot say it too many times, incarceration is the privation of liberty, but does not entail other punishments, above all not that of impairing health which would be infinitely worse than the death penalty, when the judge's intentions were that it be less severe."[84] Then he enumerated the measures to be taken to preserve the health of the prisoners and recommended Howard's *On Prisons* as very useful reading for magistrates, since it had inspired several of his own instructions on jails.[85] Insisting on cells large enough to provide pure air and exercise space for the inmates, Tissot lashed out at his critics who invoked the unhealthy conditions of the worker-dwellings to excuse worse ones in jails. "Workers can move freely out of their houses while prisoners cannot" and he refused to accept an excuse based on a bad situation, which should not be tolerated in the first place concluding: "I despise much more the harsh man who lightheartedly dismisses the sufferings of his fellowmen than I do the unfortunate criminal often led by circumstances rather than by will who would be able to feel compassion and pity for others if only he was called upon to do so."[86]

Tissot's argument for decency toward prisoners has very strong affinities with Beccaria's *Dei delitti e delle pene* published in 1764, which, however, was not listed in the catalog of his library. While in Pavia Tissot might have informed himself on the question, since under the impulse of Joseph II and the unmistakable influence of Beccaria's work, the penal code was reformed in 1783; he might have even taken part in the debate over the new regulations. Beccaria defined crime as an act against society, an act that harms society.[87] Tissot did likewise and saw the punishment in separation from society and nothing more. For this reason, arguing from his position as physician, he denounced prison as a robber of good health, if the prisoners lose theirs in its cells.

In the second part of *Médecine civile* Tissot addressed the question of the supportive agencies and professions which aim to restore health. He announced that it was not enough for the magistrates to seek and to correct any condition conducive to poor health; they also had to take active steps to provide the population with all the known means of healing and cure. It appears that Tissot had a larger project in mind than the one he left to us; for scattered throughout his voluminous notes and comments was material he could retrieve to complete the task he had set forth in his introduction to the second part. One such source was his notes for the minutes from the Collège de Médecine; others were *Du régime dans les maladies aiguës, Des cimetières, Des noyés, Sur les eaux minérales,* or *Observations sur la réforme de quelques objets importants relatifs à la santé du peuple.*[88]

Tissot intended first to treat the question of how to supply a town with good physicians, surgeons, midwives, and nurses; second, he wanted to address the respective roles of *miséricordes*, hospitals, and other resources in promoting the people health. He began with the hospital, the subject he had studied most and of which he had the widest experience. For the topic of *miséricorde*, he referred readers to his nephew's "excellent" work published in 1789.[89] His first chapter **Des Hôpitaux** dealt, in the perspective of a town-hospital, with many of the same topics he had discussed for a clinical ward: choice of location, material to be used in the construction, and the layout of the building to minimize contagion from patient to patient and to the neighborhood. He examined the appropriate size for a town-hospital, first remarking that hospitals ought to be open to everyone in need of health care and ought to be supported by public funds. Tissot insisted that the best place for recovery in case of accident and of most acute diseases was the hospital, but he added that the prejudice of the people against the hospital or even the intervention of a physician bordered on fatalism. This prevented them from calling for help on time, even for their own children for whom their love was certainly unquestionable. He wanted to see a regulation imposing a fine on parents whose children had died of disease without the physician having been called on the second day of the illness.[90] Tissot recognized that poorly fitted hospitals had been numerous well into the recent past and were still to be found, yet regretted that this situation be allowed to serve as easy slandering of an institution that was so useful when wisely managed. Because the right size for a hospital depended upon the community it would serve, he suggested consulting the civil records to ascertain the proportion of dead-to-living persons for each year, that of poor-to-affluent, and the industry and business of the city, for these facts influenced the health and proneness to accident and disease of any population.[91] He quoted Tenon's figures for Paris "one hospitalized sick to 105 and 4/5 able-bodied residents".[92] Tissot commented that this ratio was too high for most places which were smaller than Paris. He thought that for towns between 10,000 and 30,000 inhabitants the correct proportion was one sick to 150 healthy, and that for well-situated towns without large factories it should be one to 200. Yet he warned that the size of urban population was on the increase as was the number of factories, so it was wise to stay with the one-to-150 ratio. He thought that the optimum size for a hospital was seventy-two beds which would serve the needs of a community of about 10,000 souls. Very large hospitals are unmanageable and the distance between them too long for most patients. Thus, Tissot recommended that larger towns should have several small hospitals.

Out of the seventy-two beds, Tissot allotted fifty for patients with "fevers" (thirty-six for men, fourteen for women), twelve for victims of accidents who required a surgeon's attention (eight for men, four for women), and the remaining ten to be divided between a room of four beds, one of two, and four single rooms.[93] Tissot justified this distribution by the kinds of diseases that would be admitted to the hospital: only those with a quick recovery period; no venereal disease, smallpox, or scabies, because of the risk of contagion; but he saw no objection to admitting phthisis' case: "Etisis is not a contagious disease, but toward its end it is a disgusting illness ... besides it is always very long and would be better off in the countryside ... yet a precise cure in its beginning might save some, so justifying their admissions..."[94] Tissot's opinion on phthisis was shared by most of his colleagues. It took until the discovery of the tubercle bacillus by Koch in 1882 to settle the case of the contagious nature of etisis. What is of interest here is Tissot's view of the role of the hospital: a place where one receives precise treatment at the beginning of sickness, when chances of recovery were at their peak. Those with bilious and putrid fevers were to be admitted to the hospital for their healing depended on fast and exact help best found in a hospital. Tissot did not, like most of his colleagues, acknowledge the contagious nature of these diseases. He proposed that some beds in the woman ward be reserved for delivery; this would be beneficial to mothers with difficult deliveries and would provide an opportunity for training midwives properly.[95]

Tissot devoted a special paragraph to the admission of patients. The tone reveals the atmosphere of peaceful quiet confidence he wanted to establish in the hospital. After the name was registered, the patient was to be taken to a single bed; face, hands, and feet were to be washed to procure freshness and promote better perspiration. {S}he was to receive something to drink, perhaps the usual tea of the hospital or, if very feeble, nourishing broth. Afterwards, the surgeon was to examine the patient and prescribe whatever was necessary until the visit of the physician.

Then Tissot wrote: "...many would ask me, what about all the sick you reject from the hospital?" His answer was that the *miséricorde* was to provide help at home for contagious (mainly venereal) diseases and incurables, for which the hospital would do more harm than good, freeing the one from the shame of debauchery and encouraging idleness in the other. He spoke from the premises of the still prevalent mentality of helping only the "deserving poor", those that by no fault of theirs needed temporary support; nevertheless he considered provisions for the setting up of an outpatient clinic, like the one he had at Pavia.[96] To the objection that neither enough money nor a suitable location could be found for his project, Tissot simply replied: "...then do the best you can with what you have!"

In his fourth section **De la distribution des malades et des appartements**, Tissot again took up the subject of rooms for convalescents. He wrote that convalescents have different needs than sick or healthy people and deserve a special place to walk and regain their strength, plus a room in which to converse during the day and sleep undisturbed at night. Tissot reserved the four single rooms for isolation either in the case of contagion or delirium, or when a patient required more tranquility to recover. He wrote of usual heating and ventilation systems; but when it came to lighting the rooms he advocated the Argand incandescent mantle (invented in 1784) which burns almost without smoking because of the intensity and rapidity of its flame and hence reduces air pollution.[97]

In the conclusion to his chapter on hospitals, Tissot addressed the question of supplies and directorship. He advised that the supporting services be obtained outside of the hospital compound, because providing for these would increase its size and the responsibilities of its director beyond a manageable point. He wanted supplies acquired from different shops, since he generally believed that competition ensured the best quality at the fairest price.[98] For Tissot, the choice of the hospital director was of the utmost importance and difficulty because of the qualities required: foremost, he [Tissot saw this position occupied by a man and a married man at that!] should be compassionate and devoted to his task, which he should understand in all its details. No favor should determine who was chosen for this post.[99] The director and his family should live at the hospital: "one is always a stranger to a house when one is not attracted back to it by what one cherishes most, also the whole family should be animated by his zeal ... his wife should want to share his praises, her greatest pleasure should be to see joy on every face when she enters the wards..."[100] If Tissot's description appears romantic or idealistic, remember that he sought to reform an institution which did not enjoy a reputation for competence nor inspired confidence. He had to appeal to humanitarian sentiments to convince others of the rewards that would accrue from a new attitude toward the people, all too often seen as a mob of worthless idlers. His apologia of the hospital director also reveals another dimension of his thought, namely his view of the relations between husband and wife, a view in tune with the bourgeois ethos of affectionate family life.

When Tissot wrote on institutional changes, he first described their traditional aim and function, then he marshalled his arguments for change in such a manner that the reader would be drawn unsuspectingly to endorse and to agree with the revolutionary results. He followed precisely this strategy in chapter two: **Hôpitaux d'enfants trouvés**. He declared that initially the idea of a foundling hospital might appeal to those who seek to perfect the medical police. He wrote warmly of the charitable aim of the foundling home, of saving lives, of relieving suffering, of rescuing unwed mothers from shame or even from committing infanticide. Then abruptly he announced that the public had been mistaken and misled; in fact, foundling homes were the worst institutions. Experience with such establishments revealed their destroying power; it was well-known that none of these hospitals ever brought up a tenth of the infants received.[101] They were meant, wrote Tissot, for children born out of wedlock, therefore encouraging debauchery in both sexes; but more often they were used by misinformed parents who, not able to assume the burden of an extra birth, were lured to leave their offsprings at a foundling home in the hope of insuring them a better life, when in fact they assured only their death.[102] He rejected any suggestions that more money, better management, or any thing else would help, even giving as reason that mothers had just enough milk for their own child and none to spare if they took their role seriously. He knew that in his day no reliable substitute for woman's milk had been found, not to speak of an adequate implement to feed an infant artificially. Proper (sufficient and clean) nourishment meant a chance of survival, its absence sure death. Tissot was categorical: foundling homes were to be dismantled rather than built. Public measures were to be taken to relieve the poverty which forces the abandonment of children. For him it was the political authorities' duty to provide enough food at prices that even the most deprived people could afford: "No mother is such a monster as to abandon her nursling when she herself has enough to eat without selling her milk."[103] Earlier he had warned: "a starving people is a people in uprising."[104]

In his chapter three **Des personnes chargées du soin de conserver la santé et de la rétablir,** Tissot addressed the means to recruit well-trained people for the many tasks of preserving and restoring health. He did not deal with the problem of staffing the hospital, but that of providing villages and towns with qualified medical personnel. Since medicine dealt with life and death, its regulation ought to be a matter of High Police and, like others of its kind, should emanate from the Prince; Tissot first wrote sovereign, but crossed it out and substituted prince. With the French Revolution raging, sovereign could mean the people, and he intended no confusion about the fact that he only entrusted the highest authority of the land to control the quality of the practitioners; even if the Magistracy had not taken seriously the task as demonstrated by the number of quacks, ignorant physicians and midwives, and sellers of universal drugs, who ran through towns and coutryside, sowing languor and desolation among the people. He insisted that integrity, rather than indulgence or favoritism, ought to determine the licensing of medical personnel. He also warned against the presence of too many practitioners in a town; none had enough work to earn a decent living and all had to resort to cunning or other devices to subsist. A delicate balance was to be reached between just enough competition to inspire good service and not so much of it as to encourage sloth and deception. For Tissot, the death toll at childbirth resulted as much from the paucity of competent midwives as from the people's lack of money for paying their services; to remedy this he advised having midwives paid by the township. He charged them to report all clandestine births. He forbade them to use instruments to help in the delivery, rather they should call immediately a surgeon if difficulty arose.

Despite the frequent neglect of dentistry, Tissot insisted that each town of 10,000 or so inhabitants should have a dentist: "Many will smile at my advice, for them teeth are just an ornament and they never care to rinse out their mouth for cleanliness; as a result they are living *mofettes*, carrying infection from place to place, and their smile does not take away a bit of the usefulness of my advice ..."105

In his section on **Apothicaires**, Tissot wrote again on the inconvenience of too many pharmacies in the same town, but would not recommend having only one in a small town, as competition would keep the quality of drugs at its peak and their price at its lowest. He thought that an apothecary for 2,500 inhabitants was a reasonable figure. He was against a list price for drugs and found the practice insulting and unfair to competent pharmacists, and not at all in the best interest of the sick. Pharmacy inspections were more useful and should be done at best once a year, but at least every other year. In any event, added Tissot, if a patient thought he has been overcharged, he could ask the physician who prescribed the drug to check with the pharmacist and lodge a complaint with the judge if necessary. "But why would an apothecary be less honest than any other merchant? Why do we use the expression 'comptes d'apothicaire' for an inflated and complicated bill? It is because once cured by the drug one forgets its virtue only to remember its price."[106] He remarked that one does not often see a pharmacist become rich swiftly, which he took as a sign of honesty.[107] As a last argument for free trade in drugs, Tissot wrote that regulated prices would normally be higher than market price, placing drugs out of reach of most people, throwing the sick into the hands of quacks and sellers of secrets. Charlatans were always too expensive for their {dis}services.

The last section of *Médecine civile* was to be about nurses; only its title **Des gardes malades** and where to find its content was indicated on the last page of the manuscript. The reference was to the end of *Du régime dans les maladies aiguës*.[108] This circumstance seems to confirm that Tissot planned a larger work and would have used many of his other writings to complete *Médecine civile*. Illness prevented him from accomplishing his goal.

Nonetheless, this manuscript is a tribute to Tissot's vision of public hygiene and a witness to his times. It is an attempt to bring reason rather than coercion into the picture of better health for everyone. *Médecine civile* is also a call to be responsible addressed first, to the magistrates to provide means to preserve or restore health; second, to the citizens to seek on their own these means of better health, as a right and a duty of all human beings. In writing *Médecine civile* Tissot attempted to extend the microcosm of private health into the macrocosm of public health. His concern for the individual rendered him aware of the link between single human being and society, even more so after his sojourn in Pavia and his travels across Italy where he visited large cities such as Naples. The manuscript shows him mainly concerned with the urban setting, potential seat of morbidity and restlessness: the "laborious/dangerous" classes spawned by nineteenth-century industrialization and urbanization already loomed large in Tissot's mind as he was writing in the 1790s.[109] The work exhibits tensions between paternalist and liberal attitudes, between an ideal vision and a repressive situation. Tissot tried not to lose sight of private liberties when dealing with the commonweal, but he was not consistently successful. Amidst the reports on the French Revolution upheavals, Tissot clung to a utopian rational achievement of a just and healthy situation brought about by radical, but peacefully achieved, measures. Tissot certainly recognized the tensions in his drive to be physician to the society. With his health failing, he never again had the strength to face the task and to resolve these tensions in a completed treatise. Tissot did not publish *De la médecine civile*, hence never fully brought to the public attention his social conception of health as a right of the citizentry and a responsibility of the government.

Conclusion

The life, career, and writings of Samuel-Auguste Tissot provide an arresting case-study of medicine in the Era of the *Encyclopédie*, of enlightened medicine not merely as progress toward modernity, but also as a whirlpool of cross-currents. Tissot's attitude of mind, conduct in medical practice, and writings about health and disease were well within what has come to be called modernization. His appeals for better health — private and public — were to be achieved through individual and collective actions in conjunction with physicians. His calls for personal and social responsibility toward the state of one's own body and living environment were distinctively modern in their drive to tap new discoveries; they aimed to surpass the present conditions; and they strived to develop the full potential in each life. Yet, the thrust of his argument for medical reforms was far from an unbroken ascending line away from obscurantism toward enlightenment. His reasoning exhibited the stresses of grappling with novel endeavors in the existing context; of wedding the old and the new in order to usher an acceptable present. Tissot's career, which spanned almost the entire second half of the eighteenth century, exemplified the best and the worst of the era — the polite policing.[1]

Tissot's medical concerns are mirrors of the trends and lines of force within the wider reflection of the Philosophes. On the same token, these currents are manifestations of the hiatus and fragility of their program. Tissot believed the individual to be capable of proper judgement, once presented with the means for his or her own betterment. He supposed governments to be driven by the good of their people. Was not Voltaire or Diderot lured to believe the same from the great Frederick or Catherine? The optimism of the Era might very well have been its demise, and Tissot shared both. The Philosophes and the doctor failed to see the egotism spawned by self-interest. And selfishness proved omnipotent.

Tissot was no lonely prophet crying in the desert. He was a sturdy companion to the cohort of medical reformers and social critics whose repeated advocacies for new pursuits, for reaching further in every directions (e.g. agriculture, industry, medicine, politics, science) were by their sheer numbers to move Europeans toward modernity and perhaps also toward a destroying self-confidence. Yet, much as Rousseau did, Tissot brought to the common enterprise the special touches of Calvinism and democracy.

Tissot began his career by defending the practice of inoculation for which he used experimental data and new mathematical methods to buttress a case for defying fatalism. The inoculation battle encapsulated the Enlightenment spirit which emphasized accomplishments over speculations, daring deeds over inertia. With no theory of immunization to justify their conduct, the inoculators were sustained by their initial results; true believers blind to danger, they pursued happiness in a world where inoculation meant banning ugliness and early death. His choice of audience for his first book, the starting point of his long battle for an improved medicine, foreshadowed many of his succeeding quests. In his writings about inoculation, Tissot especially sought to convince women. Already in the early 1750s, he had perceived the new role women were being called to play in the ascendency of domestic economy which paralleled the male sphere of capital economy.[2] Throughout his career, Tissot propounded this new role for women and appealed to their rationality in order to enlist them in his program.

With his second subject, onanism, Tissot entered the arena of medicalization and secularization, at best transforming a sin into a malady to be cured, at worst introducing repression of sexuality and deviance into the medical discourse. Taken out of context by subsequent moralists, it seems that only the worst part of Tissot's argument persisted down to our time.[3] But the appraisal should not stop here; the question intellectual history should ask is: what was it in onanism that so fascinated the Enlightenment in its struggle for the unfettered pursuit of happiness? The eighteenth-century fixation with onanism, of which Tissot is only a much cited representative, rested on a deeper yearning for redefining sexual relations which was directly linked to the newly discovered affectionate family. Happiness was to be found there, in the intimacy of the home, away from the artificiality of public life, rather than in the individual alone. Onanism was a threat to conjugal love, either as solitary enjoyment or homosexual pleasure. This dimension of the fight is easily lost, because the nuclear family became the "norm" of the Victorian era and because domesticity (as unsophisticated home economics) is today looked upon with suspicion. For Tissot, onanism was an obstacle to equal partnership of men and women in the considerate family; a partnership meant to liberate both from the shackles of tradition. Perhaps because his own marriage, at first, was not without tensions, he was better able to feel the under-currents of the fight against masturbation. Onanism is a flagrant example of the stresses of the era. It created an imbalance, a clash—which still baffles— between priorities in the Enlightenment.

Physicians, population theorists, and governmental agencies had, in the second half of the eighteenth century, declared a renewed war of decrees upon charlatans and the superstitions on which they peddled their secret drugs.[4] Thus medical and political authorities hoped to expose and eradicate quackery, but these spokesmen of modern medicine too often failed to propose a viable substitute for the medical deeds of the quacks or the "disgusting" folklore of the medicine of the poor. Tissot participated in this effort with *Avis au peuple sur sa santé*, transcending not only the repressive edicts with a book which offered direct medical advice, but also with a call for action to the educated section of the population, and in particular women, to serve as dispensers of enlightened medical care. This call for responsibility toward health-care for the people by the elite was (in Tissot's plan) to offer the dual possibility of improving the understanding of hygienic rules and medical treatment, for the elite who dispensed the care as well as for the people who received it. Tissot expanded on this theme of education, so dear to his time and so close to his faith, in *De la santé des gens de lettres* and *Essai sur les maladies des gens du monde*. Thereafter, Tissot denounced both idleness and credulity, and he offered in the medical sphere a radical—if not even revolutionary—chastisement of indulgence and selfishness, almost writing a class, the leisured arrogant well-to-do, out of the ranks of those who could be cured and, hence, who could be useful. Tissot associated decent health with a purposeful life and, later advocated good health as an unalienable right, as a

real property which enable its owner to earn a decent living. Therefore, Tissot challenged citizens and magistrates to provide, under
the direction of physicians, the right and fair environment for
everyone's health.

Tissot, in his stress on a healthy life as a purposeful life, was
particularly aware of the link between psyche and soma. Furthermore, his extensive use of the Galenic non-naturals in explaining
ills and health led him to consider "passions" as underlying causes
for nervous troubles. In *Traité des nerfs et de leurs maladies*, under
the heading of passions, Tissot took a hard look at polite expectations and conformity, and denounced the constraints a genteel
society was pressing on its female and male members alike, the
culprit behind many escapes into psychic disorders. Tissot advocated individual search and responsibility for one's happiness,
which included facing one's calling. His work was seminal for the
re-directing of much thought about insanity, hypochondria, and
hysteria.[5] *Traité des nerfs* stemmed directly from concerns for the
well-being of the whole person, anchored in the adequate understanding of the effects the non-naturals have on proper mental and
physical hygiene, and hence on health. Whether Tissot's recourse
to passions for explaining nervous diseases was prophetic or not is
a question raised by post-Freudian sensibilities; for him it was a
matter of using correctly all of the non-naturals to attain the best
possible health.

Within the main current of professionalization and education
that deeply marked Encyclopedist thought, Tissot takes his place in
the re-thinking of the training and task of the physician. His
formative book on the reform of medical studies, *Essai sur les
moyens de perfectionner les études de médecine*, addressed the
problem of educating a physician for the task, of replacing the
priest in a society evolving with its new dominant class — the secularized bourgeoisie, and of social critic and mentor to the political
authorities. Tissot's choice of the Magistracy for an essential role
in providing and insuring public health also disclosed his awareness
of the secularizing trend in society and his commitment to further
it. Tissot, in tune with the mood of his time, identified the hospital
as the starting point of medical reform. He envisioned transforming its purpose of poor-relief and occasional healing into the most
suitable means for the training of doctors and the curing of

patients. He insisted on the importance of extensive medical observation and experience in the education of physicians, well in step with the Neo-Hippocratism professed by the Montpellier School, his Alma Mater. His plan for bettering medical studies relied heavily on clinical training to provide physicians early in their careers with the unique experience of numerous bedside and *post mortem* case-studies. His influence was openly acknowledged by Pinel,[6] and implicitly by Frank, the master of assimilating the thoughts of others without proper attribution.

Tissot's published works record his contribution to the general re-consideration of medicine and medical care. In this general context, he made his distinctive contribution by challenging individuals to improve their health by a better understanding of hygiene under the guidance of a physician. His emphasis on the individual exemplifies the emerging mentality which called for intervention and education to replace apathy and ignorance. Tissot's call for reform of the hospital and for the clinical teaching of medicine was central to the preoccupations of the closing years of the Ancien Régime, to that drive to improve institutions which ultimately led to revolution in politics as well as in medicine.

Tissot's unpublished works reveal him to be even more attuned to the tensions of his age, torn between benevolent paternalism and challenging liberalism. Tissot restricted himself to the realm of medicine, indeed to a medicine which on the surface seemed old-fashioned in its extensive use of the humoral physiology model and of the Galenic non-naturals, but which in practice was intended as a powerful vehicle for introducing the lay public to the innovative tenets of the expectant medicine and to the newly introduced attitude of the vitalist thought of the Montpellier School.

Tissot hoped that the dispensing of appropriate medicine to all levels of society was to transform society and promote a social environment in which each life was to be respected and no life wasted by the caprice of the few. He envisioned a society in which good health was to be recognized as a natural right. Consequently, such a vision of the social contract led him towards the formulation of a social conception of health and health-care. He left the blueprint for such a liberal enterprise under the most paternalistic of titles: *De la police de la médecine.*

Tissot, in various published and unpublished treatises, inter-twined several existing lines of thought. Specifically, his combining Reformed faith, Neo-Hippocratism, vitalism, humoralism, theories of irritability and of fiber, with each reinforcing the others, produced quite an original and explosive result. The Reformed faith appealed to the Creation's purpose and to final causes. Neo-Hippocratism put forward bedside observation. Vitalism brought trust in Nature healing power. Humoralism combined with irritability and fiber theory prompted new experiments and under-standings. These lines of thought tended to emphasize hygiene over therapeutics, social justice and a fair society over absolute decrees.

Greek ethos and Reformed faith both called for a just society, which could not exist without insuring the health and happiness of all its members. From Hippocrates Tissot inherited: "Health is to the body what justice is to a righteous soul or to the city, result of an equilibrium at the same time as the cause of this equilibrium."[7] From the Bible he received the Decalogue stipulations for a just society and from Calvinism the responsibility of governments for the common good.[8] Tissot wedded these themes to his knowledge of medicine and moved forward to a new concept of social justice premised first on the individual right to the best possible health, second on comprehensive public health. In this perspective, it is only natural that Tissot looked at the individual as the focus of his medical concern: God through the Scriptures declared the worth of each individual, and the Enlightenment magnified individuality. However, individuals are not alone; they interact in society. God had given {wo}man a rule for a just society, and the Philosophes had also advocated a just society ordered by natural rights. Tissot, faithful to his religious upbringing and dedicated to enlighten, labored in the field where he was best qualified —medicine and public health.

Tissot, in his march toward a social conception of health, took two logical leaps from his usual way of dealing with medical matters. First, in the same way that he had merged the individual into the group to extend the reach of medical care and hygiene, he considered the different groups within the whole of society and he translated private hygiene into public hygiene. One group alone could neither starve nor thrive without affecting the entire population. His second leap was to move out of the peculiarism of the Pays de Vaud or Pavia to the world-at-large in order to define rules and plans that were to befit a universal mold.

The same concern for service, compassion, and especially for education, which informed his writings on the health of the individual, permeated his studies of medical matters in the public sphere. The new physician, whose training Tissot had addressed in his book on medical studies, had now to expand his services from what might be called a "directeur de conscience" into the role of a social critic and a reformer of the state apparatus, to be consulted in all questions of health, hygiene, city-planning, and public well-being.

Tissot had portrayed one of the roles of his new physician as that of teaching individuals to listen to their body's signs of health or disease in order to establish a partnership between patients and doctor. Now he promoted a further development that carried far-reaching implications. His new physician was to become the mentor of the political authorities, to educate them to read in the environment and in the weaknesses of the population the deeds of pollution, contagion, and malnutrition, and to instruct them on how to prevent or counteract the unhealthy results of societal life.

If Tissot's motivations derived from his Calvinist background, they also meshed tightly with eighteenth-century ideologies of reason, reform, and education. From Calvin's *Institutes* Tissot drew his justification for his physician to be the conscience of the Magistracy in matters of health.[9] The Encyclopedist movement gave him the secular support to advocate rationality in the use of all resources for the commonweal.

The beginning physician, who with youthful ardor reached out to women for persuading them of the usefulness of inoculation, aimed in his maturity at implementing a social conception of health to which the political authorities were to be alerted as the representatives of the public's concerns with the general good. His social conception of health, which encompassed private and public contributions, pointed to a democratization of health care and medicine. Tissot's liberated hospital was the embodiment of this conception of a hospital open to all, from poor to wealthy, with patient and physician embarking together on the road to recovery and discovery of the true meaning of health.

Thus, Tissot pertinently echoes and exemplifies the "tournant des mentalités" in his call for action, education, partnership, and responsibility of each member of society to bring forth a new and better state of affairs in his or her own field of expertise. He lent his voice to the chorus of medical reformers. He tried to the best of his abilities and in conformity with his conscience to fulfill his calling in the realm of medicine. However, when political happenings and his own declining health robbed him of the stamina to pursue, he took heart from the fact that he was but one worker in the field, for others shared his vision of reform. Always driven by the desire to serve the common good, Tissot left us a vivid picture of what hope arising from a changed mentality can try to accomplish for the pursuit of happiness through a healthier life.

Notes

Preface

1 Miller (1957): 205.

Introduction

1 Staum (1980): in particular, Chaps. 1-6.

2 *Dix-huitième siècle 9* (1977) "Le sain et le malsain".

3 Chaussinand-Nogaret (1985); Groethuysen (1927).

4 *Avis au peuple sur sa santé.* Lausanne: Grasset, 1761; *De la santé des gens de lettres.* Lausanne: Grasset, 1768; *Essai sur les maladies des gens du monde.* Lausanne: Grasset, 1770.

5 *Des maladies des femmes*; *Des maladies et de l'éducation physique des petits enfants* in PP-BCU-L.

6 *Essai sur les moyens de perfectionner les études de médecine.* Lausanne: Grasset, 1785; *De la médecine civile* in PP-BCU-L.

7 Kuhn (1977): chapter 3 for details on Pascal's thought experiment.

8 Fox-Genovese (1976).

9 Bernoulli, D. "Essai d'une nouvelle analyse" in *Histoire de l'Académie royale des sciences*, année MDCCLX: 1-45.

10 *L'Onanisme.* Lausanne: Grasset, 1758.

11 This is the view of Tissot given in standard textbooks in the history of medicine and based on reading only *Avis au peuple sur sa santé*, e.g. Rosen (1958). This attitude can be traced back to Goethe: *Aus mein Leben, Dichtung und Wahrheit* in *Samtliche Werke*, Bd 10 Zurich: Artemis, 1950: 305. Johann Wolfgang von Goethe (1749-1832), German writer.

12 see Tissot's definition of a country surgeon in *Essai sur les moyens de perfectionner les études de médecine* and compare with the officier de santé of Consulate France.

13 Hoffmann (1977); also the reprintings of *Onanisme* in 1980 and 1991; and of *De la santé des gens de lettres* in 1981 and 1991; each time with scholarly introductions.

14 Frank (1779-1817), English edition (1976). Johann-Peter Frank (1745-1821), German physician.

15 Greenbaum (1971, 1972, 1973, 1974, and 1976).

Chapter I

1 Uri, Schwyz, and Unterwald: the three founding states of Switzerland. For a history of Switzerland see: Martin (1971). 1536, year of adoption of the Reformation in Geneva by a vote of the Conseil Général, composed of all adult male citizens.

2 See the article about Switzerland in the Table analytique et raisonnée des matières de l'*Encyclopédie*. Paris: Panckouke, 1770, tome second: 719.

3 For an appraisal of eighteenth-century Switzerland's cultural achievement, consult: Sorell (1972) or Muller (1837-1851).

4 See also Durand (1973).

5 Gay (1971): 65-89. This is a good, succinct description of the political situation in Geneva in the eighteenth century. See also: Palmer (1959): vol I, Chapt. 5.

6 Guillaume Farel (1489-1565), French Reformer; Pierre Viret (1511-1571), Swiss Reformer. For a history of the conquest by Bern, see: Gilliard (1935).

7 Eynard: *Essai sur la vie de Tissot* (Lausanne: Ducloux, 1839): 10. Charles Eynard (1808-1876), a Swiss writer, used Tissot's personal papers and conversations with Tissot's nephew Marc d'Apples to document his study. His account is largely biographical, with some appraisal of Tissot's achievements but with no interpretation of the medical or intellectual significance of Tissot's written works, especially the unpublished material. He often quoted from Tissot's father "livre de raison", now unfortunately lost.
Tissot is often mistakenly first-named Simon-André.

8 Leith (1977): 72.

9 Monter (1976).

10 Charles Bonnet (1720-1793), naturalist and philosopher; Jean-Louis Calandrini (1703-1758), mathematician; Jean Jalabert (1712-1768), physicist; Horace-Bénédict de Saussure (1740-1799), geologist; Augustin-Pyramus de Candolle (1778-1841), botanist; Gabriel Cramer (1704-1752), mathematician; — all of Geneva. Tissot wrote in his *Lettre à M. Zimmermann*: "...ayant été disciple de deux grands mathématiciens, MM. Calendrini (sic) et Cramer,

dont on doit chérir à jamais la mémoire..." in *Oeuvres complètes* (1807): tome 4, 192.

11 Eynard (1839): 14.

12 PP-BCU-L Q120/69.

13 Tissot to Zimmermann, letter dated 21 February 1758, Johann-Georg Zimmermann (1728-1795), Swiss physician, student of Haller, established at the court of Hanover. Albrecht von Haller or Albert de Haller (1708-1777), Swiss physiologist and poet. Original letters of Zimmermann to Tissot in Bern; Original letters of Tissot to Zimmermann in Hanover. For more details on Zimmermann, see Bouvier (1925) or Ackerknecht (1978).

14 Dewhurst (1966): 36. Thomas Sydenham (1624-1689), English physician.

15 For example, in *Lettre à M. Haller* in *Oeuvres complètes*, (1807): tome 4, 204.

16 Théophile de Bordeu (1722-1776), French physician and a member of the Encyclopedists' circle; one of the proponants of vitalism. See: *Correspondance de Bordeu.* (Fletcher ed. 1978); also: Benoit (1862).

17 François Boissier de Sauvages de la Croix (1706-1767), French physician and botanist. For the importance of Sauvages, see: King (1966); or Dulieu (1969).

18 Tissot to Zimmermann, letter dated 21 February 1758.

19 in FE-BPU-G.

20 O'Malley (1970): 89; Garrison (1960): 198. François Rabelais (1490-1553), French physician and writer.

21 Astruc: *Mémoires pour servir à l'histoire de la Faculté de Médecine de Montpellier* (1767); or Delmas (1929). Jean Astruc (1684-1766), French physician.

22 Guillaume Rondelet (1507-1566), French surgeon.

23 Gelfand (1982); Imbault-Huard (1973).

24 Hermann Boerhaave (1668-1738), Dutch physician; François de la Boë or Sylvius (1616-1672), French Huguenot physician. See: Lindenboom (1968); O'Malley (1970): 257 & 223; and Risse (1989). The twelve-bed model for clinical teaching is as much emulation of the six-men-and six-women-bed wards of Boerhaave as it is traditional use of the dozen.

25 These combinations of surgery/pharmacy and anatomy/botany might seem a little strange, but they are due to the adaptation of the curriculum to the seasons. Surgery and anatomy were taught in the fall, pharmacy and botany in the spring.

26 Castan (1878).

27 Tissot to Zimmermann, letter dated 21 February 1758. "En 7bre 1745, j'allais à Montpellier, c'est la période la plus triste de ma vie. Une université composée de Professeurs ignorants et mercenaires, pas un homme de génie, pas une leçon intéressante, point d'émulation, point de goût pour les sciences, voilà l'état où était l'université. Rien ne pouvait intéresser un étudiant qui sortait d'une académie si différente et une foule de compagnons livrés au plaisir ne pouvaient qu'entrainer un jeune homme de 17 ans, aussi je fus entrainé."

28 Eynard (1839): 17.

29 Eynard (1839): 241-242. After the reprimand for lavish entertaining, Colonel Tissot-Grenus moved to Geneva and dissipated a large part of his own fortune on unworthy friends and lawsuits. Hallé, in his edition of the *Oeuvres complètes de Monsieur Tissot*, has some enigmatic words about a member of Tissot's family in need of money, for whom he (Hallé) is giving up part of the revenue from that edition. Could it have been the unpecunious Colonel? Or was it Clément Joseph Tissot (1750-1826), a French surgeon-physician, who took advantage of S.A.A.D. Tissot's fame and claimed to be one of his relatives, a claim that was only a boast. C.J. Tissot tried all kinds of schemes to make money, including asking the Treasurer of the restored Bourbon King for arrears owed for his services to the revolutionary armies. (I owe this last information to Dr. Samuel X. Radbill, who owned the original letter of C.J. Tissot.)

30 Tissot to Zimmermann, letter dated 21 February 1758.

31 Gerald Fitzgerald (died 1748), probably of Catholic Scottish descent.

32 Germain (1879).

33 See below, Chapter XII.

34 Delauney (1935): 95.

35 Eynard (1839): 19.

36 Tissot to Zimmermann, letter dated 21 Novembre 1794 and his *Traité de l'étisie*, PP-BCU-L: Q120/I46: 345-352.

37 Rosen (1975) and Brunnert (1984).

38 Starobinski (1961) and (1962).

39 *Encyclopédie*: volume VIII: 120a and Suppl IV: 60a.

40 Starobinski (1963).

41 Tissot: *Oeuvres complètes*, (1807): vol. 4, 189: "...les végétaux ont aussi leur nostalgie (que nos adversaires en prennent occasion, s'ils le veulent de

ridiculiser les Suisses)..." For the Swiss as more prone than others to nostalgia, see: Gusdorf (1976).

42 Tissot: *Oeuvres complètes*. (1807): vol. 4, 409: "Etant de retour dans ma patrie, en 1749, je trouvai que ma mère, que je chérissais, et qui était d'une constitution délicate et mobile, était incommodée de plusieurs symptômes qui faisaient craindre avec raison une hydropisie prochaine: mais il faut reprendre de loin, et dès les commencements, l'histoire de cette maladie. D'autres médecins, voulant y remédier, avaient déjà conseillé depuis longtemps des purgations fréquentes, et des infusions en guise de thé à prendre plusieurs fois par jour; mais tout cela n'avait réussi qu'à faire empirer le mal de jour en jour. Je proscrivis sans retour l'un et l'autre de ces remèdes, et je prescrivis des pillules anti-hystériques à prendre régulièrement deux fois par année [sic] pendant quelques semaines: je suis ainsi parvenu, grâce à l'Etre Suprême, à rendre la santé à ma mère, en sorte qu'elle en jouit encore actuellement (10 mai 1761) autant que sa constitution peut le permettre et sans avoir rien à craindre de l'hydropisie; danger qui a cessé en même temps que l'usage des purgatifs." This may seem like a very long quotation for the purpose, but it so well exemplifies Tissot's style that it seemed a pity to cut it short.

Chapter II

1 See Chapter I, note 14.

2 Théodore Tronchin (1703-1781), Genevan physician; see: Tronchin (1906).

3 Eynard (1839): 29-30; the original letters are in FE-BPU-G.

4 see below, this chapter; also Emch-Dériaz (1982).

5 See Chapter I, notes 40 and 41.

6 Olivier (1962).

7 See the "autobiography of J.P. Frank" translated by George Rosen (1948); see also: Russell (1981).

8 Dupont de Nemours in *Idées sur les secours à donner aux pauvres malades dans une grande ville*, handwritten copy at Euletherian Mills Historical Library (document W2 4682): 16-17 and also published in Philadelphia in 1786; see also Fox-Genovese (1984). Pierre-Samuel Dupont de Nemours (1739-1817), French publicist, political and economist theorist.

9 "Quand on n'a pas vu soi-même de malades, il n'est pas aisé de dire quelque chose d'exact, même en copiant de bons auteurs." Sauvages to Tissot in 1751. Eynard: (1839): 20; the original letter is in FE-BPU-G.

10 François Marie Arouet de Voltaire (1694-1778), French writer and philosopher. For more details, see: Mason (1981).

11 Edward Gibbon (1737-1794), British historian. For more details, see: Craddock (1982) and (1988).

12 See: Sévery (1911) and Morren (1970).

13 Charlotte d'Apples (1724-1797).

14 Tissot to Zimmermann, letter dated 10 December 1754.

15 Tissot to Zimmermann, letter dated 26 December, 1758.

16 Suzanne Curchod (1739-1794); Jacques Necker (1732-1804), Genevan banker and Comptroller of Finances to Louis XVI. See: Harris (1979) and (1986).

17 The original letters are in FE-BPU-G.

18 *Avis au peuple sur sa santé in Oeuvres complètes* (1803-1807): vol. 2, 179.

19 See below, Chapter IV.

20 Emch-Dériaz (1985); also Minder-Chappuis (1974). The original letters from Tissot to Haller are in Bern.

21 Emch-Dériaz (1982). Charles Marie de La Condamine (1701-1774), French mathematician. The original letters are in FE-BPU-G.

22 Matthieu Maty (1718-1776), Huguenot physician, settled in London and editor of the *Journal Britannique*. See: Janssens (1981).

23 John Pringle (1707-1782), Scottish physician, student of Boerhaave, first physician to the King of England; James Kirkpatrick (1696-1770), English physician, practiced first in the Thirteen Colonies, then in England; George Baker (1722-1808), English physician, first physician to the King and Queen of England. All of their original letters are in FE-BPU-G.

24 Maty to Tissot, letter dated 29 May 1760 in FE-BPU-G.

25 Anton de Haen (1704-1776), Dutch physician, student of Boerhaave, famous clinician established in Vienna, councillor to the Emperess Maria-Theresa; Count Francesco Parolino de Roncalli (1692-1763), Italian surgeon. Their original letters are in FE-BPU-G.

26 Emch-Dériaz (1986).

27 Jean-Antoine Butini (1723-1810), Genevan physician; Charles Chais (1701-1788) Huguenot minister, refugee in Holland.

28 Voltaire: *Letters Concerning the English Nation*. London, 1733 or *Lettres philosophiques*, 1734.

29 Tissot to Haller, letter dated 22 February 1754 in Minder-Chappuis (1974): 15-17.

30 Haller to Tissot, letter dated 24 March 1754 in Minder-Chappuis (1974): 18 and Hintzsche (1977): 26.

31 *Encyclopédie*: Vol. VIII, 755-771.

32 Tronchin to Tissot, letter dated 4 May 1759, in FE-BPU-G.

33 Voltaire to Tissot, letter dated 22 March 1755, signed Le malade Voltaire in FE-BPU-G.

34 La Condamine to Tissot, letter dated 6 January 1760.

35 La Condamine to Tissot, letter dated 2 June 1762. Jean Le Rond d'Alembert (1717-1783), French mathematician; Daniel Bernoulli (1700-1782), Swiss mathematician, "Essay d'une nouvelle analyse" in *Histoire de l'Académie des sciences*, année MDCCLX. See Bradley (1971) or Daston (1988): 83-86 for the controversy and Wilson (1972): Vol. I, 432 for the attitude of d'Alembert at the Académie royale des sciences, vis-à-vis La Condamine.

36 King (1976): 1205.

37 Robert Sutton (1707-1788) and his son Daniel (1735-1819); Thomas Dimsdale (1712-1800); William Watson (1715-1787); to name only a few. For more details, consult: Klebs (1913): 69-83 and 1914.

38 See below chapter V.

39 Eynard (1839): 27.

40 Edward Jenner (1749-1823), British physician. For the history of inoculation and vaccination, see Baxby (1981) or Darmon (1986).

Chapter III

1 Bilious fever = typhoid fever or petechial typhus.

2 Tissot to Zimmermann, letter dated 10 December 1754.

3 Eynard (1839): 34. Since the Reformation, divorce had been legal in Lausanne.

4 Eynard (1839): 35 and Tissot to Zimmermann, letter dated 6 Septembre 1755. "C'est que d'un *médecin galant* j'ai fait un mari tendre dans le mois de juillet dernier."

5 *De la santé des gens de lettres* (1768): 91.

6 PP-BCU-L Q120/71.

7 To Tissot, ancient medicine meant anything written in the ante-Harvey era. William Harvey (1578-1657), British physician; Galen (c. 130-200 AD), Graeco-Roman physician; Hippocrates (c. 460-377 or 359 BC), Greek physician; the School of Salermo most famed book is the *Regimen Sanitatis Salernitanum*, a manuscript dating from the twelfth century, the School most flourishing period; Julius Caesar (100 or 102-44 BC), Roman writer, military officer, and emperor; Homer (c. 850-800 BC), Greek writer; Lucretius (c. 99-55 BC), Roman writer; Tacitus (c. 55-120 AD), Roman historian; Virgil (70-19 BC), Roman writer.

8 Alexander Monro Primus (1697-1767), Alexander Monro Secondus (1733-1817), Alexander Monro Tertius (1773-1859), Donald Monro (1727-1802), John Monro (1715-1791), Percival Pott (1714-1788), all British physicians.

9 For example, in English: Aiken (1786); Amstrong 1767); Bribane (1769); Bubillard (1767); Fothergil (1783); Home (1762); Mead (1773); Pemberton (1771); Stephen (1791); Whyte (1767) and in Italian: Algarotti (1764); Basetti (1786); Marcheroni (1793); Razori (1793); Rezia (1784); Volta (1788).

10 Marc d'Apples (1760-1840), Swiss physician, Tissot's nephew; see below chapter VI.

11 Howard: *The State of Prisons in England and Wales* (London: 1777) and *An Account of the Principal Lazarettos in Europe* (London 1780); Tenon: *Mémoires sur les Hôpitaux de Paris.* (Paris: 1788); Poyet: *Mémoire sur la nécessité de transfèrer et de reconstruire l'Hôtel-Dieu de Paris.* (Paris: 1785); Frank: *A System of Complete Medical Police* (English Translation Baltimore: 1976; German edition 1779-1821); Tissot owned its 1786 Italian translation. John Howard (1726-1790), British philanthropist; Jacques Tenon (1724-1816), French surgeon; Bernard Poyet (1742-1824), French architect.

12 Antoine de Lavoisier (1743-1794) French chemist; Joseph Priestley (1733-1804), British Presbyterian minister and chemist; Carl Wilhelm Scheele (1742-1786), Swedish chemist. For more on Lavoisier, see Guerlac (1975) or Duveen and Klickstein (1955).

13 Philippe Peu (died 1707), French physician; William Cadogan (1711-1797), British physician; Jean-Louis Fourcroy de Guillerville (1717-1799), French publicist; Jean-Jacques Rousseau (1712-1778), Genevan writer.

14 Pierre-Samuel Dupont de Nemours, editor of François Quesnay: *Physiocratie ou Constitution naturelle du gouvernement le plus avantageux au genre humain.* Leyden, Paris: Merlin, 1768. François Quesnay (1694-1774), French royal surgeon and economist.

15 Tissot: *De morbis ex usu secalis cornuti ad illustrem Baker.* London: Philosophical Transactions, 1765. Baker wrote on inoculation and lead poisoning.

His famous work of 1767 on the Devonshire Distemper is a model of detective medical inquiry.

16 *Tissot: Avis au peuple sur sa santé.* Lausanne: Zimmerli pour Grasset, 1761; see below chapter V.

17 Benjamin Rush (1745-1813), American politician and physician.

18 Benjamin Franklin (1706-1790), American statesman and scientist.

19 Samuel von Puffendorf (1632-1694), German jurist; Jean-Jacques Burlamaqui (1694-1748), Genevan political theorist; John Locke (1632-1704), British philosopher and physician; David Hume (1711-1776), British philosopher and historian; Charles Bonnet (1720-1793), Genevan philosopher and naturalist: *Réponses sur l'Amérique.* (Lausanne: 1795).

20 William Paley (1743-1805), British theologian.

21 Charles Maurice de Talleyrand-Périgord (1754-1838), French bishop, politician and diplomat.

22 Balthazar Louis Tralles (1707-1797), German physician; personal physician to the King of Poland Stanislas Augustus Poniatowski (1732-1798) after Tissot declined the post; see below chapter V.

23 *Courrier Suisse*, 2 décembre 1842; *Nouvelles vaudoises*, 3 janvier, 1843.

24 *Dissertatio de febricus biliosis, anni 1755.* Lausanne: Bousquet, 1758.

25 Emch-Dériaz (1988).

26 see below, Chapter XI,

27 Eynard (1839): 202 and 214.

28 Tissot to Zimmermann, letter dated 6 September 1755. The French adjective "habituel" is here to be understood as meaning "that which has turned into a habit", Gattel: *Dictionnaire universel de la langue française* Lyon: 1819

29 Tissot to Zimmermann, letter dated 14 July 1756.

30 See below, Chapter VII and Appendix II: 333.

31 *Discours préliminaire du traducteur de la Dissertation sur les parties irritables et sensibles des animaux par M. de Haller.* Lausanne: Bousquet, 1755.

32 see Appendix II: 323-324.

33 *Dissertatio de febricus biliosis*: 269.

34 *Dissertatio de febricus biliosis*: 197.

35 PP-BCU-L Q120/130.2 and Emch-Dériaz (1982): 71.

36 *Lettre à M. de Haen en réponse à ses questions sur l'inoculation.* Lausanne: Grasset, 1759; *De variolarum inoculatione ad illustrissimo Roncalli.* Lausanne: Grasset, 1759; *Observationes de Colica saturnina.* Bern: Haller, 1759; *Zimmermanno epistola, de morbo nigro.* Lausanne: Grasset, 1760; *Alberto Hallero epistola, apoplexia e hydrope.* Lausanne: Grasset, 1761; *Lettre à M. Hirzel sur quelques critiques de M. de Haen.* Lausanne: Grasset, 1762; *De morbis ex usu secalis cornuti ad illustrem Baker.* London: Philosophical Transsactions, 1765; *Lettre à M. Zimmermann sur l'épidemie courante.* Lausanne: Grasset, 1765; *Seconde lettre à M. Zimmermann sur l'épidemie de 1766.* Lausanne: Grasset, 1766. Gaspard Hirzel (1725-1803), Swiss physician.

37 Julien Offray de La Mettrie (1709-1751), French physician and philosopher.

38 Haller to Tissot, letter dated 12 June 1756 in Hintzsche (1977): 52.

Chapter IV

1 see Appendix II: 324-326.

2 Flandrin (1976); Leroy-Ladurie (1977): 3e partie.

3 Biéler (1963) and Fuchs (1979).

4 Père Féline. *Cathéchisme des gens mariés.* Caens, 1782; See: I Cor. 7: 3-5; Flandrin (1970) and Lebrun (1975).

5 Tissot to Rousseau, letter dated 8 July 1762; Tissot to Zimmermann, letter dated 14 November 1764.

6 which is not the reading of Jordanava (1987).

7 Edition Le Sycomore, Paris (1980).

8 There is a vast scholarly literature from which the followings are only a sample: Ariès and Bejin (1985); Bullough (1976), (1981), & (1987); *Eighteenth-Century-Life* (3/1985); *Dix-huitième siècle* (1980); Engelhard (1974); Fishman (1982); Foucault (1976) & (1987); Gay (1980); Goulémot (1980); Hare (1962); Jordanava (1987); MacCubbin (1987); McDonald (1967); Rosenberg (1975): Part I, Chapter 3; Rousseau and Porter (1988); Stengers et van Neck (1984); Tarczylo (1980),(1983) & (1983).

9 Tarczylo (1983) and Flandrin (1981).

10 *Avis au peuple sur sa santé.* Lausanne: 1761: 144.

11 Tissot to Zimmermann, letter dated 12 September 1758.

12 Boisseau, François-Gabriel. "Notice sur l'auteur" in *De la santé des gens de lettres.* Paris: Baillière, 1826: iij. "Il mourût célibataire..."

13   Sévery (1911), (1925), & (1928).

14   Bonnard (1945): 60.

15   de Morsier (1965): 21.

16   Boys were to sleep with their hands outside their covers in a French boarding school in the late 1940s and still in the mid 1950s Catholic Youth organizations promoted the idea of the wasting of the body through masturbation.

17   *Encyclopédie*. vol. XII: 922.

18   *Encyclopédie*. vol. X: 51.

19   Traer (1980); Mitterauer and Reinhard (1982).

20   PP-BCU-L Q120/144.

21   Tissot to Zimmermann, letter dated 30 May 1768.

22   FE-BPU-G, in his old age, La Condamine had become deaf. PP-BCU-L Q120/12: Des maladies des oreilles.

23   *Onanisme*. Lausanne: Grasset, 1788: XVI & XVII.

24   MacCubbin (1987): 122-131 and 179-191.

25   Charlton (1984): chapters 7 & 8.

26   Ariès and Bejin (1985): chapter 3.

27   Azouvi (1981): 22-36.

28   Rey in MacCubbin (1987).

29   *Onanism*. New York: Collins & Hannay, 1832: 51.

30   *Onanism*. (1832): 30.

Chapter V

1   *Avis au peuple sur sa santé*. (1761); *De la santé des gens de lettres*. (1768); *Essai sur les maladies des gens du monde*. (1770); *Des maladies des femmes*. PP-BCU-L Q120/47 *De l'éducation physique et des maladies des petits enfants*. PP-BCU-L Q120/49 or /122.

2   Emch-Dériaz (1992).

3   See below Chapter X and XI.

4   *De la santé des gens de lettres* (1768): 117.

5   Tarczylo in Preface to *Onanisme* & (1983); Benaroyo (1988); Jolivet (1980); Olivier (1928): 259ff; Azouvi in 1981 Preface to *De la santé des gens de lettres*; Calame in 1991 Preface to *De la santé des gens de lettres*; Daremberg (1865): 353-396; Godoumêche (1974); Saisselin (1979): 140-143; Bucher (1958).

6   The English translation of titles is even more revealing: *Advice to the People in General with Respect to Their Health; An Essay on Diseases Incident to Literary and Sedentary Persons; An Essay on the Disorders of People of Fashion.*

7   Ramazzini: *De morbis artificium diatriba.* Modena: 1700; Bernardino Ramazzini (1633-1714), Italian physician.

8   Biéler (1961) & in English (1964) and Graham (1971).

9   This idea can be founded in the writings of Francis Bacon (1561-1626), English philosopher, which are listed in the catalog of Tissot's library.

10 Hooykaas (1972): 40.

11 See Frank's *Medical Police* where he reported the fact and played the naive at not knowing why. Also see: Risse in Bell (1982).

12 Tissot. *Traité de la catalepsie.* Lausanne: Grasset, 1784; tome neuvième des oeuvres complètes de M. Tissot: 72. Harvey: *De motus cordi.* London: 1628. Tissot often wrote on the same subject that Hippocrates, for example: Hippocrates: *On the Sacred Disease* / Tissot: *Traité de l'épilepsie*; Hippocrates and Tissot: *On Regimen During Acute Illnesses.*

13 For opium, he succeeded; nevertheless, he still tended to abuse the prescription of quinine.

14 See: *Annales ESC.* (1977); *Dix-huitième siècle* (1980); Laget (1982); Mousnier (1975); Park (1976); Rosen (1958); Rosenberg (1983); Shryock (1974) (first edition 1936).

15 Tissot to Zimmermann, letter dated 14 March 1760.

16 PP-BCU-L Q120/130.3; see below: chapter X.

17 see Appendix II: 327-329.

18 See Eynard (1839): 77 and letters in FE-BPU-G.

19 Jean-Baptiste Senac (1693-1770), French physician; the letter is in FE-BPU-G.

20 See above, chapter I: notes 39 and 40.

21 Tissot to Haller, letter dated 22-24 July 1762 in Hintzsche (1977): 143.

22 Tissot to Zimmermann, letter dated 13 July 1762.

23 *Des maladies des femmes*. PP-BCU-Q120/66: 421.

24 François (1911), also Barth (1949): 123-133.

25 see below, Chapter VI.

26 see below, Chapter VI and FE-BPU-G.

27 Tissot to Haller, letter dated 4 February 1766 in Hintzsche (1977): 226.

28 *De la santé des gens de lettres* was re-edited in 1981 (facsimile of the 1768 edition) and 1991 (re-edition of the 1788 version). See Appendix II: 331-332.

29 see below, Chapter VI.

30 Leopold Auenbrugger (1722-1809), German physician; Giambattista Morgagni (1682-1771), Italian physician; for more details see: Garrison (1929): 352-354; Shryock (1936, 1974): 66; Lesky (1959); Ackerknecht (1968): 133-134; Reiser 1978: 18ff; Jarcho (1961).

31 Tissot to Zimmermann, letter dated 13 March 1761; *Avis au peuple sur sa santé*. Nancy: Leclerc, 1780: 92.

32 see below, chapter VIII.

33 *Lettre à M. Haller* in Oeuvres de Tissot (1855): 624.

34 Yverdon: de Felice, 1779; 3 volumes.

35 Typical titles, but not an exhaustive list of them are: *Avis au public* (1763); *Avis sur le commerce des grains* (1764); *Avis aux mères qui veulent nourrir leurs enfants*, Le Rebours (1767); *Avis au peuple sur son premier besoin*, Baudeau (1768); *Avis aux honnêtes gens qui veulent faire le bien*, Baudeau (1768); *Avis au peuple concernant le parlement* (1787); *Avis au public, surtout le Tiers-Etat, surtout l'armée*, Servan (1790); Nicolas Baudeau (1730-1792), French political economist; Marie Angélique Anel Le Rebours (1731-1821), French midwife; Joseph Michel de Servan (1737-1807), French politician.

36 Gay (1969): Vol. II, Chap. 1.

37 Braudel (1981): vol. I, 70-92, 108-145, and 163-172.

38 Fohlen (1971): 125.

39 Chevallaz (1949).

40 Mathias (1969): 76ff.

41 For quinine, see: Dousset (1985): 161; McGrew (1985): 298; first mention of Peruvian bark, Jesuit bark, or cinchona, in 1643 by Heyden in "Discours et

avis sur les flus de ventre douloureux"; inoculation was introduced in Western Europe around 1720, Miller (1981): 2-16; Herman van der Heyden (1572-1650), Flemish physician.

42 Ackerknecht (1982); Chap. 11; Reiser (1978): Chap. 1; Shryock (1936, 1974): Chap. IV.

43 Riley (1987).

44 *Avis au peuple sur sa santé* (1761): 13-14.

45 Coleman (1977).

46 Spengler (1954): 311 on Rousseau and Linguet; Simon Nicolas Linguet (1736-1794), French writer, for more details, see Levy (1980).

47 Lawrence (1975); Rosenberg (1983). Buchan: *Domestic Medicine*. Edinburgh: 1769; Gunn, John C.: *Domestic Medicine*. Knoxville, TN: 1830.

48 Coleman (1974).

49 *Essai sur les maladies des gens du monde* (1770): 35.

50 Spengler (1942); Rosen (1976).

51 *Avis au peuple sur sa santé* (1761): 21 & 25; see also *Missionscope* 6 (8) (1982): "pastor to combine duties with medicine" for the persistance of the idea (and the need).

52 *Avis au peuple sur sa santé* (1761): 27.

53 *Avis au peuple sur sa santé* (1761): 24.

54 *Avis au peuple sur sa santé* (1761): 516.

55 *Avis au peuple sur sa santé* (1761): 23.

56 Sévery (1928): 139.

57 *Avis au peuple sur sa santé* (1761): 511.

58 *Avis au peuple sur sa santé* (1761): 507.

59 *Avis au peuple sur sa santé* (1761): 13.

60 *Avis au peuple sur sa santé* (1761): 518.

61 *Essai sur les maladies des gens du monde* (1770): 11-13.

62 *Avis au peuple sur sa santé* (1761): 511.

63 *De la santé des gens de lettres* (1768): 71.

64 *De la santé des gens de lettres* (1768): 241-242.

65 Shryock (1974): 189.

66 *An Essay on the disorders of People of Fashion.* translated by Francis Bacon Lee. London: Richardson and Urquhart, 1771: vi.

67 *Essai sur les maladies des gens du monde* (1770): 125.

68 *Essai sur les maladies des gens du monde* (1770): 123.

69 see Appendix II: 332.

70 *Essai sur les maladies des gens du monde* (1770): 1.

71 *Essai sur les maladies des gens du monde* (1770): 121.

72 *De la santé des gens de lettres* (1758): 139, 141, 142.

73 Rousseau and Mirabeau among others shared the same vision; Victor Riqueti, Marquis de Mirabeau (1715-1789), French political economist.

74 *Essai sur les maladies des gens du monde* (1770): 45.

75 FE-BPU-G Madame Necker to Tissot, Paris 10 March 1773.

76 *Essai sur les maladies des gens du monde* (1770): 38. Tissot is denouncing a state of affairs others were also e.g. Montesquieu and Saint-Simon; Charles-Louis de Secondat, Baron de Montesquieu (1689-1755) French writer; Louis de Rouvroy, Duc de Saint-Simon (1675-1755), French writer.

77 *Essai sur les maladies des gens du monde* (1770): 126. *De la santé des gens de lettres* (1758): 238-239.

78 *Essai sur les maladies des gens du monde* (1770): 127.

79 Emch-Dériaz (1992).

80 see below chapter XII.

81 Tronchin (1906): Chap. 2.

82 Tronchin dixit, February 1778; cited in Braudel (1981): Vol. 2, 234; Miller (1957): 205.

83 Daremberg (1865): 352-396; Charles Daremberg (1817-1872), French physician and critic.

84 reforms of the grain trade, of the royal finances, of parlements and representatives bodies in the decades prior to the French Revolution by Turgot, Malesherbes, Necker; Chrétien-Guillaume de Lamoignon de Malesherbes (1721-1794), French stateman; Jacques Turgot (1727-1781), French economist and royal minister.

85 Tissot to Zimmermann, letter dated 2 April 1763.

86 PP-PBU-L,Q120/144; Bonnet to Tissot, letter dated 12 June 1769 in FE-BPU-G.

87 Daremberg (1865): 383.

88 Daremberg (1865): 359 and 379, note 1; 386, Brigham, A.: *Remarks on the Influence of Mental Cultivation and Mental Excitement upon Health.* London: 1844.

89 Claude Bernard (1813-1878), French physiologist.

90 On the health of children, see: *Avis au peuple sur sa santé* (1761): 384-404; *De la santé des gens de lettres* (1768): 107-122; *Essai sur les maladies des gens du monde* (1770): 135-147; on the health of women, see: *Avis au peuple sur sa santé* (1761): 364-383. The manuscripts are: *De l'éducation physique et des maladies des petits enfants.* Q120/49 is a copy with notes by Tissot; Q120/122 is the manuscript in Tissot's hand, and it is 345 pages long, all references will be to this copy; *Traité des maladies des femmes* PP-BCU-L Q120/47bis in Tissot's hand; PP-BCU-L Q120/47 is a copy with additions in Tissot's hand, 975 sheets in 5 volumes, all references will be to this copy.

91 Ariès (1973); Flandrin (1976) & (1981); Hunt (1970); MacFarlane (1985); Ozment (1983); Pollock (1983); Shorter (1975); Stone (1977).

92 Abt and Garrison (1923); Ackerknecht (1967); Ulmann (1967); Still (1931); Teysseire (1982); and Bloch (1974).

93 Cadogan: *An Essay upon Nursing and the Management of Children* (1748); Brouzet: *Essai sur l'éducation médicale des enfants* (1754); Des Essartz: *Traité de l'éducation corporelle des enfants en bas-âge ou réflexions pratiques sur les moyens de procurer une meilleure constitution aux citoyens* (1760); Ballexserd: *Dissertation sur l'éducation physique des enfants* (1762); Rousseau: *Emile* (1762); Raulin: *De la conservation des enfants* (1763); Le Rebours: *Avis aux mères qui veulent nourrir leurs enfants* (1765); Fourcroy de Guillerville: *Les enfants élevés dans l'ordre de la nature* (1774); Venel: *De l'éducation des filles destinées au mariage* (1784); Jacques Ballexserd (1726-1774) Genevan physician, for more details see Morsier (1974); Jean-Charles Des Essartz (1729-1811), French physician; Joseph Raulin (1708-1784), French physician; Jean-André Venel (1740-1791) Swiss physician and pioneer in orthopedy, see Olivier in Saudan (1987).

94 Rosen (1974): 163; Garrison (1960): 273; Edmond Halley (1656-1742), English astronomer and mathematician; Sir William Petty (1623-1687), English economist.

95 This view of demographical trends was soon to be reversed: from depopulation, the concerns shifted to over-population already by the nineteenth century; see e.g. Malthus: *Essay on the Principle of Population as it Affects the Future Improvements of Society* (1798); see Flinn (1981) and Post (1985).

Thomas Robert Malthus (1766-1834), English economist and demographer, best known for his remark that population increases faster than the means of subsistence.

96 Abt and Garrison (1965): 37.

97 Shryock (1936, 1974): 136; Darmon (1986): 1ere partie; Emch-Dériaz (1982 & 1985); paediatrics is a 19th-c. word.

98 Flandrin (1976): 217ff; also Bergues (1960); Fox and Quitt (1980); McLaren (1985).

99 Tissot to Zimmermann letter dated 20 April 1768.

100 Ulmann (1967): 29.

101 Q120/122: 224; Michael Ettmüller (1644-1683), German physician.

102 For *De la médecine civile*, see below Chapter XII; and for the *Traité des maladies des femmes*, below this chapter.

103 Q120/122: 93.

104 The Lausanne Collège de Médecine was founded in 1787, see below, chapters IX and X.

105 Q120/122: 2; 301; 282; 307; 333   Buchan: *Domestic Medicine* (1769); Catogan: *An Essay upon Nursing and the Management of Children* (1748); Hunter: *Treatise on the diseases of the teeth* (1778) or *Lettres sur les preuves de l'infanticide* (1786); Journal encyclopédique 1784, one example among many; William Hunter (1718-1783), Scottish anatomist and obstetrician; John Hunter (1728-1793), Scottish surgeon physiologist and surgeon.

106 Q120/122: 20.

107 Q120/122: 51.

108 Mercier (1961). Tissot had already written against the practice of swaddling cloth in *Avis* (1780): tome 2, 80.

109 Q120/122: 3. Locke: *Thoughts on Education* (1693).

110 Badinter (1980; Knibiehler & Fouquet (1980).

111 Flandrin (1976): 228 for a similar point about wives teaching their husband about infant welfare.

112 Q120/122: 155.

113 Q120/122: 5; Q120/49: 6; see note 93.

114 Professionalization was a serious issue in the late eighteenth century; it would become even more so in the nineteenth century. See the special issues of *Réflexions historiques* (1982); or Hamilton (1951).

115   Q120/122: 11ff.

116   Q120/122: 127 and 221.

117   Q120/122: 139.

118   Q120/122: 141.

119   Q120/122: 237.

120   Q120/122: 247; no wine nor meat until the child is inoculated when around five years old.

121   Q120/122: 121, 139, and 157.

122   see below this chapter and chapter XII.

123   Q120/122: 243.

124   Q120/122: 43; Rousseau wrote the same thing in *Emile*.

125   Sussmann (1982):   Chapter 2; Hufton (1975):   1-22; Fox-Genovese (1984): 17 and 113-115.

126   Q120/122: 211.

127   Q120/122: 201.

128   Sussmann (1982): 3.

129   Joubert: *Des erreurs populaires en médecine* (1587) is listed in the catalog of Tissot's Library; Laurent Joubert (1529-1583), French physician.

130   "Car le laict eschauffé d'une femme passionnée d'amour est pire de beaucoup et plus nuisant que celuy d'une femme enceinte...je ne donne point de conseil autres que je ne prenne pour moy." Joubert dixit.

131   Rosen (1976): 305. The "overlay" question should be re-examined in view of the evidences accumulated from the contemporary cribdeath occurrences.

132   Q120/122: 303.

133   Sussmann (1982):   77 and 93.   Different explanations are given, even a Freudian one.

134   Q120/122: 321.

135   Q120/122: 341.

136   Q120/122: 113.

137   Rousseau: *Oeuvres complètes* (1959-69); *Confessions* tome I: 575 and 1556; *Emile*'s Preface tome IV: lxi.

138 Helvétius: *De l'esprit, discours quatrième*. (1758); Claude Adrien Helvétius (1715-1771), French Philosophe.

139 Plumb (1975).

140 Raulin: *De la conservation des enfants*. Paris: 1763.

141 *Traité des maladies des femmes* PP-BCU-L Q120/47 (975 sheets); or *Traité des fièvres* PP-BCU-L Q120/41 (193 sheets) /101(257 sheets) /120 (38 sheets); *Traité de l'inflammation* PP-BCU-L Q120/98 (288 sheets); *Traité de l'étisie* PP-BCU-L Q120/46 (531 sheets).

142 *Vie de Zimmermann*. Lausanne: Fischer & Luc Vincent, 1797; Jacques Necker thanked Tissot for the gift of the book in a letter dated 25 February 1797 in FE-BPU-G.

143 Roussel: *Système physique et moral de la femme ou Tableau philosophique de la constitution des moeurs et des fonctions propres au sexe* (1775); last reprinted in 1869. Pierre Roussel (1742-1802), French physician.

144 Q120/47. 540 and 938

145 Table of content of *maladies des femmes*:

Chapitre I:	des maladies des femmes en général	1
Chapitre II:	structure de l'utérus	12
Chapitre III:	des règles	20
Chapitre IV:	des anomalies des règles	84
Chapitre V:	de l'inflammation de la matrice	101
Chapitre VI:	de l'érésypelle de l'utérus	138
Chapitre VII:	de l'inflammation chronique de l'utérus	146
Chapitre VIII:	de l'ulcère de la matrice	151
Chapitre IX:	du cancer de l'utérus	219
Chapitre X:	des hémorragies de l'utérus (pertes de sang dans les grossesses)	228
Chapitre XI:	des dépôts laiteux ou des maladies occasionnées par le lait épanché	293
Chapitre XII:	des engorgement des seins	428
Chapitre XIII:	du choix d'une nourrice et de la substitution du lait de femme	446
Chapitre XIV:	de la suppression des règles	497
Chapitre XV:	de la conduite que l'on doit tenir par rapport aux règles dans la maladie	624
Chapitre XVI:	des pâles couleurs	636
Chapitre XVII:	des pertes blanches	707
Chapitre XVIII:	des maladies des ovaires	777
Chapitre XVIIIbis	de l'hydropsie de l'utérus	894
Chapitre XIX:	de la tympanite de l'utérus	925
Chapitre XX:	des calculs de la matrice	942
Chapitre XXI:	des polypes de la matrice	955

146 Q120/47: 10. see below chapter XI.

147 Q120/47: 580.

148 Q120/47: 594.

149 Q120/47: 600.

150 Q120/47: 621.

151 Q120/47: 391.

152 Q120/47: 474. For an historic perspective on the subject of infant feeding, see Fildes (1986).

153 Q120/47: 496.

154 Hudson (1977).

155 Q120/47: 674bis and 677.

156 Starobinski (1981).

157 Siddall (1982).

158 Figlio (1978).

159 *Avis au peuple sur sa santé* (1761): 371.

160 Q120/47: 682.

161 Q120/47: 702.

162 For a view of physicians and male-midwives as intrusive, immodest, perhaps lascivious, to which Tissot might be reacting; see: Rousseau and Porter (1988): chapter 8.

163 Azouvi (1981).

Chapter VI

1 *Onanisme* (1760) and *Avis au peuple sur sa santé* (1761).

2 Tissot to Zimmermann, letter dated 19 september 1794.

3 Tissot to Zimmermann, letter dated 6 September 1755.

4 Tissot to Zimmermann, letter dated 12 September 1758.

5 Tissot to Zimmermann, letter dated 8 September 1762.

6 see below Chapter X and above Chapter V.

7 PP-BCU-L Q120/62: 445-472.

8 The root of de Haen's attack might be in Tissot *Discours préliminaire* to Haller's *Dissertation sur les parties irritables et sensibles des animaux* (1755) in which Tissot disclaimed any role or rule of the Church over medicine. For Tissot's reaction to de Haen's attack, see: *Lettre à Hirzel* (1762): 136ff; also Lesky (1959).

9 La Mettrie: *L'homme-machine.* Leyden: 1748; for more details see: Vartanian (1960).

10 Georges Leclerc de Buffon (1707-1788), French naturalist and writer; Denis Diderot (1713-1784), French writer.

11 See Leith (1977): 22.

12 *Encyclopédie*, vol. VII: 578-a,b,c,d.

13 See *Lettre à Hirzel* (1762): 137.

14 Hooykaas (1972): 9-26.

15 Biéler (1959): 152-161.

16 See below chapter VII.

17 See below chapter XII.

18 Müller: *Histoire de la Suisse.* Genève: Cherbullier, 1846; tome XV, Chap. I: 51ff. To compare with what was done elsewhere, see: Gutton (1974): in particular, Chap. III; Chisick (1981); Jean de Müller (1752-1809), Swiss historian and writer.

19 PP-BCU-L Q120/62.

20 PP-BCU-L Q120/130.3.

21 The Société économique had been organized in 1759.

22 Zimmermann to Tissot, letter dated 21 June 1766.

23 Stanislas-Augustus Poniatowski (1732-1798) was king of Poland from 1764 to 1795, his letters are in FE-BPU-G.

24 see above this chapter, also Emch-Dériaz (1982).

25 FE-BPU-G.

26 Tissot to Haller, letter dated 24 January 1766 in Hintzsche (1977): 223.

27 Haller to Tissot, letter dated 26 January 1766 in Hintzsche (1977): 223.

28 Eynard (1839): 135.

29 Tissot to Zimmermann, letter dated 31 January 1766; for a comparison of this offer with others in the period, see Garrison (1929, 1960): 391-392.

30 For more details on Stanilas-Augustus see: Fabre (1952).

31 See, for example in Delauney (1935) the adventure of another physician at the Polish Court.

32 FE-BPU-G.

33 Chevallaz (1949); Babaiantz (1961).

34 Tissot to Zimmermann, letter dated 6 January 1769.

35 Emch-Dériaz (1984): Appendix III; Six letters from Pringle to Tissot in FE-BPU-G. Haller had been professor of anatomy, physiology, and botany at the University of Goettingen from 1736 to 1753.

36 Tissot to Haller, letter dated 24 January 1766 in Hintzsche (1977): 223.

37 Eynard (1839): 155-157.

38 Tissot/Zimmermann correspondence passim; Tissot: *Vie de Zimmermann* (1797); Emch-Dériaz: (1986).

39 Haller to Tissot, letter dated 2 April 1768 in Hintzsche (1977): 283.

40 Letters from the Princes of Anhalt-Dessau; Hesse-Darmstadt; Mecklemburg-Schwerin; Zweibrücken; Hohenlohe-Waldenburg in FE-BPU-G.

41 Morren (1970): 18.

42 Sévery (1911, 1978), vol. II: 161.

43 Claude Piarron de Chamousset (1717-1773), French philanthropist, credited with the ideas of the mutual help society and of social insurance; see Rosen (1944); Etienne François de Choiseul (1719-1785), French stateman

44 Sévery (1928) for the Golowkin/Tissot relations. Alexandre de Golowkin (1732-1781), ambassador of Russia to Paris and to the Hague, retired in the Pays de Vaud; Wilhelmina de Golowkin, born de Moshein, married in 1796 the Duke of Noailles d'Ayen and died in 1823.

45 Tissot to Zimmermann, letter dated 8 December 1770.

46 see below: chapter X; Chamousset to Tissot, letter in FE-BPU-G.

47 At the instigation of Voltaire, who loved to meddle in the affairs of the Republic and who saw in the agitation between Natifs, Habitants, and Bourgeois a way to weaken the industry of the city, Choiseul developed a rival town at Versoix, a small French village about 10 miles from Geneva on the right bank of the lake. Discontented watchmakers and jewelers left the city

for Versoix but soon returned to Geneva. Choiseul and the French Court had been delighted with the prospect but could not come up with the funds to build houses and factories. All that is left of the enterprise today is a name for a pleasure boat harbor called Port Choiseul; see Martin (1951): Vol. I, 458.

48 Eynard (1839): 218-221.

49 Tissot to Zimmermann, letter dated 13 April 1771.

50 Tissot to Zimmermann, letters dated from Spa on 18 June and 9 July 1772; letters to his wife PP-BCU-L Q120/131.

51 Letters to his family PP-BCU-L Q120/131.

52 Tissot to Pidou, his brother-in-law who was a minister in PP-BCU-L Q120/131.1.

53 see below Chapters X and XII.

54 Tissot to Zimmermann, letter dated 13 October 1772.

55 Eynard (1839): 236.

56 see below Chapter X.

57 Eynard (1839): 205-215.

58 Haller to Tissot, letter dated 13 June 1769 in Hintzsche (1977): 310.

59 Gavard (1898): 28.

60 Haller to Tissot, letter dated 16 February 1769.

61 Leith (1977): 104. See also: *Traité des nerfs* in vol. X *Oeuvres complètes* (1790): 194.

62 Tissot to Zimmermann, letter dated 16 February 1774.

63 Tissot to Zimmermann, letter dated 19 December [1759?].

64 see below Chapter VII.

65 Girolama Fabrizio d'Acquapente (1537-1619), Italian physician; Andreas Vesalius (1514-1564), Flemish physician; see: *Les siècles d'or de la médecine à Padoue XVe-XVIIIe*, special exhibition in Paris 1989.

66 FE-BPU-G; Joseph Lieuthaud (1703-1780), French physician.

67 Eynard (1839): 249; original letter in FE-BPU-G.

68 Tissot to Haller, letter dated 23 May 1775 in Hintzsche (1977): 416.

69 See below, chapter VIII.

70 For more details on Joseph II (1741-1790), see: Blanning (1970).

71 FE-BPU-G; Felix de Vicq d'Azyr (1748-1794), French physician.

72 Gillipsie (1980): 33 and 194-203.

73 Hannaway (1972): 257-273; (1977): 431-447.

74 PP-BCU-L Q120/62: 907-909; "...j'ai vu en septembre 1779, une femme...je partis le cinquième jour de sa couche pour un assez long voyage, mais de retour au bout de dix mois..." Tissot came back on 6 August 1780; "Arrivé seulement depuis douze jours de Paris, mon plus cher ami, j'ai eu le plaisir de trouver chez moi votre excellente lettre du 15 juin." Tissot to Zimmermann, letter dated 18 August 1780.

75 PP-BCU-L Q120/131.

76 Sévery (1911) vol II, Chapter VI; Sévery (1928): 255ff.

77 Sévery (1911): vol. II: 181.

78 Jean-Louis Gallatin of the same family as the American stateman Albert Gallatin (1761-1849) who also left Geneva in the early 1780s. The city was going through a very dark period of social strife and foreign interventions, which ended with the "Edit noir", as the Edict of Pacification of 1783 was nicknamed. Imposed from outside, mainly by France, the 1783 edict left a false and forced peace in the city, which burst out in revolutionary troubles about five years later. Necker had done his best to minimize France's intervention in the affairs of the Republic. Many Genevan left the city at that time. For more details on the rebellions in Geneva and their relevances to European history, see Palmer (1959).

79 See below, chapter XI; also Greenbaum (1971): 317-350; (1972): 651-675; and (1975): 43-56.

80 Robinet to Tissot, letter dated 28 Mai 1771: "Personne n'est plus en état que vous de nous donner du neuf et de l'excellent." In six different letters Robinet requested articles with such titles as "éducation physique, diète, diètétique, médecine, médecin, maladie, médecin des pauvres," all in FE-BPU-G. Tissot dragged his feet and seemed never to have obliged because of Robinet's editing method. Jean-Baptiste Robinet (1735-1820), French writer.

81 see below Chapter VII.

Chapter VII

1 Gay (1967) vol. 1: 53; Fontenelle: *Entretiens sur la pluralité des mondes.* (1686); Rousseau: *La Nouvelle Héloïse.* (1761); Bernard Le Bovyer de

Fontenelle (1657-1757), French author, perpetuel secretary of the Académie des sciences.

2 FE-BCU-L Q120/75, "Lettre sur le Heimweh", "Lettre sur l'hystérie", /125 "Lettre sur les maladies nerveuses"; see above chapter III.

3 see above chapter V.

4 Tissot to Zimmermann, letter dated 25 Septembre 1779.

5 see below chapter VIII.

6 see the last two pages of tome neuvième of the *Oeuvres de Monsieur Tissot* Lausanne: Grasset, 1790.

7 FE-BCU-L Q120/4 de l'apoplexie; /5 de la paralysie; /7 des spasmes ou convulsions; /8 de la folie; /9 de la rage; /10 des vapeurs; /74 des insomnies; /77 de la mobilité.

8 Philippe-Rodolphe Vicat (1742-1781), Swiss physician, residing in Payerne (Pays de Vaud), studied at Goettingen and took his M.D. in Basel. See Appendix II: 335.

9 see appendix II: 333.

10 *Traité de l'épilepsie*. Tome huitième of *Oeuvres de Monsieur Tissot*. Lausanne: Grasset, 1790: 193 & 198. All references will be to this edition.

11 Temkin (1971): 229.

12 *Traité de l'epilepsie*: 24.

13 *Traité de l'epilepsie*: 147.

14 *Traité de l'epilepsie*: 27.

15 *Traité de l'epilepsie*: 28.

16 *Traité de l'epilepsie*: 44ff.

17 *Traité de l'epilepsie*: 207.

18 *Traité de l'epilepsie*: 223.

19 *Traité de l'epilepsie*: 98.

20 *Traité de l'epilepsie*: 154ff.

21 see below this chapter.

22 *Traité de l'épilepsie*: 138-139.

23 *Traité de l'épilepsie*: 403.

24 *Traité de l'épilepsie*: 403.

25 *Traité de l'épilepsie*: 215.

26 *Traité de l'épilepsie*: 315.

27 see below Chapter X.

28 *Traité de l'épilepsie*: 377.

29 *Traité de l'épilepsie*: 229.

30 *Traité de l'épilepsie*: 367.

31 *Traité de l'épilepsie*: 394.

32 *Traité des nerfs et de leurs maladies*. Tome neuvième of *Oeuvres de Monsieur Tissot*. Lausanne: Grasset, 1790: iv; see also Canguilhem (1978).

33 Monter (1976); Olivier (1962): vol. III, 493-521.

34 *Traité des nerfs et de leurs maladies*: IX-liii.

35 *Traité des nerfs et de leurs maladies*: IX-liv; in line with the Hippocratic Oath which Tissot followed.

36 *Traité des nerfs et de leurs maladies*: IX-xxiii-xxiv.

37 *Traité des nerfs et de leurs maladies*: IX-passim. Thomas Willis (1621-1673), British physican; Robert Whytt (1714-1766), Scottish neurologist; George Cheyne (1671-1743), Scottish physician; Friedrich Hoffmann (1660-1742), German physician; Raymond Vieussens (1641-1715), French physician.

38 *Traité des nerfs et de leurs maladies*: IX-xix, note c).

39 *Traité des nerfs et de leurs maladies*: IX-134.

40 *Traité des nerfs et de leurs maladies*: IX-140.

41 *Traité des nerfs et de leurs maladies*: IX-215. Louis de Jaucourt (1704-1780), French physician and Encyclopedist, studied in Geneva and in Leyden with Boerhaave; for more details, see Morris (1979); Schwab (1958); or Zeiler (1934).

42 *Traité des nerfs et de leurs maladies*: IX-271.

43 *Traité des nerfs et de leurs maladies*: tome dixième des *Oeuvres de Monsieur Tissot*. Lausanne: Grasset, 1790: 99.

44 *Traité des nerfs et de leurs maladies*: IX-298.

45 *Traité des nerfs et de leurs maladies*: Edition Hallé, (1811), vol. 7: 81; and the so-called Edition Hallé (1855), a reprint of the *Encyclopédie des Sciences médicales*' volume 10: 34.

46 *Traité des nerfs et de leurs maladies*: X-91 & X-208.

47 *Traité des nerfs et de leurs maladies*: X-97.

48 *Traité des nerfs et de leurs maladies*: X-91-94.

49 *Traité des nerfs et de leurs maladies*: IX-264.

50 *Traité des nerfs et de leurs maladies*: X-103.

51 *Traité des nerfs et de leurs maladies*: IX-296.

52 *Traité des nerfs et de leurs maladies*: X-158.

53 *Traité des nerfs et de leurs maladies*: X-154.

54 *Traité des nerfs et de leurs maladies*: X-158.

55 *Traité des nerfs et de leurs maladies*: X-176.

56 *Traité des nerfs et de leurs maladies*: X-190.

57 *Traité des nerfs et de leurs maladies*: X-193-194.

58 Johann Kaspar Lavater (1741-1801), Swiss physiognomist and theologian, *Physiognomische Fragments* (1778) English translation *Physiognomics* (1793).

59 *Traité des nerfs et de leurs maladies*: 1855-193.

60 *Traité des nerfs et de leurs maladies*: 1855-85.

61 *Traité des nerfs et de leurs maladies*: 1855-96.

62 *Traité des nerfs et de leurs maladies*: 1855-97.

63 Pomme: *Traité des vapeurs*. Lyon: 1769; Raulin: *Traité des affections vaporeuses du sexe*. Paris: 1768; Pierre Pomme (1735-1782), French physician.

64 *Traité des nerfs et de leurs maladies*: 1855-141.

65 *Traité des nerfs et de leurs maladies*: 1855-158.

66 *Traité des nerfs et de leurs maladies*: 1855-212 & 214.

67 *Traité des nerfs et de leurs maladies*: 1855-223-224.

68 Ellenberg (1970).

69 *Traité des nerfs et de leurs maladies*: 1855-159 & 161.

70 Anders Celsius (1701-44), Swedish astronomer & physicist.

71 *Traité des nerfs et de leurs maladies*: 1855-226 and 255.

72 Hoffmann (1977): 198; Philippe Pinel (1745-1826), French physician.

Chapter VIII

1 Tissot to Zimmermann, letters dated 18 August 1780 and 9 June 1781. Louis-Jean-Marie de Daubenton (1716-1800), French naturalist.

2 Lazzaro Spallanzani (1729-1799), Italian naturalist; Jacobus Rezia (1745-1825), Italian anatomist.

3 Giambattista Borsieri de Kanifeld (1725-1785), Italian physician; Andrew Duncan the elder (1744-1828), Scottish physician. See: Garrison (1929): 399 or Risse (1989).

4 Official letter of appointment dated 16 December 1780 and formal acceptance letter dated 9 June 1781 in PP-BCU-L Q120/144(6).

5 Portmann (1980).

6 Sévery (1911): volume 2, 165 and Sévery (1928): 302.

7 PP-BCU-L Q120/144.6: the first letter dated 7 September 1780 is a request to see Tissot; a second letter dated from Bern 30 October 1780 gives more details about the appointment: in particular that no professor in Pavia is so well paid.

8 The censor is perhaps Colonel Tissot-Grenus himself, who, according to Eynard, annotated his father's "livre de raison" about his brother the doctor.

9 Lüthy (1959-1961).

10 Lüthy (1959-1961): volume 2, 136-141 and 619-647.

11 Rudolf Emmanuel Haller (1747-1833) third son of Albrecht, lived to serve Napoleon Bonaparte as purveyor of the armies in Italy and died in Switzerland, quite poor and forgotten.

12 Lüthy (1959-1961): volume 2, 620.

13 Tissot to Zimmermann, letter dated 9 October 1781: "Je pars dans quelques heures,..."

14 Eighty letters from the Italian sojourn are deposited in PP-BCU-L Q120/131.3; see also Guisan (1931).

15 Tissot to Zimmermann, letter dated 28 August 1784 mentioning a letter from December 1781.

16 Tissot to his wife, letter dated 27 November 1781.

17 Tissot to his wife, letter dated 8 December 1781.

18 At the end of the century Frank, who succeeded Tissot at Pavia in 1785, had to bow to intrigues and moved to Vienna; he complained of this in a letter to Tissot dated 22 February 1793 in FE-BPU-G.

19 Spallanzani to Bonnet, letter dated 31 December 1781, cited in Eynard (1839): 288-290.

20 Eynard (1839): 292.

21 PP-BCU-L Q120/75 & *Essai sur les moyens de perfectionner les études de médecine*. Lausanne: Mourer Cadet, 1785. It saw two Lausanne editions in 8° and 12°, one each in Bern, Basel and Paris in 1785. It was translated into German and into Italian for two editions each in 1785 and 1786. It was not reprinted in the so-called complete works edited by Hallé at the beginning of the nineteenth century. The 8° edition, which is at the Bibliothèque publique et universitaire in Geneva, is dedicated in Tissot's handwriting to Doctor Butini, an early advocate of inoculation; see Emch-Dériaz (1982). The 12° edition, which is my reference edition, has printed on its last page the certificate from the censor which read as follows: "Cet ouvrage offert à la Censure est une nouvelle preuve du zèle infatigable de son célèbre Auteur, pour le bien de l'humanité, & de son habileté consommée dans la science qu'il professe. De Bons, Censeur, Lausanne, le 17 Mars 1785." My reconstruction of the inaugural lecture and of Tissot's attitude at the bedside is based on his description in *Etudes de médecine* and on his personal notes.

22 *Etudes de médecine* (1785): 139.

23 *Etudes de médecine* (1785): 144. Scholastic medicine is meant here as the medicine of discourse and definition not based on precise information and scientific observation, i.e. unscientific speculative medicine.

24 Leroy-Ladurie (1973): quatrième partie; Gillispie (1980): chapter III; Corbin (1986); Hannaway (1972); Riley (1987)

25 *Etudes de médecine* (1785): 146. For the importance of the Montpellier School in directing medicine toward clinical observation and away from iatromechanical or iatrochemical theorizing, see Moravia (1972); Bordeu: *Recherches sur le pouls par rapport aux crises* (1756); Paul Joseph Barthez (1734-1806), French physican.

26 *Etudes de médecine* (1785): 152. The quote is worth giving completely: "surtout, il est important de n'en humilier aucun; il n'y a que l'ignorance présomptueuse qui mérite ce terrible châtiment."

27 *Etudes de médecine* (1785): 153.

28 *Etudes de médecine* (1785): 158. I translated the French pronoun *en* by him or her, since Tissot taught in male and female wards, the French usage of the masculine is always inclusive.

29 Troehler (1988).

30 PP-BCU-L Q120/75.

31 Tissot to his wife, letter dated 25 October, 1781.

32 PP-BCU-L Q120/75.

33 PP-BCU-L Q120/75: 11.

34 PP-BCU-L Q120/75: 5.

35 Tissot to his wife, letter dated 15 December 1781.

36 Joseph Frank (1771-1842), German physician, the son of Johann Peter Frank.

37 See Kondratas (1977): 125.

38 PP-BCU-L Q120/75: 45.

39 Weiner (1980): 18.

40 Tissot developed this point in his personal notes on clinical teaching; PP-BCU-L Q120/75.

41 In fact, at some point, Tissot's personal papers at the BCU in Lausanne were thinned out; some sort of cataloguing was done at the turn of the century and many letters recorded at the time have since disappeared. Eynard himself possessed a large set of documents on Tissot, all of which have been deposited at the BPU in Geneva in bound volumes; but the diary is not there. Notes Eynard took with a view to writing his own book on Tissot are in the BCU in Lausanne. But again no diary. Dr. Antoine Curchod in Geneva, a descendent of Marc d'Apples, told me (in a private communication in June 1984) that in the 1930s what was left of Tissot's personal papers in the hands of the family was divided among three sisters (one of them Dr. Curchot's mother). Tissot's desk was emptied of his content and divided at random in equal piles... One "pile" stayed in Switzerland and part of it has since then been given to the Fonds Tissot in Lausanne, the other "piles" were taken to Germany by the aunts. If they still exist, they are now in the eastern part of Germany or in Poland left there by their owners fleeing from the Soviet armies.

42 Eynard (1839): 298.

43 Tissot to his wife, letter dated 8 November 1781. Potatoes were introduced in Switzerland in the early eighteenth century; see Chevallaz (1949).

44 Sévery (1911): volume 2, chapter 2. 4

45 Louisa, Countess of Albany (1752-1824), she was the wife of the Stuart pretender; Maria-Carolina (1752-1814), daughter of Empress Maria-Theresa (1717-1780).

46 Tissot to his wife, letter dated 30 November 1782.

47 Tissot to his wife, letter dated 7 January 1783.

48 Maria Anna Angelica Kaufmann (1741-1807), Swiss painter, made her career in London and Rome.

49 Eynard (1839): 304. Giovanni Angelo Braschi (1717-1799), Pope under the name of Pius VI from 1775 to 1799.

50 Tissot to his wife, letter dated 27 October 1782.

51 Tissot to his wife, letter dated 1 March 1783.

52 Sévery (1911): volume 2, 191.

53 Tissot to his wife, letter dated 22 March 1783. "J'ai dû voir plus de malades que je ne l'aurai voulu."

54 PP-BCU-L Q120/64 *Du régime dans les maladiës aigues*: 30; and as part of professional attitudes, see Ramsey (1988).

Chapter IX

1 see below chapter X, XI, and XII.

2 see below for his involvement with the Collège de Médecine.

3 *Vie de Zimmermann*. Lausanne: Fischer et Vincent, 1797.

4 see Appendix II: 335-336.

5 PP-BCU-L Q120 /34 *Traité de l'inflammation*; /41 *Traité des fièvres*; /47 *Traité des maladies des femmes*; /49 & /122 *Essai sur l'éducation physique des petits enfants*; /46 *Traité de l'étisie*.

6 PP-BCU-L Q120/112 and 115. Marc d'Apples: *Instruction pour les personnes qui gardent les malades*. Lausanne: Pott, 1788 and *Parallèle entre les miséricorde et les hôpitaux*. Lausanne: Pott, 1789.

7 Tissot to Zimmermann, letter dated 28 August 1784.

8   PP-BCU-L Q120/128.12.

9   Gibbon: *Miscellaneous Works* (1796): vol. I: 410-412. "Your taxes, moder-
    ate as they are, exhaust the country ... While the great kingdoms of Europe,
    loaded with expenses and debts, are driven to expedients ... Bern is the only
    state which has amassed a large treasure ... the Canton enriches itself by the
    simple means of receiving much and expending little. It spends far less than it
    receives ... revenues that in other countries would be devoted to an army or a
    court, expenses likened to dew on the earth from which the revenues were
    pulled, here are buried in the State coffers or dispersed through the banks of
    Europe, to become one day a prey to the knavery of a clerc or the ambition of
    a conqueror. This continual loss of species extinguishes industry ... and
    gradually impoverishes the country."

10 Calvin (1560): II.ii.13-14.

11 Tissot to Zimmermann, letter dated 15 September 1792. Necker was
    dismissed on 11 July 1789.

12 Tissot to Zimmermann, letter dated 15 September 1792.

13 Olivier (1962): 2e partie, tome premier, chapitre II.

14 Perrochon (1971): 55-57.

15 Bonnet to Tissot, letter in FE-BPU-G; Friedrich Franz Anton Mesmer
    (1734-1815), Austrian physician; see Azouvi (1982), Darnton (1968), and
    Schenk (1959).

16 Eynard (1839): 325ff.

17 Tissot to Zimmermann, letter dated 31 July 1790.

18 J.P. Frank autobiography published in English (1948): 35.

19 J.P. Frank to Tissot, letter in FE-BPU-G.

20 J.P. Frank autobiography published in English (1948): 301

21 Frank: *De vertebratis columnae in morbis dignitate* (1792)

22 Nicole (1934): 367-374.

23 *Traité de l'étisie* [tuberculosis]. PP-BCU-L Q120/46; Tissot to Zimmermann,
    letter dated 21 Novembre 1794.

24 *Traité de l'étisie*: 345-352.

25 Tissot to Zimmermann, letter dated 19 September 1794. Kermès minéral or
    poudre des Chartreux, an oxysulfur of antimony is an expectorant for bron-
    chitis or emphyzema, when prescribed in a dosage of 0.05g to 0.3g, an emetic
    at a higher dosage. *Larousse médical illustré* (1923).

26 Spengler (1942).

27 Coleman (1977): 91-100.

28 i.e. foundation of the Société royale de médecine and its preoccupation with epidemic and epizootic or creation of the Commission of the Académie royale des sciences on hospitals or the *Encyclopédie*'s articles on medicine, hygiene, physical exercise, etc. See *Annales ESC* (1977).

29 PP-BCU-L Q120/124 & 130.11a,b,c,d,e; see below chapter XI

30 see above Chapter V.

31 Tenon's expression & a book title by Foucault's school. *mouroir*: place where one dies easily.

32 PP-BCU-L Q120/66; see below, chapter XII.

33 Eynard (1839): 384.

34 Olivier (1928): 286-287. One can read in the minutes of the Société vaudoise des sciences médicales of 12 May 1842 meeting: "Le Président fait lecture des questions proposées par le Comité, dont on élimine celle relative a l'influence qu'a produite les ouvrages de Tissot."

35 Jean-Noël Hallé (1754-1822), French physician and hygienist, who published an annotated edition of Tissot's complete works, see appendix II: 335-336.

Chapter X

1 See above Chapter VI.

2 Payne (1976); Chisick (1981).

3 Boschung (1986).

4 Olivier (1962): 2e partie, tome I, chapitre II.

5 Olivier (1962): 2e partie, tome I, chapitre I and in particular page 13.

6 see above Chapt. VI.

7 Ramsey (1982): 118-135 or (1987); Raeff (1983): 53.

8 *Réflexions historiques* (1982): Nos. 1 and 2.

9 Saudan (1987): 55-106.

10 Laget (1982), Rousseau and Porter (1988): chapter 8.

11 Béné (1957): 4-6.   Victor-Amadeus III (1726-1790) became King of Sardinia-Piedmont in 1773; he resided in Turin and was also the Duke of Savoy.

12 PP-BCU-L Q120/62 & /130.3.

13 By the time of the publication of *De l'instruction des chirurgiens pour les campagnes*, the champion of midwifery was Venel; Tissot played a supporting role in Venel's campaign to train better midwives.   In the 1780s the two reformist physicians worked in harmony, each where he thought he could best accomplish his task.   Venel lived and worked in Yverdon, a town close to village life, hence his interest in midwifery; Tissot lived and practiced in Lausanne among well-to-do, hence his awareness of their changing needs and of their desires for male midwives, i.e. physicians trained in obstetrics.

14 La Berge (1975), (1977) & (1984);   Weiner (1970).

15 *Etudes de médecine* (1785): 187. "qu'ils connussent très bien leur religion;"

16 For similar views, see Ramsey (1988).

17 *Etudes de médecine* (1785): 158.

18 Private communication from Dr. Y. Saudan of Lausanne.

19 *Etudes de médecine* (1785): 199. Stoeck: *Precepta medico-practica*. Vienna: 1777; Buchan: *Domestic Medicine*. London: 1772;   Dionis: *Cours d'opération de chirurgie*. Bruxelles: 1708; La Motte: *Traité de chirurgie*. Paris: 1771; Verdier: *Abrégé d'anatomie*. Paris: 1747; I established this list from the catalogue of Tissot's library, since in typical eighteenth-century style he gave only the names of the authors, not the titles of the works; Anton von Stoerck (1731-1803), Austrian physician, famous for his pharmaceutical research; Pierre Dionis (died 1718), celebrated French surgeon; La Motte (1655-1737), French surgeon; César Verdier (1687-1759), French anatomist.

20 Ramsey (1988): 77-78.

21 *Encyclopédie*. 7th edition: Vol. 11, J.L. Pellet, Genève (1779).   Gillispie (1980):   Chapter III, section 4. Louis-Anne Lavirotte (1725-1759), French physician.

22 *Encyclopédie*, Vol. 11: 183.

23 *Encyclopédie*, Vol. 11: 183.

24 *Etudes de médecine* (1785): 120.

25 *Etudes de médecine* (1785): 18.

26 *Etudes de médecine* (1785): 122.

27 *Etudes de médecine* (1785): 41.

28 *Etudes de médecine* (1785): 49.

29 PP-BCU-L Q120/24: *Des intestins*; PP-BCU-L Q120/48: *De morbis infantum*; PP-BCU-Q120/54: *Diaetetica*; to cite a few.

30 Theophratus Bombatus von Hohenheim (1493-1541), Swiss physician, nicknamed himself Paracelsus; is said to have ostentatiously burned treatises by Galen and Avicenna while he was on the Faculty at Basel. Avicenna or Ibn Sina (980-1037), Persian physician.

31 Giorgio Baglivi (1688-1707), Italian physician; see King (1976); Zimmermann (1764).

32 *Etudes de médecine* (1785): 157, footnote m.

33 *Etudes de médecine* (1785): 15.

34 Tissot to Zimmermann, letter dated 2 April 1763.

35 *Etudes de médecine* (1785): 84.

36 See: appendix II: 334.

37 See: Gelfand (1977) & (1981) and Keel (1984) & (1985) for Paris; Risse (1986) for Edinburgh and (1989) for Vienna and Pavia; Swick and Antuono (1983) for Florence.

38 Andrew Duncan in Edinburgh; Anton de Haen in Vienna; Johann Peter Frank in Pavia and later in Vienna; or Philippe Pinel in Paris.

39 For a description of the licensing procedure in Geneva, see: Gautier (1906); for the Collège, see above Chapt. IX.

40 PP-BCU-L Q120/130.11.

41 PP-BCU-L Q120/130.5.

42 PP-BCU-L Q120/130.11: 1.

43 PP-BCU-L Q120/130.11: 2 & 3.

44 PP-BCU-L Q120/130.11: 4.

Chapter XI

1 Jetter (1986): Teil C; Murken (1988).

2 Hufton (1974); Fairchilds (1976); Gutton (1971); for the revolutionary period: Forrest (1981).

3 Thompson and Goldin (1975): 105ff.

4 It is this hospital for which on the eve of the French Revolution, Tissot formulated a plan for its transformation into a curing hospital; *Notes sur l'Hôpital de Lausanne*, PP-BCU-L Q120/124; see below this chapter, also Emch-Dériaz (1988).

5 Yet, in Vienna, de Haen used the pool of patients of the Algemeinde Hospital for a program of bedside teaching at the small Burgerspital.

6 The expression is in Tenon (1788); see the following list which is not even exhaustive: *Mémoire de l'Académie* (années 1786, 1787, & 1788); Alkin: *Observations sur les hôpitaux relatives à leur construction* (1787); Cabanis: *Observations sur les hôpitaux* (1790); Chambeau: *Moyens de rendre les hôpitaux utiles à la Nation* (1787); Chamousset: *Exposition d'un plan proposé pour les malades de l'Hôtel-Dieu* (1757); Colombier: *Instruction sur la manière de gouverner les insensés et de travailler à leur guérison dans les asyles qui leur sont destinés* (1785); Coqueau: *Essai sur l'établissement des hôpitaux dans les grandes villes* (1787); Du Laurens: *Moyens de rendre les hôpitaux utiles et de perfectionner la médecine* (1787). Howard: *Etats des prisons et des hôpitaux* (1788); Le Roy: *Précis d'un ouvrage sur les hôpitaux* (1787); Petit: *Projet et mémoire sur la meilleure manière de construire un hôpital de malades* (1774): Poyet: *Mémoire sur la nécessité de transférer et reconstruire l'Hôtel-Dieu de Paris, suivi d'un projet de translation de cet hôpital* (1785); Tenon: *Mémoires sur les hôpitaux de Paris* (1788).

7 Gelfand (1973).

8 Tenon (1788).

9 Ackerknecht (1967): 25; Temkin (1951): 248-259.

10 Thompson and Goldin (1975): 128.

11 Murken (1988): Chapt. 8.

12 Labasse (1980).

13 Abraham (1958); Greenbaum (1971), (1972), (1973), (1974), (1975); and Jetter (1986): 199-219.

14 Foucault (1963); Foucault et al. (1979); Gelfand (1982).

15 By Dupont de Nemours for example, see below note 18); Greenbaum (1976); Emch-Dériaz (1987). *Miséricorde*: a charitable institution.

16 Weiner (1972); Greenbaum (1979) & (1981).

17 Freidson (1963): 24.

18 Dupont de Nemours: *Sur les secours à donner aux pauvres malades dans les grandes villes.* (Paris and Philadelphia: 1786); also as a manuscript at Eleutherian Mills Library, W2 4683, this first draft is from 1773.

19 see the report on the Hôtel-Dieu by Tenon.

20 Ignaz Philipp Semmelweiss (1818-1865), Austro-Hungarian physician.

21 For example the studies of Pinel; see Foucault (1972); Rosen (1969).

22 See above chapter V.

23 Labasse (1980).

24 For example the work of Lavoisier on respiration to determine hospital room size.

25 For Cabanis and the circle of the Idéologues, see: Staum (1980); Rosen (1946); Pierre-Jean-Georges Cabanis (1757-1808), French physician.

26 Bluche (1980).

27 Ackerknecht (1975): 40.

28 PP-BCU-L Q120/112.

29 see above note 17).

30 See below in this chapter for the Lausanne Hospital; charities were of two main types: first through the *miséricordes* of the *bannières* [neighborhood], second through specialized organizations such as *La bourse française* which took care of the population of French descent, but not with bourgeois status; for the Inselspital, see: Olivier (1962).

31 Olivier (1962): 2e partie, tome second, 801; Gibbon traveled to Bern in 1758 and gave his views on the Inselspital, see: Craddock (1982): 83-84.

32 Tenon (1788); Jetter (1986): 203-204.

33 Tronchin (1906).

34 Kondratas (1977); Belloni in O'Malley (1970).

35 PP-BCU-L Q120/75; the word "blueprint", here and elsewhere in this book, is used freely although, stricto senso, it is an anachronism since the process was only developed in 1842 by Sir John Herschel (1792-1871), English astronomer and pioneer of photography.

36 Tissot owned the book entitled: *Observations on Duties and Offices of the Physician*. London: Stradan and Cadell, 1770 by the Scottish physician John Gregory (1724-1773), and showed in his emphasis on kindness toward patients a strong affinity to Gregory's thought. See also Risse in Bell (1982).

37 *Etudes de médecine* (1785): 162-181.

38 *Etudes de médecine* (1785): 164.

39 See above Chapter V: note 146)

40 one toise = six feet.

41 As used in Northern Europe or Great Britain; presumably the warmer climate did not require fireplaces; the Sutton's machine was a device used aboard ships to ventilate the lower decks.

42 *Etudes de médecine* (1785): 178.

43 *Etudes de médecine* (1785): 166.

44 *Etudes de médecine* (1785): 171.

45 *Etudes de médecine* (1785): 179.

46 see below Chapter XII: note 108).

47 *Etudes de médecine* (1785): 151. See also Risse (1986): 274-275; Emch-Dériaz (1984).

48 Olivier (1962): 780-795 and Archives cantonales vaudoises registre de la commission, manuals of the Town Council.

49 Bridel (1928): 313-318.

50 Morren (1970): 105ff.

51 Olivier (1962): 782. The heads of family received to the bourgeoisie that single year accounted for more than the half of those received during the whole eighteenth century, see Olivier (1962): 782, note 5).

52 Olivier (1962): 786 and Manual B44: 90.

53 PP-BCU-L Q120/124.

54 Tissot's eleven points:

"**First**, the hospital building is to be rid of dampness as soon as feasible by cross-ventilation and proper sewage.
Second, the first floor rooms, which are vaulted, are to be used as cellars and warehouses, nevermore for the purpose of lodging, except for an occasional raving mad person whose isolation is necessary to ensure the peace of the other patients. There are enough rooms on the second floor to house all the confined poor, never two to a bed.
Third, all the rooms of the second floor should be panelled with wood, fitted with heating stoves or fireplaces. This floor could then easily house the fourteen paupers, and the capacity could be raised to twenty-four if the paupers were to be boarded two-to-a-room.
Fourth, consequently, the *Miséricordes* should look into the number of poor kept on the dole at home, and have them moved to the Hospital for a more efficient use of the poor fund and of the hospital building.

Fifth, the servants of the Hospital should perform their duties with more exactitude to improve the cleanliness of the Hospital.

Sixth, a decent dormitory for the transient poor should be set up. This is a urgent necessity; meanwhile the actual dormitory should be closed and two other rooms should be allocated for this purpose. There are rooms on the second floor, even those of the first floor would be infinitely better than the dormitory as it exists.

Seventh, a common dining-room should be created to ease the service and improve the life of the confined poor.

Eighth, the cellar entrance should be improved to render storage more efficient.

Ninth, a better room for the Boys School should be found.

Tenth, two windows should be opened in the blind room of the workhouse to improve its hygienic conditions.

Eleventh, all the empty and unused apartments of the Hospital should be converted into rooms for patients with acute diseases; and when they are sick confined poor they should be transported there to be treated."

55 Olivier (1962): 786 and manual B44.

56 Olivier (1962): 786 and manual B44.

57 This is the last sentence of his manuscript entitled: Parallèle entre les miséricorde et les hôpitaux: PP-BCU-L Q120/112: "Hâtons-nous de ne plus refuser à ceux de nos semblables qui gémissent en même temps sous le poids de la douleur et de l'indigence un des plus grand privilèges que la richesse puisse donner, celui d'être soigné dans la maladie avec exactitude, servi avec intelligence, et secouru par tous les moyens qui peuvent être mis en usage!"

58 PP-BCU-L Q120/66, 176 manuscript pages.

59 For Tissot, this meant twenty-one to twenty-three days, while Tenon considered up to six months as a usual stay in the hospital for cure.

60 Ackerknecht (1968): chapter 8, Numbers and Amundsen (1986).

61 PP-BCU-L Q120/64: 31. *Du régime dans les maladies aiguës* is in a copyist hand with many additions by Tissot's.

62 PP-BCU-L Q120/64: 32.

63 Huard et Imbault (1975); Keel (1984), (1985), (1986), & Keel in Bynum and Porter (1985); Lesky in O'Malley (1970); Risse (1974), (1986) & (1989); Weiner (1980).

Chapter XII

1 *De la médecine civile or De la police de la médecine.* PP-BCU-L Q120/66, 66bis, 66ter, 66ter is the first draft in Tissot's hand, 366 pages recto + 45 pages verso; 66bis is in a copyst's hand with numerous corrections in Tissot's,

166 sheets; 66 is the "final" version in a copyst's hand with some corrections in Tissot's, 176 sheets in quarto, bound in cardboard. All reference will be to this copy. It received no mention by Tissot's two previous biographers. This silence is especially surprising for Eynard who had full access to Tissot's papers. Maybe the word "police", which too directly evoked Ancien Régime, muted his curiosity. Cochet's study which depended heavily on Eynard's has no new information or interpretation and reads like an abstract of its predecessor.

2 Brown in Lipkin (1982).

3 Rosen (1958): 118, 135, 162. and (1974): 156. Viet Ludwig von Seckendorff (1626-1692), German statemen; Franz Anton Mai (1742-1814), German physician.

4 Raeff (1983).

5 Riley (1987).

6 Calvin: *Institutio religionis christiane*. Basel: Platter, 1536. I use the revised French edition established by Calvin in 1560; Part IV, Chapter XX: du gouvernement civil.

7 It is interesting to note that the Scottish physician Andrew Duncan treated the subject with the same approach as Tissot, i.e. the non-naturals in *Heads of Lectures on Medical Police*. Edinburgh: Adam Neil & Co., 1801.

8 Heller (1979).

9 A common explanation in eighteenth-century medicine; see also Corbin (1986).

10 Frank edited by Lesky (1976): vol. 1, part 1, section 1.

11 Foucault (1976): 35.

12 Frank: *Sistema compinto de polizia medica*. Milano: 1786. PP-BCU-L Q120/71: 65.

13 Kondratas (1977): 140; Frank/Rosen (1948); Nicole (1934). See also above Chapter IX.

14 FE-BPU-G. Tissot to Zimmermann, letter dated 31 Mai 1768 which emphasized the importance of forensic medicine.

15 In Solothurn, Zweibrücken, and Venice, for example.

16 See above Chapters IX and X.

17 PP-BCU-L Q120/66: 1.

18 PP-BCU-L Q120/66: 1. "la médecine des citoyens pris en gros."

19 PP-BCU-L Q120/66: 2.

20 PP-BCU-L Q120/66: 1.

21 PP-BCU-L Q120/66: 1.

22 PP-BCU-L Q120/66: 3.

23 PP-BCU-L Q120/66: 4; Frank (Milano: 1786): tome 1, preface: 24. The English translation given in the text is taken from Frank (Baltimore: 1976): 10.

24 François (1911): 19-40. Rousseau to Tissot, letter dated Môtier 1st April 1765. "Combien dans ma dernière maladie ne voudrais-je pas avoir un Tissot à mon chevet, afin que, quand il n'y aurait plus rien à faire au corps, il fut encore le médecin de l'âme. Je vous embrasse."

25 PP-BCU-L Q120/66: 5.

26 PP-BCU-L Q120/66: 5, well within the Hippocratic Corpus.

27 See: *Lettre à M. Baker sur les maladies causées par le seigle ergoté* (1768), first Latin version published in *Philosophical Transactions*, London 1765, and *Lettre à M. Hirzel sur le bled et le pain* (1779).

28 PP-BCU-L Q120/66: 10 & 12.

29 PP-BCU-L Q120/66: 16. For just one successful example, in Goettingen, the townwalls were transformed in such a way.

30 The same widening of streets was advocated on the grounds of ease of traffic and later in the nineteenth century on the premises of security and riot's repression.

31 PP-BCU-L Q120/66: 16.

32 PP-BCU-L Q120/66: 17 & 18. Jan Inghen-Houze (1730-1799) Dutch physician who lived in England.

33 PP-BCU-L Q120/66: 19. Spams, asthma, convulsions,...

34 PP-BCU-L Q120/66: 21; *Observatio de colica saturnina* (in *Excerpto literaturae helveticae*, Bern, 1759: 142-150, *Observations sur la colique de plomb* (1761); Lavoisier, *Opuscules*. (Paris, 1774): 143.

35 See: Franklin (1887-1901), volume on Hygiène.

36 PP-BCU-L Q120/66: 25.

37 PP-BCU-L Q120/66: 26. Tissot never treated the subject in this manuscript; he wrote a small tract entitled: *Des cimetières*, PP-BCU-L Q120/83.

38 Corbin (1986): 30.

39 PP-BCU-L Q120/66: 28a, Journal de Paris 20 février 1797.

40 PP-BCU-L Q120/66: 29.

41 PP-BCU-L Q120/66: 30.

42 PP-BCU-L Q120/66: 31.

43 see above Chapter V.

44 PP-BCU-L Q120/66: 37.

45 PP-BCU-L Q120/66: 38 & 39. John Ferriar (1761-1815), British physician.

46 PP-BCU-L Q120/66: 43.

47 PP-BCU-L Q120/66: 44. Here Tissot is concerned with health matter, evidently not with the new weights and measures introduced in France in 1795, although some of the motivations for their introduction were related to public health. For another kind of administrative and medical concern, see Raeff (1983): 133.

48 PP-BCU-L Q120/66: 46ff.

49 Tissot had treated the problem in *Traité des nerfs*, vol. 6, Chapitre XXIII, article III: des maladies produites par le seigle ergoté; des maladies gangrèneuses.

50 PP-BCU-L Q120/66: 54.

51 PP-BCU-L Q120/66: 57.

52 PP-BCU-L Q120/66: 59.

53 PP-BCU-L Q120/66: 59. Tissot did not foresee the increase in standard of living the Industrial Revolution was to bring.

54 Guisan (1931): 116.

55 Chevallaz (1949).

56 PP-BCU-L Q120/66: 63. He was right on the lack of nutritive value, but over-pessimistic about the digestive problem.

57 His mention of forty years of practice gives a clue to estimate the date (1789) at which Tissot was already at work on *Médecine civile* since he graduated in 1749.

58 PP-BCU-L Q120/66: 68.

59 PP-BCU-L Q120/66: 69.

60 PP-BCU-L Q120/66: 70.

61 See: Leroy-Ladurie (1977): le climat de la France.

62 See: Emch-Dériaz (1984): appendix III. Baker: *Essay Concerning the Cause of the Endemic Colic of Devonshire* (London: 1767); Tronchin: *De colica pictorum* (Genève: Cramer, 1757). Their letters are in FE-BPU-G.

63 PP-BCU-L Q120/66: 74.

64 PP-BCU-L Q120/66: 75.

65 PP-BCU-L Q120/66: 79; Tronchin (1757). William Heberden (1710-1801), British physician; Thomas Percival (1740-1804), British Physician.

66 PP-BCU-L Q120/66: 84. Tissot cited an article in the *Bibliothèque physico-économique* (Paris 1791), tome 2: 422 .

67 PP-BCU-L Q120/66: 85.

68 PP-DCU L Q120/66: 86; such a bench at "Les Bougeries" in the Canton of Geneva/Switzerland, is now a registered national historical monument.

69 PP-BCU-L Q120/66: 88.

70 PP-BCU-L Q120/66: 88; this was particularly important in Lausanne where most of the streets are steep and many alleys are in fact stairs. See, Heller (1979).

71 See above Chapter VII.

72 Thomas (1983).

73 Thomas (1983): 180.

74 PP-BCU-L Q120/66: 94 & 95.

75 Thomas (1983): 112 & 117.

76 See: Spengler (1942): chapters IV and IX, section V. Jean-Baptiste Colbert (1619-1683), chief minister of Louis XIV (1638-1715).

77 PP-BCU-L Q120/66: 98.

78 PP-BCU-L Q120/66: 99.

79 PP-BCU-L Q120/66: 101.

80 PP-BCU-L Q120/66: 103; *Aphorismi de politia medica*. Pest: Kilian, 1795: 283; Franz Schraud (1761-1806), Hungarian physician.

81 PP-BCU-L Q120/66: 103.

82 PP-BCU-L Q120/66: 104.

83 Tissot did not say how he learned of the Philadelphia jail; see Ignatieff (1978): 58, 59, & 69-70.

84 PP-BCU-L Q120/66: 110.

85 PP-BCU-L Q120/66: 106.

86 PP-BCU-L Q120/66: 111.

87 See: Gay (1969): 443; Foucault (1975); Maestro (1942); Cesare Bonesana di Beccaria (1738-1794), Italian political and philanthropist writer.

88 PP-BCU-L Q120/130.5 & 11; PP-BCU-L Q120/130.3; PP-BCU-L Q120/64; PP-BCU-L Q120/83 & 130.15; PP-BCU-L Q120/72; PP-BCU-L Q120/73; PP-BCU-L Q120/130.4

89 see above Chapt. IX, note 6.

90 PP-BCU-L Q120/66: 113.

91 PP-BCU-L Q120/66: 120.

92 PP-BCU-L Q120/66: 127.

93 PP-BCU-L Q120/66: 136.

94 PP-BCU-L Q120/66: 132. Phthisis = etisis = tuberculosis.

95 PP-BCU-L Q120/66: 133.

96 PP-BCU-L Q120/66: 134.

97 PP-BCU-L Q120/66:   149; François Pierre Ami Argand (1750-1803), Genevan chemist and physicist.

98 PP-BCU-L Q120/66: 155

99 PP-BCU-L Q120/66: 156.

100 PP-BCU-L Q120/66: 157.

101 PP-BCU-L Q120/66:   158; for corroborative figures and opinions, see Rosen (1976): 303.

102 PP-BCU-L Q120/66: 160.

103 PP-BCU-L Q120/66: 160 verso.

104 PP-BCU-L Q120/66: 20.

105 PP-BCU-L Q120/66: 166; *mofette*: noxious gas emanations.

106 PP-BCU-L Q120/66: 167.

107 PP-BCU-L Q120/66: 171.

108 PP-BCU-L Q120 /66: 176; PP-BCU-L Q120/64: 30ff, and above chapter XI.

109 Chevalier (1958).

Conclusion

1 Elias (1978).

2 Fox-Genovese & Genovese (1983): chapter 11.

3 As witnessed by the many "enlarged" reprintings of the book and the paraphernalia included to control the habit. See: Viallaneix et Ehrard (1980): 307-314, 345-356, and 471-478; Bullough (1987); Tarczylo (1983).

4 Ramsey (1987).

5 Hoffmann (1977).

6 Weiner (1980).

7 Ulmann (1967); 34.

8 Skinner (1980).

9 Calvin: *L'Institution chrétienne* (1560): Livre IV, Chapitre XX.

Bibliography

Manuscript Sources (used with permission)

Bibliothèque cantonale et universitaire, Lausanne/Switzerland Fonds Tissot, IS 3748 (Q120/1-145): personal papers and correspondence; referred as PP-BCU-L; Fonds Olivier and Fonds Bousquet.

Bibliothèque publique et universitaire, Geneva/Switzerland Fonds Eynard, MSS. Suppl. (1908-1909): letters addressed to Tissot; referred as FE-BPU-G.

Burgerbibliothek, Bern/Switzerland MSS. Hist. Helv. XVIII: letters from Tissot to Haller; letters from Zimmermann to Tissot; letters from Haller to Tissot.

Zentral Bibliothek, Zurich/Switzerland Hirzel Family Nachlass, letters from Tissot to Hirzel.

Niedersächsischelandesbibliothek, Hanover/Germany Zimmermann Nachlass.

Universitaet Bibliothek, Goettingen/West-Germany Haller Nachlass.

Eleutherian Mills Historical Library, Wilmington/Delaware Pierre-Samuel Dupont de Nemours' personal papers and correspondence.

American Philosophical Society, Philadelphia/Pennsylvania Eighteenth-century documentation on hospitals.

Printed sources

Books by Tissot, listed in chronological order of first edition; see appendix II for a list of consecutive editions and translations.

L'inoculation justifiée	1754
Essai sur la mue de la voix	1754
Dissertatio de febricus biliosis	1758
Tentamen de morbis ex manustupratione ortis	1758
Lettre à M. de Haen	1759
De variolum inoculatione (to Count Roncalli)	1759
Observatione de colica saturnina	1760
De morbo nigro (to Zimmermann)	1760
L'Onanisme	1760
De variolis, apoplexia et hydrope (to Haller)	1761
Avis au peuple sur sa santé	1761
Quatre observations sur l'insensibilité des tendons	1762
Lettre à M. Hirzel (sur des critiques de M. de Haen)	1762
De morbis ex usu secalis cornuti (to Baker)	1765
Lettre à M. Zimmermann (sur l'épidemie courante)	1765
Seconde lettre à M. Zimmermann	1766
Sermo inauguralis de valetudine litteratorum	1766
De la santé des gens de lettres	1768
Essai sur les maladies des gens du monde	1770
Traité de l'épilepsie	1770
Traité des nerfs et de leurs maladies (4 volumes)	1778-80
Lettre à M. Hirzel sur le bled et le pain	1779
Traité de la catalepsie, de l'extase et de la migraine	1780
Essai sur les moyens de perfectionner les études de médecine	1785
Vie de Zimmermann	1797

Other pre-twentieth-century printed sources

Alembert, Jean Le Rond d'. *Opuscules mathématiques, onzième mémoire: sur l'application du calcul des probabilités à l'inoculation de la petite vérole*. Paris: 1762: 26-95.

Apples, Marc d'. *Instruction pour les personnes qui gardent les malades*. Lausanne: Pott, 1788. *Parallèle entre les miséricordes et les hôpitaux*. Lausanne: Pott, 1789.

Augenbrugger, Leopold. *Inventum novum expercussione thoracis humani*. Vienna: 1761.

Ballexserd, Jacques. *Dissertation sur l'éducation physique des enfants*. Yverdon: 1763.

Beccaria, Cesare. *Dei delitti e delle pene* (1764). Turin: Einaudi, 1973.

Benoit, Justin. "La Faculté de Médecine de Montpellier au point de vue de l'histoire du protestantisme français" in *Bulletin de la société du protestantisme français 11* (1862): 445-461.

Bernoulli, Daniel. "Essai d'une nouvelle analyse..." in *Histoire de l'Académie royale des sciences*. Année MDCCLX. Paris: Imprimerie royale, 1766.

Bienville, J.D.T. de. *La nymphomanie*. Amsterdam: Rey, 1778; reedition Paris: Le Sycomore, 1980.

Bordeu, Théophile de. *Correspondence* edited by Martha Flechter. Montpellier: 1977-1979, 4 volumes; *Recherches sur le pouls par rapport aux crises*. Paris: de Dures l'aîné, 1756; *Recherches sur quelques point d'histoire de la médecine*. Paris: 1764.

Brouzet, N. *Essai sur l'éducation médicale des enfants*. Paris: 1754.

Buchan, William. *Domestic Medicine*. Edinburgh: Balfour, Auld and Smellie, 1769.

Butini, Jean-Antoine. *Traité de l'inoculation*. Paris, Genève: 1752.

Cadogan, William. *An Essay upon nursing and the Management of children*. London: J. Roberts, 1748.

Calvin, Jean. *L'institution chrétienne* (1560). Genève: Labor et Fides, 1955.

Castan, Alfred. *Coup d'oeil sur l'histoire de la Faculté de Médecine de Montpellier.* Montpellier: 1878.

Chais, Charles. *Essai apologétique sur la méthode de communiquer la petite vérole par l'inoculation, où l'on tâche de faire voir que la conscience ne saurait être blessée ni la religion offensée.* La Haye: 1754.

Daremberg, Charles. *La médecine, histoire et doctrines.* Paris: Baillières, 1865; *Histoire des sciences médicales.* Paris: Baillières, 1870.

Des Essartz, Jean-Charles. *Traité de l'éducation corporelle des enfants en bas-âge ou réflexions pratiques pour les moyens de procurer une meilleure constitution aux citoyens.* Paris: Hérissant, 1760.

Diderot, Denis, ed. *Encyclopédie ou Dictionnaire raisonné des arts et des sciences.* Paris: 1757.

Du Laurens, Joseph-Michel. *Moyens de rendre les hôpitaux utiles et de perfectionner la médecine.* Paris: 1787; *Essai sur l'établissement des hôpitaux dans les grandes villes.* Paris: 1787.

Duncan, Andrew (the elder). *Heads of Lectures on the Theory and Practice of Medicine.* Edinburgh: Malfarquar and Elliot, 1781; *Heads of Lectures on Medical Jurisprudence.* Edinburgh: 1795; *Heads of Lectures on Medical Police.* Edinburgh: Adam Neil & Co. 1801.

Dupont de Nemours, Pierre-Samuel. *Idées sur les secours à donner aux pauvres malades dans les grandes villes.* Paris, Philadelphia: 1786.

Eynard, Charles. *Essai sur la vie de Tissot.* Lausanne: Bousquet, 1839.

Fourcroy de Guillerville, Jean-Louis. *Les enfants élevés dans l'ordre de la Nature.* Paris: 1774.

Frank, Johann Peter. *System einer vollstandige medizinischen Polizey*. Mannheim: Schwann, 1777-1788; English edition by Erna Lesky, Baltimore: The Johns Hopkins University Press, 1976; "The People's Misery: mother of disease (Pavia 1790) in *Bulletin of the History of Medicine 9* (1941): 81-100; *De vertabratis columnas in morbis dignitate*. Ticini: 1792; "Autobiography" translated by George Rosen in *Journal of Medical History 3* (1948): 11-46 and 279-314.

Franklin, Alfred Louis Auguste. *La vie privée d'autrefois*. Paris: Plon-Nourit, 1887-1901, 23 volumes.

Gavard, Alexandre. *Histoire de la Suisse au XIXe siècle*. La-Chaux-de-Fonds: Kahn, 1898, in particular chapter 1.

Germain, Alfred. *Le "Cérémonial"*. Montpellier: 1879, *L'école de Montpellier: ses origines, sa constitution, son enseignement*. Montpellier: 1880.

Gunn, John C. *Domestic Medicine*. Knoxville: 1830; reprinted with an introduction by C.E. Rosenberg, Knoxville: University of Tennessee Press, 1896.

Helvétius, Claude-Adrien. *De l'esprit* (1758). Paris: Editions sociales, 1968.

Howard, John. *Etats des prisons et des hôpitaux*. Paris: 1788; *On Principals Lazarettos*. London: 1789.

Kirkpatrick, James. *The Analysis of Inoculation*. London: 1754.

La Condamine, Charles de. "Premier mémoire sur l'inoculation" in *Histoire de l'Académie royale des sciences, année MCXXLIV*; "Deuxième mémoire sur l'inoculation" in *Histoire de l'Académie royale des sciences, année MCXXLVIII*; "Troisième mémoire sur l'inoculation" in *Histoire de l'Académie royale des sciences, année MCXXLXV*; *Histoire de l'inoculation*. Amsterdam: 1773.

Le Rebours, Angélique Anel. *Avis aux mères qui veulent nourrir leurs enfants.* Paris: 1765.

Morgagni, Giambattista. *De sedibus et causis morborum, per anatomen indagatis* (1761). With a preface by Tissot, Yverdon: 1779.

Müller, Jean de. *Histoire de la Confédération Suisse.* Genève: Cherbuliez, 1837-1851, 18 volumes.

Petit, Antoine. *Projet et mémoire sur la meilleure manière de construire un hôpital de malades.* Paris: Callot, 1774; *Projet de réforme sur l'exercice de la médecine en France.* Paris: 1791.

Pomme, Pierre. *Traité des vapeurs.* Lyon: 1769.

Poyet, Bernard. *Mémoire sur la nécessité de transférer et reconstruire l'Hôtel-Dieu de Paris, suivi d'un projet de translation de cet hôpital.* Paris: 1785.

Raulin, Joseph. *De la conservation des enfants.* Paris: 1763; *Traité des affections vaporeuses.* Paris: 1768.

Rousseau, Jean-Jacques. *Oeuvres complètes.* Paris: Gallimard, 1959-1969, 4 volumes; *Correspondance complète.* London, Geneva: Voltaire Foundation, 1965-1982, 40 volumes.

Roussel, Pierre. *Système physique et moral de la femme ou Tableau philosophique de la constitution, des moeurs et des fonctions propres au sexe.* Paris: Vincent, 1775.

Tenon, Jacques. *Mémoires sur les Hôpitaux de Paris.* Paris: 1788.

Venel, Jean-André. *De l'éducation des filles destinées au mariage.* Yverdon: 1784

Zimmermann, Jean-Georges. *Traité de l'expérience en médecine.* Paris: 1774, 3 volumes.

Twentieth-century secondary sources

Abrahams, H.J. "A summary of Lavoisier's proposals for training in science and medicine' in *Bulletin of the History of Medicine 32* (1958): 389-407.

Abt, Arthur F. and Garrison, Fielding H. *History of Pediatrics.* (1923) Philadelphia: Saunders, 1965.

Ackerknecht, Erwin H. *Grands médecins suisses.* Paris: 1966; *Medicine at the Paris Hospitals, 1794-1848.* Baltimore: The Johns Hopkins University Press, 1967; *A Short History of Medicine.* (1968) Baltimore: The Johns Hopkins University Press, 1982; *Kurze Geschichte des grossen Schweizer Aertze.* Bern: Huber, 1975. "Johann Georg Zimmermann" in *Gesnerus 35* (1978): 224-229; "From barber-surgeon to modern doctor" in *Bulletin of the History of Medicine 58* (1984): 545-553.

Annales ESC. Médecins, médecine et société (1977).

Ariès, Philippe. *L'enfant et la vie familiale sous l'Ancien Régime* (1960). Paris: Seuil, 1973;

Ariès, Philippe and Bejin, André eds. *Western Sexuality, Practice and Precept in Past and Present Times.* New York: Basil Blackwell, 1985.

Azouvi, François. "Woman as a model of pathology in the eighteenth century" in *Diogenes* (1981): 22-36; "Irritabilité et magnétisme animal" *in Dix-huitième siècle 14* (1982): 191-197.

Babaiantz, Christophe. *L'organisation bernoise des transports en Pays romand au XVIIIe siècle.* Lausanne: Bibliothèque vaudoise, numéro XXVIII, 1961.

Badinter, Elizabeth. *L'amour en plus. L'histoire de l'amour maternel du XVIIIe au XXe siècles.* Paris: Flammarion, 1980;

Barth, Karl. *Images du XVIIIe siècle.* Neuchâtel: Delachaux et Niestlé, 1949.

Baxby, Derrick. *Jenner's Smallpox Vaccine.* London: Heinemann, 1981.

Bell, M.K. ed. *Who Decides: conflicts of rights in health care.* Clifton, NJ: Humana Press, 1982.

Benaroyo, Lazare: *"L'avis au peuple sur sa santé" de Samuel-Auguste Tissot (1728-1797): la voie vers une médecine éclairée.* Zurich: Juris, 1988.

Béné, Raymond. *Jean-Jacques Dussaix (1722-1797), maître-chirurgien et bourgeois de Saint-Jeoire.* Académie du Faucigny: 1957.

Bergues, Hélène et al. *La prévention des naissances dans la famille; ses origines dans le temps.* Paris: Presses universitaires de France, 1960.

Biéler, André. *La pensée économique et sociale de Calvin.* Genève: Georg, 1959; *L'humanisme social de Calvin.* Genève: Labor et Fides, 1961, English translation: *The Social Humanism of Calvin.* Richmond, VA: John Knox Press, 1964; *L'homme et la femme dans la morale calviniste.* Genève: Labor et Fides, 1963.

Blanning, T.C.W. *Joseph II and Enlightened Despotism.* London: Longman, 1970.

Bloch, Jean. "Rousseau's reputation as an authority on children and physical education in France before the Revolution" in *Paedagogia historica XIV* (1974): 5-33.

Bluche, François. *La vie quotidienne au temps de Louis XVI.* Paris: Hachette, 1980.

Bonnard, Georges, ed. *Le journal de Gibbon à Lausanne.* Lausanne: Librairie de l'Université, 1945.

Boschung, Urs. "Médecine et santé au XVIIIe siècle à travers la correspondance d'Albert de Haller et Auguste Tissot" in *Revue médicale de la Suisse romande 106* (1986): 35-46.

Bouvier, Auguste. *J.G. Zimmermann: un représentant du cosmopolitisme littéraire au XVIIIe siècle.* Genève: Georg, 1925.

Bradley, L. *Smallpox Inoculation: an eighteenth-century mathematical controversy.* University of Nottingham: 1971.

Braudel, Fernand. *The Structure of Everyday Life.* New York: Harper and Row, 1981, 3 volumes.

Bridel, G.A. "Les demeures de Tissot à Lausanne" in *Revue historique vaudoise 36* (1928): 313-318.

Brunnert, Klaus. *Nostalgie in der Geschichte des Medezin.* Dusseldorf: Trittsch, 1984.

Bucher, Heinrich Walter. *Tissot und sein Traité des nerfs.* Zurich: Juris Verlag, 1958.

Bullough, Vern, L. *The Development of Medicine as a Profession.* Basel: Krager, 1966 (for a comparison between the Middle-Age and the eighteenth-century professionalization); *Sex, Society, and History.* New York: Science History Publications, 1976; "Sex and Mythology" in *Comparative Civilization Review* (1981): 40; "Technology for the prevention of 'les maladies produites par la masturbation'" in *Technology and Society* (1987): 828-832.

Bynum W.F. and Porter, Roy. eds. *William Hunter and the Eighteenth-Century Medical World.* New York: Cambridge University Press, 1985.

Charlton, D.C. *New Images of the Natural in France.* New York: Cambridge University Press, 1984.

Chaussinand-Nogaret, G. *The French Nobility in the Eighteenth Century*. New York: Cambridge University Press, 1985.

Chevallaz, Georges A. *Aspects de l'agriculture vaudoise à la fin de l'Ancien Régime*. Lausanne: Rouge, 1949.

Chevalier, J.L. *Classes laborieuses, classes dangereuses*. Paris: Plon, 1958.

Chisick, Harvey. *The Limits of Reform in the Enlightenment*. Princeton, NJ: Princeton University Press, 1981.

Cochet, Emile. *Etude sur S.A. Tissot (1728-1797)*. Paris: Boyer, 1902.

Coleman, William. "Health and Hygiene in the Encyclopédie" in *Journal of the History of Medicine XXIX* (1974): 399-421; "The people's health, medical theme in eighteenth-century French popular medicine" in *Bulletin of the History of Medicine 51* (1977): 55-74; "L'hygiène et l'Etat selon Montyon" in *Dix-huitième siècle 9* (1977): 91-100;

Corbin, Alain. *The Foul and the Fragrant*. Cambridge, MA: MIT Press, 1986.

Coury, Charles. *L'enseignement de la médecine en France des origines à nos jours*. Paris: L'expansion scientifique française, 1968.

Craddock, Patricia B. *Young Edward Gibbon, Gentleman of Letters*. Baltimore: The Johns Hopkins University Press, 1982; *Edward Gibbon: luminous historian (1772-1794)*. Baltimore: The Johns Hopkins University Press, 1988.

Darmon, Pierre. *La longue traque de la variole*. Paris: Perrin, 1986.

Darnton, Robert. *Mesmerism and the End of the Enlightenment in France*. Cambridge, MA: Harvard University Press, 1968.

Daston, Lorraine. *Classical Probability in the Enlightenment* Princeton, NJ: Princeton University Press, 1988.

Delauney, Paul. *La vie médicale au XVIe, XVIIe et XVIIIe siècles.* Paris: Edition Hippocrate, 1935.

Delmas, Paul. *Les étapes de l'enseignement clinique à Montpellier.* Montpellier: Chanteclair, 1929; *La Faculté de Médecine de Montpellier.* Montpellier: Publications du Jubilé, 1929.

Dewhurst, Kenneth. *Dr. Sydenham (1624-1689).* Berkeley: University of California Press, 1966.

Dix-Huitième Siècle, volumes 1-23, in particular volumes 9 (Le sain et le malsain), 12 (Représentations de la vie sexuelle), 15 (Aliments et cuisine), and 23 (Physiologie et médecine).

Dousset, Jean-Claude. *Histoire des médicaments.* Paris: Payot, 1985.

Dulieu, Louis. "Le mouvement scientifique montpelliérain au XVIIIe siècle" in *Revue d'histoire des sciences 11* (1958): 227-249; "La contribution montpelliéraine à l'Académie des sciences" in *Revue d'histoire des sciences 11* (1958): 255-262; "François Boissier de Sauvages (1706-1767)" in *Revue d'histoire des sciences 29* (1969): 303-32.

Durand, Yves. *Les républiques au temps des monarchies.* Paris: Presses universitaires de France, 1973.

Duveen Denis I. and Klickstein Herbert S. "Antoine-Laurent de Lavoisier's contributions to medicine and public health" in *Bulletin of the History of Medicine 29* (1955): 164-179.

Eighteenth-Century Life IX (3) (1985), special issue.

Elias, Norbert. *The Civilizing Process.* London: Oxford University Press, 1978.

Ellenberg, Henri. *Discovery of the Unconscious: the history and evolution of dynamic psychiatry.* New York: Basic Books, 1970.

Emch-Dériaz, Antoinette. "L'inoculation justifiée, or was it?" in *Eighteenth-Century Life VII* (1982): 65-72; *Towards a Social Conception of Health in the Second Half of the Eighteenth Century: Tissot (1728-1797) and the New Preoccupation with Health and Well-Being.* Ann Harbor, MI: University Microfilms International, 1984. "L'inoculation justifiée, vraiment?" in *Canadian Bulletin of Medical History 2* (1985): 237-263; "L'enseignement clinique au XVIIIe siècle: l'exemple de Tissot" in *Canadian Bulletin of Medical History 4* (1987): 145-164; "The French Revolution in the Eyes and Letters of Two Swiss Physicians " in *Proceedings of the Western Society for French History 14* (1986): 184; "The eighteenth century: the chrysalis stage of the hospital" paper presented at the 1988 AAHM Annual Meeting, New Orleans; "The Non-Naturals Made Easy" in Roy Porter, ed. *The Popularization of Medicine.* London: Routlege, 1992: chapter 5.

Engelhard, H.T. Jr. "The diseases of masturbation: value and the concept of disease" in *Bulletin of the History of Medicine 48* (1974): 234-248.

Fabre, Jean. *Stanislas-Auguste Poniatowski et l'Europe des Lumières.* Paris: 1952.

Fairchilds, Cissie S. *Poverty and Charity in Aix-en-Provence 1640-1789.* Baltimore: The Johns Hopkins University Press, 1976; *Domestic Enemies.* Baltimore: The Johns University Press, 1984.

Figlio Karl M. "Chlorosis and chronic disease in nineteenth-century Britain: the social constitution of somatic illness in a capitalist society" in *Social History 3* (1978): 167-197

Fildes, Valerie A. *Breast, Bottles, and Babies: a history of infant feeding.* Edinburgh: Edinburgh University Press, 1986.

Fishman, S. "The history of childhood sexuality" in *Journal of Contemporary History 17* (1982): 269-283.

Flandrin, Jean-Louis. *L'Eglise et le controle des naissances*. Paris: Flammarion, 1970; *Familles, parents, maison, sexualité dans l'ancienne société*. Paris: Hachette, 1976, English translation: *Families in Former Times*. New York: Cambridge University Press, 1979; *Le sexe et l'Occident*. Paris: Seuil, 1981.

Flinn, Michael W. *The European Demographic System 1500-1820*. Baltimore: The Johns Hopkins University Press, 1981.

Fohlen, Claude. *Qu'est-ce que la révolution industrielle*. Paris: Laffont, 1971.

Forrest, Alan. *The French Revolution and the Poor*. New York: St Martin's Press, 1981.

Foucault, Michel. *La naissance de la clinique*. Paris; Presses universitaires de France, 1963; *Histoire de la folie à l'âge classique*. Paris: Gallimard, 1972; *Surveiller et punir, la naissance de la prison*. Paris: Gallimard, 1975; *La volonté de savoir*. Paris: Gallimard, 1976; *The History of Sexuality*. New York: Pantheon, 1980-1987, 3 volumes.

Foucault, Michel et al. *Les machines à guérir (aux origines de l'hôpital moderne)*. Bruxelles: Mardaga, 1979.

Fox, Vivian C. and Quitt, Martin H. *Loving, Parenting, and Dying*. New York: Psychohistory Press, 1980.

Fox-Genovese, Elizabeth. *The Origins of Physiocracy, Economic Revolution and Social Order in Eighteenth-Century France*. Ithaca, NY: Cornell University Press, 1976; *The Autobiography of Dupont de Nemours*. Translated and with an introduction by E.F.-G. Wilmington, DE: Scholarly Resources, Inc. 1984.

Fox-Genevose Elizabeth and Genovese, Eugene D. *Fruits of Merchants Capital*. New York: Oxford University Press, 1983, in particular chapter 11.

François, Alexis. "Correspondance de Jean-Jacques Rousseau et du médecin Tissot" in *Annales de la société Jean-Jacques Rousseau VII* (1911): 19-40.

Freidson, Eliot, ed. *The Hospital in Modern Society*. London: Collier amd MacMillan, 1963.

Fuchs, Eric. *Le désir et la tendresse* (source et histoire d'une éthique chrétienne de la sexualité et du mariage). Genève: Labor et Fides, 1979.

Garrison, F.H. *An Introduction to the History of Medicine* (1929). Philadelphia: Saunders, 1960.

Gautier, Léon. *La médecine à Genève jusqu'à la fin du XVIIIe siècle*. Genève: Julien-Georg, 1906.

Gay, Peter. *The Party of Humanity* (1959). New York: Norton, 1971; *The Enlightenment*. New York: Knopf, 1967, 2 volumes; *The Enlightenment, a comprehensive anthology*. New York: Simon and Shuster, 1973; "Victorian sexuality, old texts and new insights" in *American Scholar 49* (1980): 372-378.

Gelfand, Toby. "The hospice of the Paris College of Surgery (1774-1793): a unique and invaluable institution" in *Bulletin of the History of Medecine 47* (1973): 375-393; "A clinical ideal: Paris, 1789" in *Bulletin of the History of Medecine 51* (1977): 397-411; "Two cultures, one profession: the surgeons of France in the eighteenth century" in *Consortium on Revolutionary Europe 1978 Proceedings* (1980): 171-187; "Gestation of the clinic" in *Medical History 25* (1981): 169-180; *Professionalizing Modern Medicine: Paris surgeons and medical science and institutions in the eighteenth century*. Wesport, Conn.: Greenwood, 1982;

Giddey, Ernest. *L'Angleterre dans la vie intellectuelle de la Suisse romande au XVIIIe siècle.* Lausanne: Bibliothèque historique vaudoise, 1974.

Gilliard, Charles. *La conquête du Pays de Vaud par les Bernois.* Lausanne: Concorde, 1935.

Gillipsie, Charles C. *Science and Polity in France at the End of the Old Regime.* Princeton, NJ: Princeton University Press, 1980.

Godoumêche, Jean. "La dégradation des gens de lettres d'après Tissot" in *Comptes rendus du 99e congrès national des sociétés savantes 5* (1974): 235-242.

Goldin, Grace. "A walk through a ward of the eighteenth century" in *Journal of the History of Medicine and Allied Sciences 22* (1967): 121-138.

Goulémot, Jean-Marie. in *Dix-Huitième Siècle* 12 (1980).

Graham, W. Fred. *Constructive Revolutionary: John Calvin and his socio-economic impact.* Richmond, VA: The John Knox Press, 1971.

Greenbaum, Louis S. "The commercial treaty on humanity, la tournée des hôpitaux anglais par Tenon en 1787" in *Revue d'histoire des sciences 24* (1971): 317-350; "The humanitarianism of Antoine-Laurent Lavoisier" in *Studies on Voltaire and the Eighteenth-Century 88* (1972): 651-675; "Jean-Sylvain Bailly, le Baron de Breteuil and the four new hospitals of Paris" in *Clio Medica 8* (1973): 261-284; "Measures of civilization: the hospital thought of Jacques Tenon on the eve of the French Revolution" in *Bulletin of the History of Medicine 49* (1975): 43-56; "Health-care and hospital-building in eighteenth-century France: reform proposal of Dupont de Nemours and Condorcet" in *Studies on Voltaire and the Eighteenth Century 152* (1976): 895-930; "Nurses and doctors in conflict: piety and medicine in the

Paris Hôtel-Dieu on the eve of the French Revolution" in *Clio Medica 13* (1979): 247-267; "Science, medicine, religion: three views of health-care in France on the eve of the French Revolution" in *Studies in Eighteenth-Century Culture 10* (1981): 373-392.

Groethuysen, Bernard. *Origine de l'esprit bourgeois en France* (1927). Paris: Gallimard, 1975.

Guerlac, Henry. *Antoine-Laurent de Lavoisier, chemist and revolutionary.* New York: Scribner's, 1975.

Guisan, André. "Le livre des malades du Dr. Tissot" in *Revue médicale de la Suisse romande XXXI* (1911): 713-721; "Tissot à Pavie" in *Revue médicale de la Suisse romande* LXVIII (1931): 113-126; "Le deuxième centenaire du Dr. Tissot" in *Revue historique vaudoise XXXVI* (1928): 225-258.

Gusdorf, Georges. *Dieu, la nature, l'homme au siècle des Lumières.* Paris: Payot, 1972; *Naissance de la conscience romantique au siecle des Lumières.* Paris: Payot, 1976.

Gutton, Jean-Pierre. *La société et les pauvres. L'exemple de la généralité de Lyon (1534-1789).* Paris: Presses universitaires de France, 1971; *La société et les pauvres en Europe, XVIe-XVIIIe siècles.* Paris: Presses universitaires de France, 1974.

Hamilton, Bernice. "The medical professions in the eighteenth century" in *Economic History Review 4* (1951): 141-170.

Hannaway, Caroline C. "The société royale de médecine and epidemics in the Ancien Régime" in *Bulletin of the History of Medicine 46* (1972): 257-273; "Veterinary medicine and rural health care in pre-revolutionary France" in *Bulletin of the History of Medicine 51* (1977): 431-447; "From private hygiene to Public Health, a transformation in Western medicine in the eighteenth and nineteenth centuries" in Ogawa (1981).

Hare, E.H. "Masturbation Insanity: the history of an idea" in *Journal of Mental Health 108* (1962): 1-25.

Harris, Robert D. *Necker: reform stateman of the Ancien Régime.* Berkeley: University of California Press, 1979; *Necker and the Revolution of 1789.* Landham, MD: University Presses of America, 1986.

Heller, Geneviève. *Propre, en ordre.* Lausanne: Edition d'en-bas, 1979.

Hintzsche, Erich, ed. *Albrecht von Haller Briefe an Auguste Tissot (1754-1777).* Bern: Huber, 1977.

Hoffmann, Paul. *La femme dans la pensée des Lumières.* Paris: Ophrys, 1977.

Hooykaas, Reijer. *Religion and the Rise of Modern Science.* Grand Rapids, MI: Eermans, 1972.

Huard, Pierre and Imbault-Huart, Marie-José. "La clinique parisienne avant et après 1802" in *Clio Medica 10* (1975): 173-182.

Hudson, Robert P. "The biography of disease: lessons from chlorosis" in *Bulletin of the History of Medicine* 51 (1977): 448-464.

Hufton, Olwen H. *The Poor of Eighteenth-Century Europe.* Oxford: Clarendon, 1974; "Women and the family economy in eighteenth-century France" in *French Historical Studies IX* (1975): 1-22.

Hunt, David. *Parents and Children in History. The Psychology of Family Life in Early Modern France.* New York: Basic Books, 1970.

Ignatieff, Michael. *A Just Measure of Pain.* New York: Columbia University Press, 1978.

Imbault-Huart, Marie-José. *L'école pratique de dissection de Paris ou l'influence du concept de médecine pratique et de médecine d'observation dans l'enseignement médico-chirurgical au XVIIIe siècle et au début du XIXe siècle.* Paris: 1973.

Janssen, Uta. "Matthieu Maty and the adoption of inoculation for smallpox in Holland" in *Bulletin of the History of Medicine 55* (1981): 246-256.

Jarcho, Paul. "Morgagni and Auenbrugger in retrospect" in *Bulletin of the History of Medicine 35* (1961): 489-496.

Jetter, Dieter. *Das Europaeische Hospital, von Spaetantike bis 1800.* Koeln: DuMont, 1986.

Jolivet, Corinne. *La médecine des pauvres.* Thèse de 3e cycle, Paris: 1980.

Jordanava, Ludmilla. "The popularization of medicine: Tissot on onanism" in *Textual Practice 1* (1987): 68-79.

Keel, Othmar. "La place et la fonction des modèles étrangers dans la constitution de la problématique hospitalière de l'école de Paris" in *History and Philosophy of the Life Sciences 6* (1984): 41-73; "La problématique institutionnelle de la clinique en France et à l'étranger de la fin du XVIIIe siècle à la période de la Restauration" in *Canadian Bulletin of Medical History 2* (1985): 183-204; and *3* (1986) 1-30; in Bynum and Porter, eds. (1985); "Les rapport entre médecins et chirurgiens dans la grande école anglaise de William et John Hunter" in *Gesnerus 45* (1988): 323-341.

King, Lester S. *The Medical World of the Eighteenth Century.* Chicago: University of Chicago Press, 1958; "Boissier de Sauvages and eighteenth-century nosology" in *Bulletin of the History of Medicine 40* (1966): 43-51; *The Road to Medical Enlightenment, 1650-1695.* New York: American Elsevier, 1970; "Theory and practice in eighteenth-century medicine" in *Studies on Voltaire and the Eighteenth Century 153* (1976):

1201-1218; *Medical Philosophy, the early eighteenth century.* Cambridge: Harvard University Press, 1978.

Klebs, Arnold C. *Die Variolation am achtzehnten Jahrhundert.* Giessen: Kopelmann, 1914; "The historic evolution of variolation" in *The Johns Hopkins Hospital Bulletin XXIV* (1913): 60-82.

Knibiehler Yvonne et Fouquet, Catherine. *L'histoire des mères, du moyen-âge à nos jours.* Paris: Montalba, 1980; *La femme et les médecins.* Paris: Hachette, 1983.

Kondratas, Ramunas A. *Joseph Frank (1771-1842) and the Development of Clinical Medicine.* Unpublished dissertation, Cambridge: Harvard University, 1977.

Kuhn, Thomas S. *The Essential Tension.* Chicago: University of Chicago Press, 1977.

Labasse, Jean. *L'hôpital et la ville, géographie hospitalière.* Paris: Hermann, 1980.

La Berge, Ann F. "The Paris Health Council, 1802-1848" in *Bulletin of the History of Medicine 49* (1975): 339-352; "A.J.B. Parent-Duchâtelet: hygièniste de Paris, 1821-1836" in *Clio Medica 12* (1977): 279-301; "The early nineteenth-century French public hygiene movement, the disciplinary development and institutionalization of 'hygiène publique'" in *Bulletin of the History of Medicine 58* (1984): 363-379.

Laget, Mireille. *Naissances: L'accouchement avant la clinique.* Paris: Seuil, 1982.

Lawrence, Christopher "William Buchan: medicine laid open" in *Medical History 19* (1975): 20-35.

Lebrun, François. *La vie conjugale sous l'Ancien Régime.* Paris: Colin, 1975.

Leistikow, Dankwart. *Ten Centuries of European Hospital Architecture*. Ingelheim am Rhein: Boehringer, 1967.

Leith, John H. *Introduction to the Reformed Faith*. Atlanta: The John Knox Press, 1977.

Leroy-Ladurie, Emmanuel. *Climat, médecins, épidemies à la fin du XVIIIe siècle*. Paris: Mouton, 1972; *Le territoire de l'historien* (1973). Paris: Gallimard, 1977.

Lesky, Erna. "Leopold Auenbrugger: Schueler van Swieten" in *Deutsche medizinischen Wochenschriften 84* (1959): 1017-1022; "Albrecht von Haller und Anton de Haen im Streit um die Lehre von der Sensibilitaet" in *Gesnerus 16* (1959): 16-46; Frank's *Complete System of Medical Police.* (1976).

Levy, Darlene Gay. *The Ideas and Careers of Simon-Nicolas-Henri Linguet. A Study in Eighteenth-Ceitury French Politics*. Urbana, IL.: University of Illinois Press, 1980.

Lindeboom, Gerrit Arie. *Herman Boerhaave: the man and his work*. London: Methuen, 1968.

Lipkin, Mark L. ed. *The Use and Abuse of Medicine*. New York: Praeger, 1982, in particular, chapter 15.

Lüthy, Herbert. *La banque protestante en France de la Revocation de L'Edit de Nantes jusqu'à la Révolution*. Paris: S.E.V.P.E.N., 1959-1961, 2 volumes; *From Calvin to Rousseau, tradition and modernity in socio-economic thought from the Reformation to the French Revolution*. New York: Basic Books, 1970.

MacCubbin, Robert P. ed. *Tis Nature Fault*. New York: Cambridge University Press, 1987.

McDonald, R. "The frightful consequences of onanism: notes on the history of a delusion" in *Journal of the History of Ideas 28* (1967): 423-431.

Ogawa, Ed. *Public Health*. Proceedings of the fifth International Symposium on the Comparative History of Medicine, East and West. Tokio: Saikon, 1981.

Olivier, Eugène. "Autour de l'Avis au peuple" in *Revue historique vaudoise XXXVI* (1928): 259-294; "La visite de J.G. Zimmermann à M. Schuppach" in *Schweizerische Medizinische Wochenschriften 59* (1929): 90-99; *Médecine et santé dans le Pays de Vaud* (des origines au XVIIIe siècle). Lausanne: Payot, 1962, 2 volumes.

O'Malley, Charles D. ed. *The History of Medical Education*. Berkeley: University of California Press, 1970.

Ozment, Steven. *When Fathers Ruled*. Cambridge: Harvard University Press, 1983.

Palmer, Robert R. *The Age of Democratic Revolution*. Princeton, NJ: Princeton University Press, 1959.

Park, Roberta. "Concern for health and exercise as expressed in the writings of eighteenth-century physicians and informed laymen (England, France, and Switzerland)" in *Research Quarterly* (American Association for Health, Physical Education, and Recreation) *47* (1976): 756-767. P

Payne, Harry G. *The Philosophes and the People*. New Haven, Conn.: Yale University Press, 1976.

Perdiguero, E. and Gonzalez, A. "Los valores morales de la higiena" in *Dynamis* (1990): 10.

Perrochon, Henri. *Esquisses et découvertes*. Genève: Perret-Gentil, 1971.

Plumb, J.H. "The new world of the children in eighteenth-century England" in *Past and Present 67* (1975): 64-95.

Pollock, Linda A. *Forgotten Children* (parent-child relations from 1500 to 1900). New York: Cambridge University Press, 1983.

Portmann, Marie-Louise. "Relations d'Auguste Tissot (1728-1797), médecin à Lausanne, avec le patriciat bernois" in *Gesnerus 37* (1980): 21-27.

Post, John D. *Food Shortage, Climatic Variability, and Epidemic Diseases in Preindustrial Europe* (the mortality peak in the early 1740's). Ithaca, NY: Cornell University Press, 1985.

Porter Roy, ed. *Patients and Practitioners*. New York: Cambridge University Press, 1985.

Raeff, Marc. *The Well-Ordered Police State*. New Haven, Conn.: Yale University Press, 1983.

Ramsey, Matthew. "The repression of unauthorized medical practice" in *Eighteenth-Century Life VII* (1982): 118-135; *Professional and Popular Medicine in France 1770-1830*. New York: Cambridge University Press, 1988.

Réflexions historiques 9 (1982), special double issue "La médicalisation de la société française, 1770-1830."

Reiser, Stanley Joel. *Medicine and the Reign of Technology*. New York: Cambridge University Press, 1978, chapter 1.

Riley, James C. *The Eighteenth-Century Campaign to Avoid Diseases*. New York: St Martin's Press, 1987.

Risse, Guenter B. "Doctor William Cullen" in *Bulletin of the History of Medicine 48* (1974): 338-351; "Typhus Fever in eighteenth-century hospitals: new approaches to medical treatments" in *Bulletin of the History of Medicine 59* (1985): 176-195; "A shift in medical epistemology: clinical diagnosis, 1770-1828" in Kawakita Y. ed. *History of Diagnosis*. Proceedings of the 9th International Symposium on the Comparative History of Medicine, East and West. Japan: Taniguchi Foundation, 1987; *Hospital Life in Enlightenment Scotland*. New York: Cambridge University Press, 1986; "Clinical instruction in hospitals: the Boerhaavian tradition in Leyden, Edinburgh, Vienna, and Pavia" in *Clio Medica 21* (1989): 1-19.

Rosen, George. "An eighteenth-century plan for a national health service" in *Bulletin of the History of Medicine 16* (1944): 429-436; "The philosophy of 'Ideology' and the emergence of modern medicine in France" in *Bulletin of the History of Medicine 20* (1946): 323-339; *Four Hundred Years of a Doctor's Life*. New York: Schuman, 1947; *A History of Public Health*. New York: M.D. Publications, 1958; *Madness in Society: chapters in the historical sociology of mental illness*. Chicago: University of Chicago Press, 1969; *From Medical Police to Social Medicine: essays on the history of health-care*. New York: Science History Publications, 1974; "Nostalgia: a 'forgotten' psychological disorder" in *Clio Medica 10* (1975): 28-51, "A slaughter of innocents: aspects of child-health in the eighteenth-century city" in *Eighteenth-Century Culture 5* (1976): 293-316.

Rosenberg, Charles E. "Medical text and social context: explaining William Buchan's 'Domestic Medicine'" in *Bulletin of the History of Medicine 57* (1983): 22-42;

Rosenberg, Charles E. ed. *The Family in History*. Philadelphia: University of Pennsylvania Press, 1975; *Healing and History* (essays in honor of George Rosen). New York: Dawson, 1979.

Rosenberg, Charles E. and Vogel, Morris J. eds. *The Therapeutic Revolution*. Philadelphia: University of Pennsylvania Press, 1979.

Rousseau, G.S. and Porter, Roy. eds. *The Ferment of Knowledge*. New York: Cambridge University Press, 1980; *Sexual Underworlds of the Enlightenment*. Chapel Hill: University of North Carolina Press, 1988.

Rowbothan, A.H. "The Philosophes and the propaganda for the inoculation of smallpox in eighteenth-century France" in

University of California Publication in Modern Philology 18 (1935): 265-290.

Russel, A.W. ed. *The Town and State Physicians in Europe from the Middle Age to the Enlightenment.* Wolffenbuttel Herzog-August Bibliothek Publications, 1981.

Saisselin, Rémy G. *The Literary Enterprise in Eighteenth-Century France.* Detroit, MI: Wayne Sate University Press, 1979.

Saudan, Guy, ed. *L'éveil médical vaudois 1750-1850.* Lausanne: Publications de l'Université, 1987.

Schenk, Jerome M. "The history of electrotherapy and its correlation with Mesmer's animal magnetism" in *American Journal of Psychiatry 116* (1959): 463-464.

Schwab, Richard N. "The Chevalier de Jaucourt, physician and encyclopedist" in *Journal of the History of Medicine* (1958): 256-259; "The history of medicine in Diderot's *Encyclopédie*" in *Bulletin of the History of Medicine 32* (1958): 216-223.

Sévery, William de. *La vie de société dans le Pays de Vaud à la fin du XVIIIe siècle* (1911). Genève: Slatkine, 1978; *Madame de Corcelles et ses amis.* Lausanne: Payot, n.d. (c. 1929); *Le Comte et la Comtesse Golowkin et le médecin Tissot.* Lausanne: Payot, 1928; "Le Docteur Tissot et ses amis" in *Revue historique vaudoise 36* (1928): 295-262.

Shorter, Edward. *The Making of the Modern Family.* New York: Basic Books, 1975; *A History of Women's Bodies.* New York: Basic Books, 1982.

Shryock, Richard H. *The Development of Modern Medicine (1935).* Madison: University of Wisconsin Press, 1974;

Siddall, A. Clair. "Chlorosis-etiology reconsidered" in *Bulletin of the History of Medicine 56* (1982): 254-260.

Skinner, Quentin. "The origins of the Calvinist theory of revolution" in *After the Reformation* (Essay in honor of J.H. Hexter), edited by B.C. Malament. Philadelphia: University of Pennsylvania Press, 1980.

Sorell, Walter. *The Swiss, a cultural panorama of Switzerland.* New York: Bodds-Merrill, 1977.

Spengler, Joseph J. *French Predecessors of Malthus.* Durham, NC: Duke University Press, 1942. French translation: *Economie et population, les doctrines françaises avant 1800,* avec en appendice: *Quelques démographes ignorés du XVIIIe siècle,* par Alfred Sauvy. Paris: Presses universitaires de France, 1954, 2 volumes.

Starobinski, Jean. "La leçon de la nostalgie" in *Médecine et Hygiène* (1961): 683-685 or in *Médecine de France 129* (1962): 6-11; "La nostalgie: theories médicales et expression littéraire" in *Studies on Voltaire and the Eighteenth Century XXVII* (1963): 1505-1518; "Notes sur l'histoire des fluides imaginaires (des esprits animaux à la libido)" in *Gesnerus 23* (1966): 176-187; *L'invention de la liberté.* Genève: Skira, 1964; *Molière et les médecins.* Basel: Ciba, 1966; "Le concept de nostalgie" in *Diogenes 54* (1966): 92-115; "Sur la chlorose" in *Romantisme* 11 (1981): 113-130.

Staum, Martin S. *Cabanis: Enlightenment and Medical Philosophy in the French Revolution.* Princeton, NJ: Princeton University Press, 1980.

Still, George F. *The History of Pediatrics.* London: Oxford University Press, 1931.

Stengers, Jean et Neck Anne van. *Histoire d'une grande peur: la masturbation.* Bruxelles: Ed. de l'Université, 1984.

Stone, Lawrence. *The Family, Sex, and Marriage in England: 1500-1800.* New York: Harper and Row, 1977.

Sussmann, George. "The wet-nursing business in France" in *French Historical Studies IX* (1975): 308-328; *Selling Mother's Milk*. Urbana, IL: University of Illinois Press, 1982.

Swick, Herbert and Antuono, Piero G. "Medical reform in Florence, 1780-1790: the Santa-Maria Nuova Hospital", paper presented at the 1983 AAHM Annual Meeting, Minneapolis, MN.

Tarczylo, Théodore. *Sexe et liberté au siècle des Lumières*. Paris: Presses de la Renaissance, 1983; in *Dix-Huitième Siècle 12* (1980) & *15* (1983).

Temkin, Owsei. "The role of surgery in the rise of modern medical thought" in *Bulletin of the History of Medicine 25* (1951): 248-259; *The Falling Sickness: a history of epilepsy from the Greeks to the beginning of modern neurology*. Baltimore: The Johns Hopkins University Press, 1971; *Galenism: rise and decline of a medical philosophy*. Ithaca, NY: Cornell University Press, 1973; *The Double Face of Janus and Other Essays in the History of Medicine*. Baltimore: The Johns Hopkins University Press, 1977.

Teysseire, D. *Pédiatrie des Lumières*. Paris: Vrin, 1982. (a comparison between the Journal de Trévoux' and the Encyclopédie' views on the medicine of children)

Thomas, Keith. *Man and the Natural World*. New York: Pantheon Books, 1983.

Thompson, John D. and Goldin, Grace. *The Hospital: a social and architectural history*. New Haven, Conn.: Yale University Press, 1975.

Traer, James F. *Marriage and the Family in Eighteenth-Century France*. Ithaca, NY: Cornell Univ. Press 1980.

Tronchin, Henry. *Théodore Tronchin (1709-1781), un médecin du XVIIIe siècle*. Genève: Kundig, 1906.

Troehler, Ulrich. "To improve the evidence of medicine: arithmetic observation in clinical medicine in the eighteenth and early nineteenth centuries in *History and Philosophy of Life Sciences 10* suppl. (1988): 31-40.

Ulmann, Jacques. *Les débuts de la médecine des enfants*. Paris: Palais de la Découverte, 1967.

Vartaniam, Aram. *L'homme-machine de La Mettrie*. Princeton, NJ: Princeton University Press, 1960.

Viallaneix, P. et Ehrard, J. eds. *Aimer en France 1760-1860*. Clermond-Ferrand, France: Presses de l'Université, 1980.

Weiner, Dora B. "Le droit de l'homme à la santé — une belle idée devant l'Assemblée Nationale, 1790-1791" in *Clio Medica 5* (1970): 209-223; "The French Revolution, Napoleon and the nursing profession" in *Bulletin of the History of Medicine 46* (1972): 274-305; "Public Health under Napoléon: the Conseil de Salubrité de Paris, 1802-1815" in *Clio Medica 9* (1974): 271-284; *The Clinical Training of Doctors. An Essay of 1793 by Philippe Pinel*. Baltimore: The Johns Hopkins University Press, 1980.

Wilson, Arthur. *Diderot*. New York: Oxford University Press, 1972, 2 volumes.

Zeiler, H. *Les collaborateurs médicaux de l'Encyclopédie de Diderot et d'Alembert*. Paris: 1934.

Appendix I

A Chronology of Tissot's Life

1728 Born, March 20 at Grancy, Pays de Vaud

1734 Studied at L'Isle, Pays de Vaud, with his uncle, a minister

1741 Entered the Collège, then the Académie at Geneva

1743 Had smallpox (referred to it often in his writings)

1745 Received his Master of Arts from the Académie at Geneva; entered the Faculté de Médecine at Montpellier.

1746 Smallpox epidemic at Montpellier, devoted his time to the sick

1749 Received his medical degree from Montpellier; returned to Grancy, cured his mother of hydropsia

1749 Smallpox epidemic in Pays de Vaud, worked hard at caring for the sick; beginning of correspondence with Tronchin

1752 Appointed to the position of "médecin des pauvres" at Lausanne by their Excellences of Bern

1754 Published *L'inoculation justifiée* and *Essai sur la mue de la voix*; beginning of correspondence with Haller and with Zimmermann; had the mumps (referred to it in his writings)

1755   Published *Discours préliminaire* du traducteur (de la *Dissertation sur les parties irritables et sensibles des animaux* par M. de Haller); Married Charlotte d'Apples; epidemic of bilious fever at Lausanne, devised a new cure with success

1756   Birth and death of his only child, a daughter

1758   Published *Dissertatio de febribus biliosis, seu historia epidemiae biliosae Lausannensis, anni 1755* and *Tentanem de morbis ex manustupratione ortis* (*L'Onanisme* in its Latin version)

1759   Published *Lettre à M. de Haen en réponse à ses questions sur l'inoculation, De variolarum inoculatione ad illustrissimus Franciscum comitem Roncalli,* and *Observatione de colica saturnina*

1760   Published *L'Onanisme* (unauthorized and authorized, much enlarged, French version), *Joanni Georgio Zimmermanno espitola de morbo nigro, scirrhis, cephalaea, inoculatione, irritabilate, cum cadaverum sectionibus*; Senac tried to lure him to Paris; elected to the Royal Society

1761   Published *L'avis au peuple sur sa santé, Alberto Hallero epistola de variolis, apoplexia et hydrope*; first contact with Rousseau

1762   Published *Quatre observations sur l'insensibilité des tendons* and *Lettre à M. Hirzel sur quelques critiques de M. de Haen*; received the bourgeoisie of Lausanne; elected member of the Société économique of Bern and gratified of a medal by their Excellencies; adoption of Marc d'Apples, his wife's nephew

1765   Published *De morbis ex usu secalis cornuti ad illustrem Georg Baker* and *Lettre à M. Zimmermann sur l'épidemie courante* (i.e. new attack of bilious fever at Lausanne); asked by their Excellencies of Bern to draw a plan to improve the health of the population; death of his uncle, the Reverend David Tissot; offer by the Canton of Solothurn of the position of State physician (rejected); offer by King Stanilas-Augustus of Poland of the position of first physician (rejected)

1766 Published *Seconde lettre à M. Zimmermann sur l'épidemie de 1766* and *Sermo inauguralis de valetudine litteratorum* (*De la santé des gens de lettres* in its Latin version); appointed professor of medicine at the Lausanne Academy by their Excellencies of Bern; delivered inaugural lecture at the Academy

1767 Death of his mother, Mme Tissot-Grenus; offer of the position of first physician of the Elector of Hanover (rejected); the Prince of Wurtemberg tried to have Tissot called to Vienna to inoculate the Imperial children (refused, on the advice of Haller); Parisian unauthorized edition of *De la santé des gens de lettres*; death of Boissier de Sauvages

1768 Published the Lausanne authorized edition of *De la santé des gens de lettres*; death of his father, M. Pierre Tissot; project of a new hospital in Paris, Chamousset tried to induce Tissot to be its first director, but Choiseul's disgrace brought to an end the project; elected to the Council of Sixty in Lausanne; consulted by the Serenissima Republica of Venice on inoculation

1770 Published *Essai sur les maladies des gens du monde* and the *Traité de l'épilepsie* (Chapter XX of the *Traité des nerfs et de leurs maladies*); elected member of the Swedish Academy

1772 Travels (alone) to Strasburg, Mannheim, Aachen, Spa, Brussels, Nancy, Lyons,...; death of his brother-in-law, the Reverend Pidou

1774 Offer by Venice of a professorship at the University of Padua; sojourn at Plombières with Mme Tissot

1775   Rejected the Venetian offer after much hesitation; visit of Zimmermann

1777   Visit of the Emperor Joseph II; elected to the Société royale de médecine; death of Haller

1778   Published the *Traité des nerfs et de leurs maladies*; address to their Excellencies of Bern on inoculation prohibition; offer of the Duke of Modena to be his first physician (rejected); death of Rousseau and of Voltaire

1779   Published *Lettre à M. Hirzel sur le bled et le pain*; offer of the Margrave of Hesse-Cassel to be his personal physician (rejected); sojourn in Paris with his nephew, Marc d'Apples

1780   Published the *Traité de la catalepsie*; Marc d'Apples studied at the Jardin du Roy; offer by the Granduke Leopold of Tuscany (on the advice of his brother, the Emperor Joseph II) of a position of professor of practical medicine at the University of Pavia (long negotiations)

1781   Departure for Pavia with Marc d'Apples; death of Tronchin

1782   Travelled through Italy (Venice, Padua, Naples,...), met in Rome with the Pope and the Countess of Albany, wife of the English Pretender; Angelica Kaufmann painted his portrait; offer of the Queen of Two Sicilies to be her physician (rejected); spent the summer in Lausanne; returned to Pavia to teach

1783   Called to Turin by the Court of Savoy-Piedmont-Sardignia, cared for the Princess of Carignan; returned to Lausanne at the end of the academic year with no intention of pursuing his teaching career, in spite of pressure to retain him in Pavia

1784   Marriage of Marc d'Apples

1785   Published *Essai sur les moyens de perfectionner les études de médecine*; birth of Auguste d'Apples

1786   M. de Servan exhibited a "Mesmer bath" at Lausanne; asked by Ch. Bonnet to investigate the phenomenon; observed one session, then banned from observing another

1787   Foundation of the Collège de Médecine at Lausanne, elected its first vice-president

1789   Reported to the Council of Two-Hundred of Lausanne about the Town-Hospital

1790   Death (March 15) of Auguste d'Apples from smallpox, when, after two unsuccessful inoculations by his granduncle, he caught the disease

1791   Visit of Johann Peter Frank and of his son Joseph

1795   Death of Zimmermann

1797   Published *Vie de Zimmermann*; death of his wife at the end of May; died from tuberculosis on June 13 after of a few weeks of lethargy

Appendix II

Bibliography of Tissot's Published Works

This bibliography lists the title of the work, original language, original place, publisher, and date of publication, succeeding editions and translations.

L'inoculation justifiée, French, Lausanne: Bousquet, 1754 with *Essai sur la mue de la voix*

In *French*:   Lausanne: Grasset, 1773, 1778, 1781, 1786
                Paris: Didot, 1773
                Berne: Haller, 1781

In *German*:   Halle: Kummeln, 1756
                Langensalza: Martin, 1768
                Leipzig: Müller, 1771
                Leipzig: Schneider, 1778

In *Italian*:   Venezia: Pompeati, 1775, 1783
                Napoli: Castellano, 1778
                Venezia: Gatti, 1779, 1784

Essai sur la mue de la voix, French, Lausanne: Bousquet, 1754 (usually reprinted with *L'inoculation justifiée*)

Dissertatio de febricus biliosis, anni 1755, Latin, Lausanne: Bousquet, 1758 (together with *Tentamen de morbis ex manustupratione ortis*)

In *Latin*:   Paris: Papinot, 1758
                  Louvain: 1760
                  Venezia: 1761, 1769
                  Napoli: 1762
                  Celle: Gsellius, 1769
                  Jena: 1771
                  Lausanne: Grasset, 1780
                  Basel: Flick, 1780
                  Lausanne: Pott, 1790
                  Paris: Crochard, 1813

In *English*:   London: Wilson and Durham, 1760

In *Italian*:   Venezia: Vitto, 1772, 1782

In *French*:   Paris: Gabon et Brosson, An VIII (1800)

Tentanem de morbis ex manustupratione ortis, Latin, Lausanne:
    Bousquet, 1758 (usually reprinted together with *Dissertatio de
    febricus biliosis, anni 1755*)

Also known as *L'Onanisme*, when reprinted separately as an
enlarged French version by Tissot; see below.

In *Latin*:   see above,
                  also alone,
                  London: Wilson and Durham, 1760, 1761, 1762,
                      1775, 1797

In *German*:   translated from the Latin
                  Frankfurt: Fleischer, 1775
                  Eisenacht: Boerke, 1785
                  Cassel: Krieger, 1797
                  Marburg: 1800

L'Onanisme, French, Lausanne: Chapuis, 1760

In *French*:   Lausanne: Chapuis, 1760, 1764, 1765, 1766, 1768, 1769, 1770, 1771, 1772, 1773, 1774, 1776, 1778, 1780, 1781, 1788, 1792
Lausanne: Grasset, 1764, 1772, 1775, 1777, 1781, 1782, 1785, 1788, 1791, 1797
Louvain: 1760, 1764
Yverdon: 1765
Amsterdam: 1771
Neuchâtel: 1775
Bern: Haller, 1781
Avignon: 1792, 1794, 1817, 1825, 1842
Paris: 1778, 1802, 1805, 1810, 1817, 1818, 1819, 1821, 1822, 1823, 1826, 1827, 1828, 1830, 1831, 1834, 1836, 1846, 1856, 1869, 1870, 1874, 1875, 1877, 1880, 1884, 1886, 1905
Lyon: 1807
Coulommiers: André, 1813
Belfort: Clerc, 1835
Paris: Sycomore, 1980
Paris: Edition de la différence, 1991

In *English*:   London: Thomas, 1760
London: Becket and de Hond, 1766
London: trad. Farrer, 1767, 1772
Dublin: William, 1772, 1773
London: Bath, 1781
New York: Collins and Hannay, 1832

In *German*:   Leipzig: 1760, 1792, 1798, 1802
Frankfurt: 1760, 1775, 1781, 1792, 1798
Hamburg: 1767
Eisenach: 1771, 1785
Wien: Trattner, 1782, 1787
Augsburg: Wolf, 1789
Karlsruhe: 1803, 1832

In *Italian*:   Venezia: Grazioni, 1774, 1784, 1785
Venezia: Carcan, 1792

| | Milano: 1835, 1857, 1870 |
| | Firenze: Salani, 1890 |

In *Spanish*: Madrid: 1770, 1807, 1814, 1828, 1845, 1876, 1877

In *Russian*: Saint-Petersburg: 1845

Lettre à M. de Haen en réponse à ses questions sur l'inoculation, French, Lausanne: Grasset, 1759

In *French*: Wien: Trattner, 1759
Lausanne: Grasset, 1765, 1773

In *Italian*: Napoli: Castellano, 1778

De variolarum inoculatione ad illustrissimo Roncalli, Latin, Lausanne: Grasset, 1759

In *Latin*: Bern: 1759
Jena: 1771
Leipzig: 1771
Lausanne: 1780, 1784
Paris: 1810

In *French*: Lausanne: Grasset, 1780, 1789

In *German*: Leipzig: Müller, 1771

In *Italian*: Napoli: Castellano, 1778

Observationes de colica saturnina, Latin, Bern: Haller, 1759

In *Latin*: Louvain: 1764
Venezia: 1789

In *French*: Lausanne: Grasset, 1761, 1780

In *English*: Dublin: 1773

Zimmermanno epistola, de morbo nigro, Latin, Lausanne: Grasset, 1760

In *Latin*:   Louvain: 1764
Lausanne: Grasset, 1765, 1769, 1783
Leipzig/Jena: 1774
Rotterdam: 1788
Venezia: 1789

In *French*:   Paris: Didot, 1769

In *English*:   London: 1776

In *Italian*:   Napoli: Castellano, 1778

Alberto Hallero epistola, apoplexia e hydrope, Latin, Lausanne: Grasset, 1761

In *Latin*:   Lausanne: Grasset, 1765, 1768, 1769, 1770
Louvain: 1764, 1783
Rotterdam: 1769
Paris: Didot, 1769
Lausanne: Pott, 1783
Venezia: 1789

In *French*:   Lausanne: Grasset, 1780, 1784
Paris: 1810

In *English*:   London: 1772
Dublin: 1773

Avis au peuple sur sa santé, French, Lausanne: Zimmerli pour Grasset, 1761

In *French*:   Lausanne: Grasset, 1763, 1766, 1770, 1775, 1777,
1783, 1785, 1788, 1790, 1792, 1799
Paris: Didot, 1762, 1763, 1765, 1767, 1768, 1770,
1772, 1776, 1778, 1779, 1782
Lyon: Duplain, 1763, 1767, 1768, 1769, 1771, 1772,
1776

Genève: Pellet, 1764
La Haye: 1767
Nancy: Leclerc, 1780
Bern: Haller, 1781, 1787
Toulouse: Desclassas, 1781
Rouen: Machud et Racine, 1782
Paris: Delarain l'aîné, 1786, 1803
Blois: Manon et Durie, 1793, 1795
Rouen: Dumesnil, An III (1795)
Paris: Belin, An X (1802)
Paris: Méquignon, An XI (1803)
Paris: Allut, 1809, 1813. 1820
Paris: Corbet, 1830

In *English*: London: 1765, 1766, 1767, 1768, 1771, 1776, 1789,
1792, 1793, 1797, 1801, 1803, 1810, 1815, 1820,
1830
Wellcome or Welkom: 1765, 1766, 1768, 1771
Edinburg: 1766, 1768, 1772, Donaldson, 1778
Boston: 1766, Mein and Fleming, 1767, 1771
Bristol: Pine, 1769
Philadelphia: 1771

In *English*: as *The Family Physician: Advice with Respect to
Health* (extracted from the *Avis*)
Bristol: 1769
Welcome or Welkom: 1769
London: 1802

In *German*: Zurich: Heidegger, 1763
Frankfurt: 1766, 17786
Leipzig: 1766, 1786, 1807
Augsburg: Wolfe, 1766, 1769, 1772
Zurich: Fuessli, 1767, 1768
Hamburg: 1767
Langafalza: Martin, 1768, 1769
Mammheim: Schwan, 1772
Zurich: Orell und Gelzner, 1773, 1775, 1785, 1786
Wien: Trattner, 1780, 1792

	Munster: Coppenrath, 1789
	Augsburg: Kranzfelder, 1795
	Augsburg: Kersten, 1818
In *Italian*:	Venezia: Zatta, 1766, 1768, 1795
	Milano: 1770, 1774
	Genoa: 1767
In *Dutch*:	Amsterdam: 1763, 1764
	Rotterdam: 1764, 1765, 1767, 1780
In *Flemish*:	Bruges: 1765, 1782
In *Danish*:	Copenhagen: 1770
In *Swedish*:	Stockholm: 1764, 1768
In *Polish*:	Warsaw: 1774, 1785
In *Hungarian*:	Carolyban: 1772
In *Russian*:	Saint Petersburg: 1772, 1781
In *Spanish*:	Pamplona: 1773
	Madrid: 1774, 1776, 1778, 1781, 1790, 1795, 1815, 1855
In *Portuguese*:	Lisboa: 1774, 1777, 1786, 1831
In *Greek*:	Venice: 1780, 1785
In *Tagalog*:	San Augustin: 1831
	Manila: 1884
In *Hebrew*:	Lemberg [Lvov]: 1851

Eynard, in *Essai sur la vie de Tissot*: 79, wrote that an Arabic translation of the *Avis* had been published in Damiette around 1830, but I could not find any confirmation of it.

Quatre observations sur l'insensibilité des tendons, French, Lausanne: Grasset, 1762

Lettre à M. Hirzel, sur quelques critiques de M. de Haen, French, Lausanne: 1762

In *French*:   Lausanne: Grasset, 1763, 1765
                 Neuchâtel: 1779

In *Italian*:   Venezia: 1771, 1782

De morbis ex usu secalis cornuti ad illustrem Baker, Latin, in *Philosophical Transactions*, London, 1765: 106-126

In *Latin*:   Lausanne: Grasset, 1770
                 Leipzig: 1771
                 Jena: 1771

In *French*:   Lausanne: Grasset, 1768, 1780

In *German*:   Leipzig: Müller, 1771, 1775

Lettre à M. Zimmermann sur l'épidemie courante, French, Lausanne: Grasset, 1765

In *French*:   Paris: 1765
                 Lausanne: Grasset, 1771

In *German*:   Zurich: Fuessli, 1767

In *Italian*:   Venezia: Caroboli, 1771

Seconde lettre à M. Zimmermann sur l'épidemie de 1766, French, Lausanne: Grasset, 1766

In *German*:   Zurich: Fuessli, 1767

In *Italian*:   Venezia: Caroboli, 1771

In *English*:   London: Kearsley, 1776

Sermo inauguralis de valetudine litteratorum, Latin, Lausanne: Chapuis, 1766
Also known as *De la santé des gens de lettres*, when reprinted as an expanded French version by Tissot; see below.

In *Latin*:   Lausanne: Chapuis, 1769
            Frankfurt: Schwickel, 1769

In *French*:   unauthorized version
            Paris: Hérissant, 1767
            Paris: Journal des scavants, 1767

De la santé des gens de lettres, French, Lausanne: Grasset, 1768

In *French*:   Paris: Didot, 1768, 1769
            Genève: Pellet, 1768, 1770, 1786
            Lausanne: Grasset, 1769, 1770, 1772, 1775, 1778, 1783, 1784
            Lyon: 1769, 1775, 1789
            Bern: Haller, 1782
            Paris: Allut, 1809, 1820
            Paris: Baillière, 1826
            Paris: Techener, 1859
            Paris: Edition du centenaire, 1868
            Genève: Slatkine, 1981 (facsimile of the 1768 Lausanne edition)
            Paris: Edition de la différence, 1991

In *German*:   Leipzig: Müller, 1768, 1770, 1775
            Hamburg: 1768
            Augsburg: Wolff, 1771, 1777
            Bern: Haller, 1775
            Augsburg: Burglen, 1803

In *English*:   London: 1768, 1769
            Boston: 1769
            Wellcome or Welkom: 1769

                    Dublin: Williams, 1769, 1771
                    Edinburgh: Donaldson, 1772

In *Italian*:   Milano: Galeozzi, 1768
                    Napoli: Castellano, 1773
                    Venezia: Caroboli, 1775
                    Venezia: Zatta, 1791

In *Spanish*:   Zaragoza: Moreno, 1771

In *Greek*:   1785

In *Polish*:   Tissot knew of a translation by Karwoski

Essai sur les maladies des gens du monde, French, Lausanne: Grasset, 1770

In *French*:   Lausanne: Grasset, 1770, 1771, 1772, 17781, 1785
                    Lyon: Bruyset, 1771
                    Amsterdam: 1771
                    Paris: Didot, 1771, 1772, 1773, 1785
                    Bern: Haller, 1783
                    Paris: Allut, 1809, 1823, 1834
                    Paris: Techener, 1859
                    Paris: Edition du centenaire, 1868

In *German*:   Frankfurt: 1770, 1771, 1772
                    Leipzig: Felsecker, 1770, 1771
                    Wien: Trattner, 1770

In *English*:   London: 1770, 1771, 1772
                    Dublin: Williams, 1772
                    Edinburgh: Donaldson, 1772
                    Wellcome or Welkom: 1772

In *Italian*:   Lausanne: Pott, 1770
                    Venezia: Caroboli, 1770, 1775
                    Venezia: Pompeati, 1770, 1775
                    Napoli: Castellano, 1771

In *Spanish*:   Madrid: 1786

Traité de l'épilepsie, French, Lausanne: Grasset, 1770.
Also reprinted as chapter XX of the *Traité des nerfs et de leurs maladies*; see below.

In *French*:   Paris: Didot, 1770, 1772, 1785
               Lausanne: Grasset, 1772, 1789
               Bern: Haller, 1788

In *German*:   Berlin: Haude und Spener, 1771
               Leipzig: Müller, 1771

In *Italian*:   Venezia: Caroboli, 1772, 1775
               Napoli: Castellani, 1774

In *Dutch*:   Amsterdam: Harlingen, 1774

Traité des nerfs et de leurs maladies, French, Lausanne: Grasset, 1778-1780 (4 volumes)

In *French*:   Paris: Didot, 1778-1780
               Genève: Pellet, 1783
               Lausanne: Pott, 1780
               Paris: Barois, 1783

In *German*:   Leipzig: Jacobaer, 1781-1783, 1790-1807
               Winterthur: Steiner, 1781-1783
               Frankfurt: 1782
               Altona: 1790

In *Italian*:   Napoli: Castellano, 1782

Traité de la catalepsie, French, Lausanne, Grasset, 1780. Also reprinted as chapters XXI, XXII, and XXIII of the *Traité des nerfs et de leurs maladies*; see above.

In *French*:   Genève: Grasset, 1783, 1785
               Bern: Haller, 1783

Lettre à M. Hirzel sur le bled et le pain, French, Lausanne: Tarin, 1779

In *French*:   Neuchâtel: 1779
                 Lausanne: Pott, 1779

In *German*:   Zurich: Ziegler, 1780

Essai sur les moyens de perfectionner les études de médecine,
    French, Lausanne: Mourer Cadet, 1785

In *French*:   Lausanne: Mourer Cadet, 1785
                 Bern: Haller, 1785
                 Basel: Flick, 1785
                 Paris: Didot, 1785

In *German*:   Basel: Thurneisen, 1785
                 Wien: Graffer, 1786

In *Italian*:   Napoli: Castellano, 1785
                 Venezia: Pompeati, 1786

Vie de Zimmermann, French, Lausanne: Fischer et Vincent, 1797

In *French*:   Genève: Pachoud, 1797
                 Zurich: Orell, 1797
                 Strasburg: Koenig, 1798
                     with Zimmermann's *Traité de l'expérience en
                     médecine*
                 Avignon: Seguin, 1800
                 Paris: Gabon, 1817

In *German*:   Hannover: Hahn, 1797
                 Zurich: Orell, 1797

In *English*:   London: Dilly, 1797
                 London: Verner and Head, 1797, 1798

Collected Works:

In *Latin*:   *Epistolae medico-praticas*
                 Jena: Gollner, 1769, 1770, 1771
                 Lausanne: Pott, 1770

Lausanne: Grasset, 1771
Paris: Cavelier, 1771
Bern: Haller, 1781
Venezia: Caroboli e Pompeati, 1770

Opuscula Medica
Leipzig: 1769

In *French*:   *Dissertations de médecine pratique publiées en forme*
    de lettres
            Genève: 1767
            Yverdon: 1780
            Lausanne: Grasset, 1780 (Vicat's translation)
            Bern: Haller, 1780

In *English*:   Three Essays (translated from the French
            Onanisme, De la santé des gens de lettres, and
            Essai sur les maladies des gens du monde)
            Dublin: Williams, 1772

In *German*:   *Medizin-Praktikum Handbuch*
            Leipzig: 1785, 1786

In *Italian*:   *Lettere mediche scritte a vari amici*
            Venezia: Caroboli, 1771
            Venezia: Pompeati, 1777
            Napoli: Castellano, 1771

Complete Works:
Of all the *Complete Works*, only the Lausanne: Grasset editions of 1790 and 1795 include the *Essai sur les moyens de perfectionner les études de médecine.* The *Vie de Zimmermann* is never included.

In *French*:   Paris: Didot, 1769-1771 (5 volumes)
            Lausanne: Grasset, 1784 (13 volumes), 1788 (14
               volumes), 1790 (15 volumes), 1795 (15 volumes)
            Paris: Allut, 1809-1820 edition Hallé, (11
               volumes), 1820-1824 (11 volumes), 1820 (3
               volumes)

Paris: Delahays, 1855 (reprint of the edition Hallé)
Paris: 1824-1846, volume 10 of *Encyclopédie des sciences médicales* in 41 volumes, edited by A. L. J. Bayle, contained some of Tissot's works

In *German*:   *Sammltliche zur Arztneykunst gehorige Schriften*
Hamburg: Kerstens und Ackermann, 1774 (7 volumes)
Leipzig: Jacobaer, 1784 (5 volumes)
Leipzig: Jacobaer, 1790 (7 volumes)
Leipzig: Jacobaer, 1807 (7 volumes)
Altona: Aue, 1807 (7 volumes)

Index